Implant Surfaces and their Biological and Clinical Impact

Ann Wennerberg
Tomas Albrektsson • Ryo Jimbo
Editors

Implant Surfaces and their Biological and Clinical Impact

Springer

Editors
Ann Wennerberg, DDS, PhD
Faculty of Odontology Dept
Prosthodontics
Malmö University
Malmö
Sweden

Ryo Jimbo, DDS, PhD
Faculty of Odontology Dept
Prosthodontics
Malmö University
Malmö
Sweden

Tomas Albrektsson, MD, PhD,
ODhc, RCPSG
Division of Clinical Sciences
Department of Biomaterials
University of Gothenburg Sahlgren's
Academy
Gothenburg
Sweden

ISBN 978-3-662-45378-0 ISBN 978-3-662-45379-7 (eBook)
DOI 10.1007/978-3-662-45379-7
Springer Heidelberg New York Dordrecht London

Library of Congress Control Number: 2014958297

Printed on acid-free paper

Springer is part of Springer Science+Business Media (www.springer.com)

Preface

This book presents an overview of implant surfaces and their clinical impact. We learnt about surface impacts already in the infancy of osseointegration, but it was first with the advent of reliable topographical measurement techniques during the 1990s that a more profound knowledge of surface importance was available. Since then, research has identified a number of different surface characteristics of an assumed clinical importance; these include micro-surfaces, nano-surfaces, and chemically or physically induced surface alterations. This book includes contributions from many world-leading scientists in the implant surface discipline. Methodological overviews are coupled with reports from experimental and clinical studies. The most commonly used oral implant surfaces include acid-etched, blasted, fluoride-treated, and anodized surfaces that are summarized in several chapters. Orthodontic implants are covered in one chapter.

This book cites predominantly oral implants, since orthopedic implants, at least so far, have been characterized mainly by macro-changes of implant surfaces. A porous surface to the orthopedic surgeon is porous coated, i.e., a macroscopic surface alteration, whereas a porous surface to the dentist is a microporous surface. Few studies about hip arthroplasties have included a surface microscopic analysis. We see it as important for orthopedic surgeons to realize the clinical potential of surface microscopical alterations as well as for oral surgeons to realize aseptic loosening phenomena that in all probability are as common for dental implants as for orthopedic ones. Orthopedic and oral implants work well, but certainly not so good that one cannot have even better clinical results with understanding the nature of the oral implant surfaces. In orthopedics, clinical long-term results are commonly based on the frequency of reoperation that can be criticized for presenting somewhat idealized results, while in dentistry, osseointegration has been seen as a somewhat mystical key for success, although in reality osseointegration is but a foreign body response. Hence, both disciplines have to learn from one another to further improve clinical outcomes for the future, which is why this book may be worthwhile reading for orthopedic surgeons as well as dentists.

Gothenburg, Sweden — Tomas Albrektsson, MD, PhD, ODhc, RCPSG
Malmö, Sweden — Ryo Jimbo, DDS, PhD
Malmö, Sweden — Ann Wennerberg, DDS, PhD

Editors

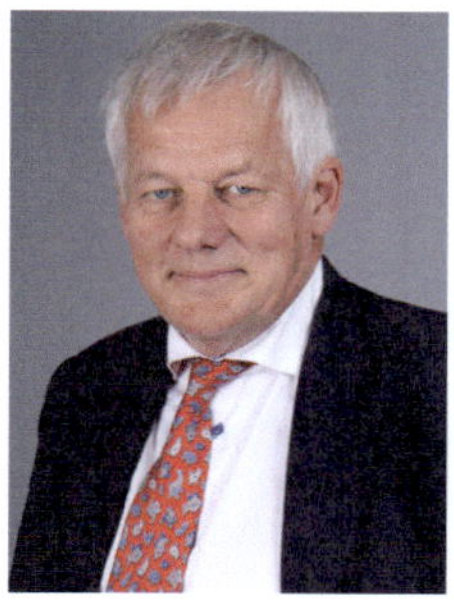

Tomas Albrektsson, MD, PhD, ODhc, RCPSG was a member of Branemark's original osseointegration team and has since worked with and patented oral implants as well as hip implants. Albrektsson has authored numerous scientific papers on implants, and he lectures frequently worldwide. He continues working as Emeritus Professor at the Department of Biomaterials, Gothenburg University, and as a Visiting Professor at the Department of Prosthodontics, Malmö University, Sweden.

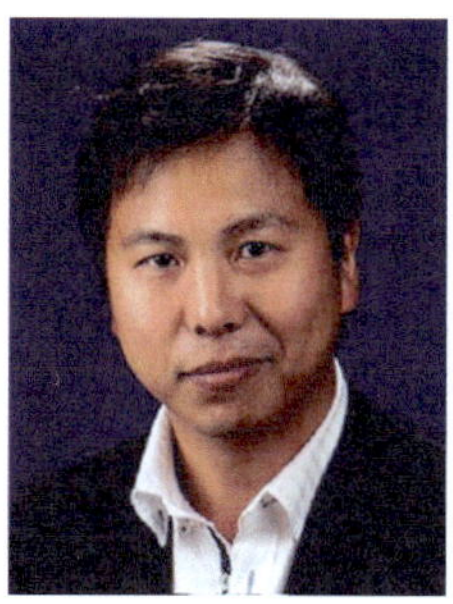

Ryo Jimbo, DDS, PhD received his DDS degree at the Nagasaki University School of Dentistry in 2004 and defended his PhD thesis at the same school in 2007. Jimbo has had specialist education in prosthodontics and has in addition worked in oral and maxillofacial surgery. He was a visiting researcher at the Department of Biomaterials, Gothenburg University, between 2009 and 2010 and is Associate Professor at the Department of Prosthodontics, Malmö University, since 2010. His current research is centered on implant basic and clinical research, with a special interest in nanotechnology applications in implant dentistry.

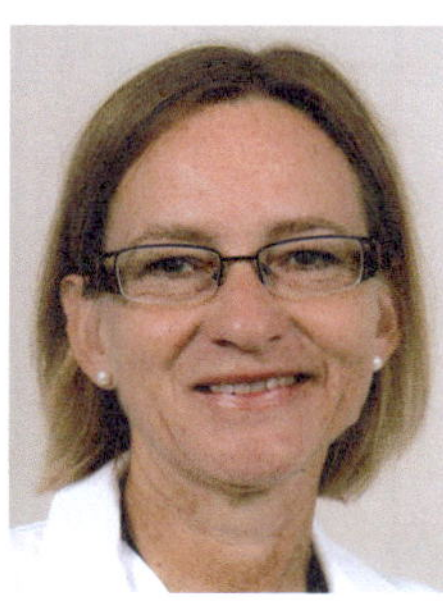

Ann Wennerberg, DDS, PhD worked 11 years in a private dental practice before she joined the Department of Biomaterials, Gothenburg University, in the late 1980s. She presented her PhD thesis *On Surface Roughness and Implant Incorporation* in 1996 and a few years later was appointed Professor and Head of the Department of Prosthodontics at Gothenburg University. She moved to the Dental School of Malmö as Head of Prosthodontics in 2008. Ann Wennerberg has published numerous papers on implant surfaces and clinical results of oral implants and is today the leader of a most active research group at her department.

Contents

Contributors

Tomas Albrektsson, MD, PhD, ODhc, RCPSG Department of Prosthodontics, Malmo University, Malmo, Sweden

Department of Biomaterials, University of Gothenburg, Gothenburg, Sweden

Martin Andersson, PhD Chemical and Biological Engineering, Chalmers University of Technology, Goteborg, Sweden

Ikiru Atsuta, DDS, PhD Section of Implant and Rehabilitative Dentistry, Division of Oral Rehabilitation, Kyushu University, Fukuoka, Japan

Estevam A. Bonfante, DDS, PhD Department of Prosthodontics, University of São Paulo – Bauru College of DentistryBauru, SP, Brazil

David L. Cochran, DDS, MS, PhD, MMSci, Drhc Department of Periodontics, The University of Texas Health Science Center at San Antonio, Dental School, San Antonio, TX, USA

Paulo G. Coelho, DDS, PhD Department of Biomaterials and Biomimetics, Department of Periodontology and Implant Dentistry, New York University, New York, NY, USA

Division of Engineering, New York University Abu Dhabi, New York, NY, USA

Hugo De Bruyn, DDS, MSc, PhD Department of Periodontology and Oral Implantology, University of Ghent, University Hospital Dental School, Ghent, Belgium

Jan Eirik Ellingsen, DDS, Dr.odont Department of Prosthodontics, Institute of Clinical Dentistry, University of Oslo, Blindern, Oslo, Norway

Klaus Gotfredsen, PhD, DDS Department of Odontology, Faculty of Health and Medical Sciences, University of Copenhagen, Copenhagen N, Denmark

Ryo Jimbo, DDS, PhD Department of Prosthodontics, Malmo University, Malmo, Sweden

Yohei Jinno, DDS, PhD Section of Implant and Rehabilitative Dentistry, Division of Oral Rehabilitation, Kyushu University, Fukuoka, Japan

Kiyoshi Koyano, DDS, PhD Section of Implant and Rehabilitative Dentistry, Division of Oral Rehabilitation, Faculty of Dental Science, Kyushu University, Fukuoka, Japan

Bo Meng, DDS, PhD Department of Periodontics, The University of Texas Health Science Center at San Antonio, San Antonio, TX, USA

Oral Implantology Center, Guangdong Provincial Stomatological Hospital, Southern Medical University, Guangzhou, Guangdong, People's Republic of China

Marta Monjo, PhD Department of Fundamental Biology and Health Sciences, Research Institute on Health Sciences (IUNICS), Instituto de Investigación Santaria de Palma (IdISPa), Palma de Mallorca, Spain

Pär-Olov Östman, DDS, PhD Department Periodontology and Oral Implantology, University of Ghent, University Hospital Dental School, Ghent, Belgium

Joana Maria Ramis, PhD Department of Fundamental Biology and Health Sciences, Research Institute on Health Sciences (IUNICS), Palma de Mallorca, Spain

Stefan K. Roehling, DDS Department of Periodontics, The University of Texas Health Science Center at San Antonio, Dental School, San Antonio, TX, USA

Department of Oral and Cranio-Maxillofacial Surgery, Hightech Research Center, University Hospital Basel, University of Basel, Basel, Switzerland

Takashi Sawase, DDS, PhD Department of Applied Prosthodontics, Graduate School of Biomedical Sciences, Nagasaki University, Nagasaki, Japan

Ikuya Watanabe, PhD Department of Biomaterials, Nagasaki University, Nagasaki, Japan

Ann Wennerberg, DDS, PhD Oral Prosthodontics, Malmo University, Malmo, Sweden

Anna Westerlund, DDS, PhD Department of Orthodontics, Sahigrenska Academy, University of Gothenburg, Gothenburg, Sweden

Overview of Surface Evaluation Techniques

1

Ann Wennerberg, Ryo Jimbo,
and Tomas Albrektsson

Abstract

Surface characterisation is necessary if we want to understand biological processes influenced by surface properties and eventually their clinical importance. In addition, we need surface characterisation if researchers want to distinguish between the components forming the implant surface, i.e. topography, chemistry, physics and mechanics. The techniques should provide objective data to decrease the possibility for subjective interpretation and biases. This chapter is a brief overview of commonly used evaluation techniques of the four different surface properties with the emphasis on topographical evaluations.

Surface Topography

Implant surface topography can be measured with three principally different techniques.

Mechanical stylus instruments: a cantilever with a tip of several microns is drawn over the surface for one profile measurement; the movements of the cantilever are registered, and data with respect to surface height and spatial variation can be achieved. Several profiles are added to achieve a 3D image and more stable numerical values of the various surface parameters. The measuring range can be several millimetres (Fig. 1.1). The resolution in height is down to the nanometre level, but in the spatial direction the resolution is only 2 μm or more due to the size of the tip. The main drawback with the technique for oral implants is that due to the small dimension of the threaded area, the tip will have great difficulties to reach the flank area; thus, measurements have to be performed on less curved areas such as the marginal portion of the implant that may not be representative for the entire implant surface.

Optical instruments: in particular interferometry has been found appropriate for measuring a

A. Wennerberg, DDS, PhD (✉)
Oral Prosthodontics, Malmo University,
Carl Gustafs Vag 34, Malmo 205 06, Sweden
e-mail: ann.wennerberg@mah.se

R. Jimbo, DDS, PhD
Department of Prosthodontics, Malmo University,
Malmo, Sweden
e-mail: ryo.jimbo@mah.se

T. Albrektsson, MD, PhD, Odhc, RCPSG
Oral Prosthodontics, Malmo University,
Carl Gustafs Vag 34, Malmo 205 06, Sweden

Dental School, Smedjegatan Malmo, Sweden
e-mail: tomas.albrektsson@biomaterials.gu.se

A. Wennerberg et al. (eds.), *Implant Surfaces and their Biological and Clinical Impact*,
DOI 10.1007/978-3-662-45379-7_1, © Springer-Verlag Berlin Heidelberg 2015

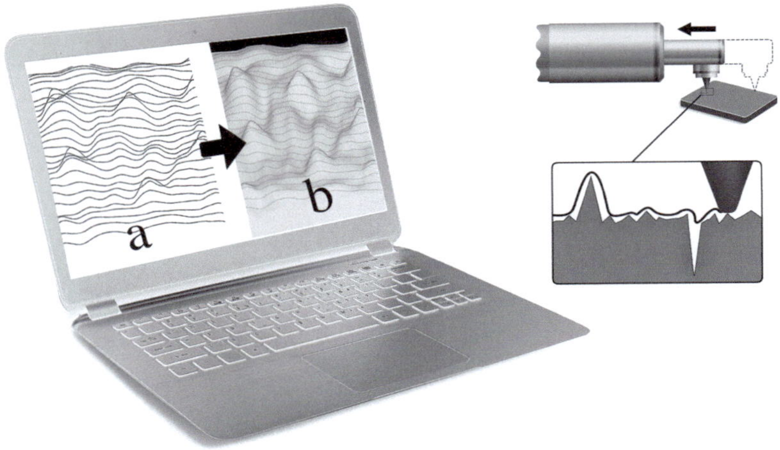

Fig. 1.1 A drawing of a mechanical stylus equipment clearly demonstrating the influence of the stylus tip. The measured profile is significantly smoother than the real surface (Figure produced by Braian Development AB, Malmö, Sweden)

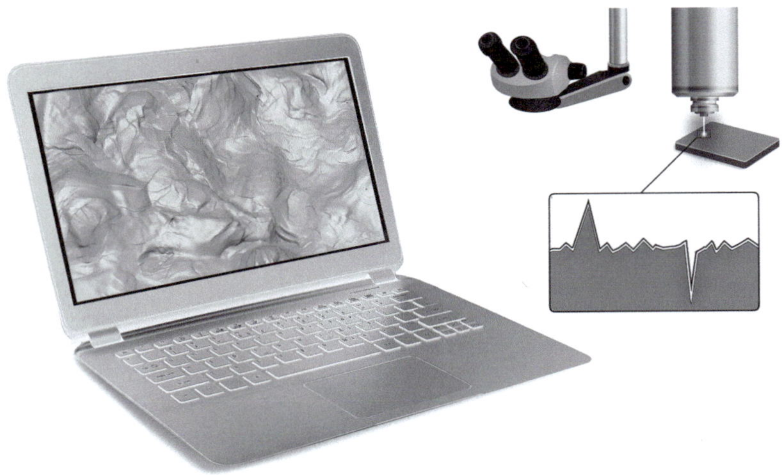

Fig. 1.2 A drawing of an optical profiler. Due to the noncontact technique, the horizontal resolution is increased. The light beam can follow the irregularities quite well (Figure produced by Braian Development AB, Malmö, Sweden)

huge variation of implant surfaces, from smooth to rough surface modifications. The technique uses reflecting light as an optical stylus (Fig. 1.2). The measuring range is within a few millimetres. The technique provides high resolution, down to the nanometre level in height direction but is limited in spatial direction to approximately 0.3 μm; thus, the technique is most appropriate for surface characterisation at the micrometre level. In relation to oral implants, one big advantage with the technique is the possibility to access all parts of the implant, even flank areas, which is important since these areas are the largest part of the implant that is in contact with the surrounding bone. One disadvantage with optical instruments is that studied objects need some reflecting capacity, at least 4 % of the incident light as a minimum.

Atomic force microscopy (*AFM*): AFM can work in principle in three different modes of operation, contact, noncontact and tapping mode. The instrument uses a tip and cantilever with similar principle as the stylus instrument but with a huge difference in size. The AFM tip is in the range of a few to approximately 20 nm in diameter. The tip can be in contact with the surface during measurements or above it with the help of van der Waals forces. The measuring area is rather small, typically in the submicron range. The resolution can approach molecular levels both in height and spatial directions which makes it possible to measure nanostructures. However, many implants have a surface that is too rough for the equipment; thus, for oral implants the application is limited to rather smooth surfaces.

Furthermore, flank areas are difficult to measure, due to the same reasons as for the stylus instrument.

Quantitative Evaluation of Measurements

Independent of measuring instruments the measuring data is used to calculate the dimensions and properties such as slope of the irregularities included in the surface. There are hundreds of different parameters; the challenge is to find descriptors that can predict the biological response to certain surface structures.

An implant surface is a geometrical combination of overlay features in different scales:

1. Overall form such as discs, cylinders or screws
2. Waviness due to, for example, machining vibration or marks from cutting tools
3. Micro features, for example, peaks, valleys, scratches, pits, ridges and porosity
4. Smaller nano-features, for example, tubes, peaks, pits and ridges

Stylus instruments originally provided information from one profile alone, i.e. 2D data. Today 3D characterisation is far more common. Needless to say 3D provides much more data; thus, the parameter values will be more reliable.

2D descriptions can be used to describe relatively simple surfaces and simple thread geometries, but very often a three-dimensional (3D) representation of a surface is required to quantify directional surface features like 'craters', 'droplets', pits, tubes, etc., features quite common on oral implants. This largely excludes 2D metrology and 2D characterisation as suitable for dental implant measurement purposes.

Before the mid-1990s, the common practice for dental implant surface geometry specification was at best the 2D profile amplitude parameters R_a and R_t describing the average and maximum amplitudes of the profile (ISO 4287:1996). Extensive research in the area resulted in a suggestion for a parameter set for dental implant characterisation based on the current EUR 15178N and ISO 25178 standards [1]. For an acceptable characterisation of implant topography, at least 1 height, 1 spatial and 1 hybrid parameter were suggested to be presented.

Height parameters describe the surfaces' deviation from an intersecting mean plane. S_q and S_a describe average height amplitudes either by the RMS method or as a simple arithmetic mean.

The shape of the amplitude distribution curve is quantified by its skewness (S_{sk}) and the kurtosis (S_{ku}).

The average amplitude parameters are very well suited for a robust characterisation of the overall roughness of the dental implants. The parameters are especially well equipped for control of isotropic implant surfaces, i.e. surfaces without a dominate direction like shot-blasted or etched surfaces, or to achieve amplitude information from turned implants (anisotropic surface) where no detailed surface feature information is required (Fig. 1.3).

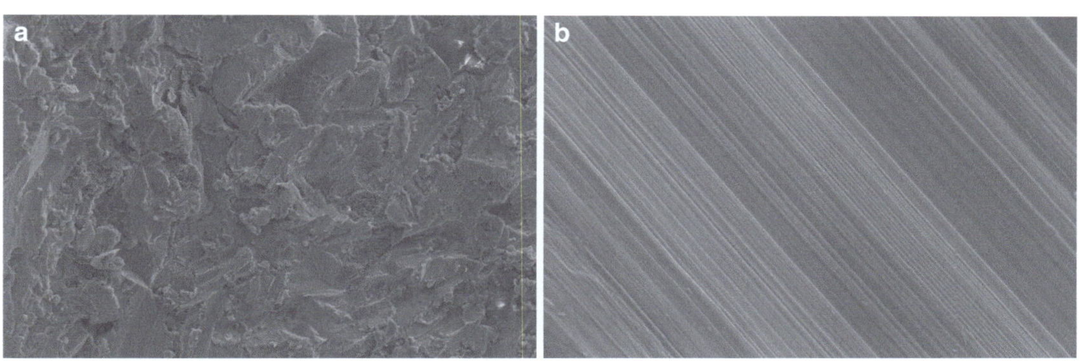

Fig. 1.3 (**a**) A SEM image of a blasted titanium implant. The imprints from the blasting media have created an isotropic surface with no dominating direction of the surface irregularities. (**b**) A SEM image of a turned implant surface. The cutting tool creates scratches with a clear direction, an example of an anisotropic surface

In addition to average calculated parameters, there are extreme height parameters, for example, S_p, S_v and S_t. Maximum peak and valley points are described by S_p and S_v, and their sum is named maximum height, S_t. These parameters are normally very sensitive to noise or spikes and are generally less stable for surface descriptions.

Spatial parameters describe the lateral property of the surface. Autocorrelation (S_{al}) indicates the starting wavelength of repeating features, while the presence of anisotropic properties is shown by the texture aspect ratio (S_{tr}), defined as a quotient between the shortest and longest autocorrelation lengths in any directions of the surface. The texture direction parameter (S_{tr}) is in ISO grouped as a 'miscellaneous' parameter but defines the direction of the largest autocorrelation length. Another spatial parameter is the description of density of summits (S_{ds}), that is, a calculation of how many peaks there are per area unit. This parameter can distinguish between dense and more structureless surfaces.

The spatial parameters have a good ability to detect anisotropy in the dental surface like underlying not removed by previous manufacturing steps or directionalities superimposed by coatings or oxidised implant layers.

Hybrid parameters describe the shape of the surface by the mean slope (S_{dq}) and the developed area ratio (S_{dr}) by a combination of amplitude and spatial properties. The latter as a measure of the total surface area compared to a nominal flat area.

The hybrid parameters have a strong potential to give numbers useful for, e.g. characterisation of active surface area (S_{dr}). The hybrid parameters are very scale sensitive and must be measured at a scale where functional wavelengths are present.

For oral implants a common parameter set is S_a, S_{ds} and S_{dr}.

SEM (Scanning Electron Microscopy)

SEM uses a high energy beam of electrons to create images of the surface. The electrons interact with the atoms on the surface, new electrons are emitted from the surface, the intensity of this signal differs in the scanned area and thus a distribution map will create the image. This image can be used for evaluation of surface morphology and chemical composition. Magnification depends on current and voltage; images can be produced with varying magnification, from 10 to 500,000 times; high-magnification SEM can provide high-resolution images and small features in the 1–5 nm range can be detected. A significant drawback for biological samples is that the samples need to be electrically conductive, which often results in a need for pretreatment with a conductive coat. A development of SEM is environmental SEM (ESEM), a technique where coating no longer is a requirement thus much more appropriate for biological samples. Previously SEM did not provide quantitative topographical data; more modern equipment have overcome this clear disadvantage, and now some surface parameters can be achieved.

Surface Chemistry XPS

Chemical composition and depth profiling can be measured with Auger electron spectroscopy (AES) and X-ray photoelectron spectroscopy (XPS). XPS provides more detailed information than AES. Information will be retrieved from the outermost 5–10 nm surface layer, and in addition the oxide layer thickness can be investigated with this technique. For evaluation of the oxide thickness and structure, Rutherford backscattering and transmission electron microscopy (TEM) can be used, but these techniques are not so common as the XPS in chemical characterisation of oral implants.

Surface Physics

Contact angle measurements are often performed as a measure of surface energy and the degree of hydrophilicity or hydrophobicity, i.e. the wettability. The sessile drop method includes a drop of liquid (for evaluating hydrophilicity/hydrophobicity, pure water is used) applied on the surface; the volume is well controlled, typically in the range of 1–6 µl. The angle between the drop and the surface is then measured. A water contact angle above 90° is considered to be hydrophobic, while less than 90° is hydrophilic. Super-hydrophilic surfaces are surfaces with a contact angle less than 10°.

Surface energy can be measured using glycol instead of water.

Surface Mechanics

The hardness of an implant surface can be measured with a Vickers or Brinell test. A pyramidal (Vickers) or a ball (Brinell) will be pressed into the implant at a certain controlled force. The imprints will be measured; soft materials will have rather big imprints and hard materials very small imprints. Today nano-indentation can be used, same principle but imprinting tip and forces at the nano-level. Nano-indentation may be a useful technique to evaluate the biological effects of implants with nano-surfaces [2].

X-ray diffraction techniques may be used to investigate residual stresses [3].

References

1. Wennerberg A, Albrektsson T. Suggested guidelines for the topographic evaluation of implant surfaces. Int J Oral Maxillofac Implants. 2000;15:331–44.
2. Jimbo R, Coelho PG, Bryington M, Baldassarri M, Tovar N, Currie F, Hayashi M, Andersson M, Ono D, Vandeweghe S, Wennerberg A. Nano hydroxyapatite-coated implants improve bone nanomechanical properties. J Dent Res. 2012;91(12):1172–7.
3. Noyan IC, Cohen JB. Residual stress measurements by diffraction interpretation. New York: Springer; 1987.

2 Overview of Surface Microtopography/Chemistry/Physics/Nano-roughness

Tomas Albrektsson, Ryo Jimbo, and Ann Wennerberg

Abstract

The implant surface has since long been recognised as important for the host response to oral implants. When the implant is inserted in the body, blood will immediately cover the implant surface. Different surface properties may trigger proteins and signalling system to enhance and speed up the healing process. The implant surface can be altered with respect to topography, chemistry, physics and mechanical properties. In particular, so far the surface topography and chemistry have gained the greatest interest from researchers and manufacturers of oral implants.

Introduction

The implant surface has since long been recognised as important for the host response to oral implants. When the implant is inserted in the body, blood will immediately cover the implant surface. Different surface properties may trigger proteins and signalling system to enhance and speed up the healing process. The implant surface can be altered with respect to topography, chemistry, physics and mechanical properties. In particular, so far the surface topography and chemistry have gained the greatest interest from researchers and manufacturers of oral implants.

Topographical Properties

The implant topographical properties may be described as alterations in the millimetre, the micrometre and the nanometre range.

Millimetre Surface Topography

The mm surface topography is normally described as the implant design. Today a screw-shaped design is dominating due to the better

T. Albrektsson, MD, PhD, Odhc, RCPSG (✉)
Department of Prosthodontics, Malmo University, Malmo, Sweden

Department of Biomaterials,University of Gothenburg, Gothenburg, Sweden
e-mail: tomas.albrektsson@biomaterials.gu.se

R. Jimbo, DDS, PhD
Department of Prosthodontics, Malmo University, Malmo, Sweden
e-mail: ryo.jimbo@mah.se

A. Wennerberg, DDS, PhD
Oral Prosthodontics, Malmo University, Carl Gustafs Vag 34, Malmo 205 06, Sweden
e-mail: ann.wennerberg@mah.se

A. Wennerberg et al. (eds.), *Implant Surfaces and their Biological and Clinical Impact*,
DOI 10.1007/978-3-662-45379-7_2, © Springer-Verlag Berlin Heidelberg 2015

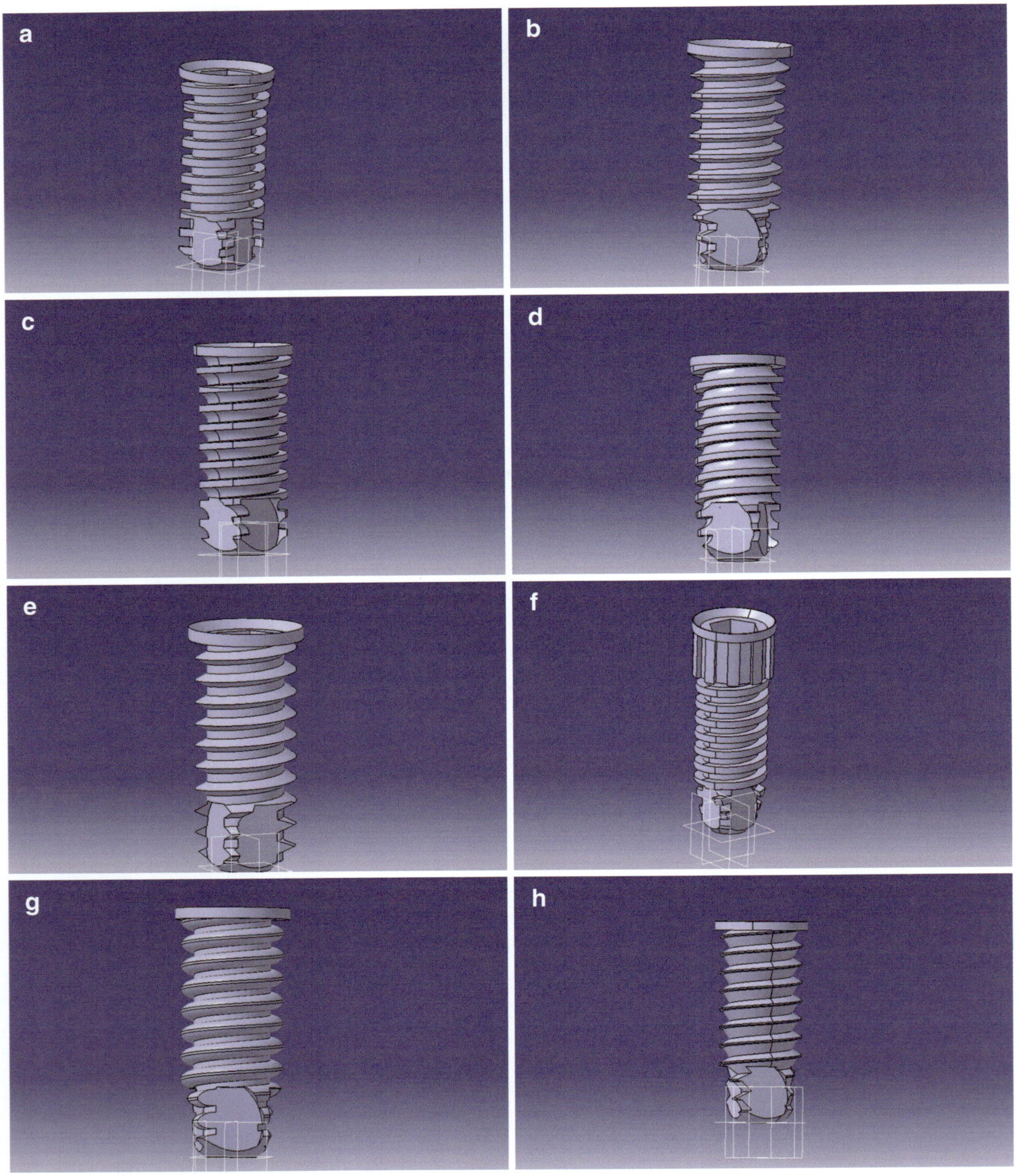

Fig. 2.1 Eight different examples of implant thread designs. (**a**) Power square thread, (**b**) power Acme thread, (**c**) buttress thread, (**d**) reverse buttress, (**e**) fixture thread, (**f**) vertical slot thread, (**g**) rounded off power thread, (**h**) Spiralock technique

primary stability such designs may provide as compared with a cylindrical model. However, the optimal thread design is still insufficiently investigated with respect to stabilisation and load-bearing capacity during function. A huge number of thread designs are available (Fig. 2.1); finite element analyses demonstrate different stress distribution of each design, but knowledge about the clinical relevance is still lacking.

Microthreads on the marginal part of the implant were introduced by the end of the 1990s. This implant design has in several controlled clinical studies been found to maintain the marginal bone levels [1–3], possibly due to the microthreads reducing peak stresses in the bone [4]. Recent research has demonstrated microthreads between larger threads positioned over the entire implant may have some bone stimulating effect too, in particularly in soft bone quality [5].

Summary Millimetre Implant Topography

Screw-shaped implant dominates the market, but the optimal design of individual treads still remains to be concluded.

Micrometre Surface Topography

The first implants used clinically were produced with a turning process; the cutting procedure leaves clear marks on the surface; thus, this surface will have a clear orientation. In addition, turned oral implants are smooth to minimally rough according to a suggested classification [6], i.e. surfaces have an Sa (average height deviation) value less than 1 μm. However, a substantial number of experimental studies performed during the 1990s clearly demonstrated potential advantages with moderately rough surfaces (an Sa value between 1 and 2 μm), whereas smoother as well as rougher implants were found to integrate less well. Today the majority of commercially available implants are produced within this range of surface topography. Common approaches to increase the roughness above the turned implants could be either by techniques that will remove materials from the surface, i.e. creating pits, or by adding material, i.e. creating bumps on the surface. The major techniques that remove material are etching, blasting, combination of blasting and etching and oxidation. Although it should be noted, etching alone removes cutting marks from the turning process and leaves a surface with high-frequency irregularities; thus, the technique produces an enlarged surface area but the Sa value will not be significantly increased. Therefore, acid etching is not sufficient to produce a moderately rough surface. Moderately rough surfaces are most commonly manufactured by blasting, a combination of blasting and etching or oxidation. The roughness achieved with blasting depends on the blasting media (e.g. TiO2, Al2O3 sand and corundum particles), the size and shape of the particles, pressure during blasting and distance from blasting equipment to target (the implant). The reason for a combination of blasting and etching is that this will provide a moderately rough surface with rather long wave components due to imprints from blasting media and small pits due to etching contributing high-frequency components.

In unselected patient materials the old turned implants have demonstrated very good long-term clinical results with survival rates above 90 % after 10–15 years. However, for more compromised patients with poor bone quality and quantity due to various reasons, moderately rough surfaces have significantly improved the clinical results compared to the old turned implants, for example, when inserted in posterior regions, in the maxillary bone, in smokers or in transplanted bone [7].

Summary Micrometre Topography

Moderately rough implants dominate the market today. The clinical results have been improved with these implants compared to smoother, turned implants in particular for some groups of patients.

Nanometre Surface Topography

The latest generation of implant surfaces includes nano-modifications. One of the most common hypotheses behind nanotopography for improvement of implant incorporation in bone is that the nano-irregularities will form attachment sites for proteins important during the healing process. Thus, the blood proteins first to attach to the implant surface during insertion in the bone which governs further biological events through signalling systems, selection of adhered cells and further bone-forming processes. Nanostructures

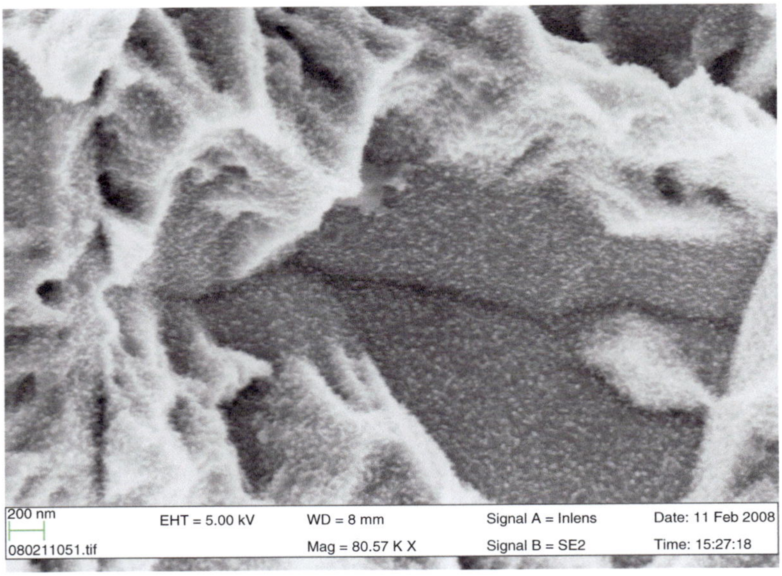

Fig. 2.2 Nanoparticles densely and evenly distributed on an SLActive surface

have even been speculated to improve marginal soft tissue adherence to implant components, which may have potential for maintaining marginal bone levels and a healthy surrounding mucosa.

The definition of nanostructures has been suggested as the range of 1–100 nm [8]. Nanostructures can be coated on the surface. Common coats are hydroxyapatite or titanium dioxide. In particular the former has been evaluated in many experimental and clinical studies.

Nanostructures may, in addition to coating procedures, be spontaneously formed during manufacturing. It seems like etching procedures in combination with storage in liquid will lead to reorganisation of the outermost titanium oxide layer into nanostructures [9]. A possible hypothesis may be that the hydride layers, which are formed due to the etching [10], will act as nucleation centres. Furthermore, the dissociative adsorption of water is expected to play a crucial role, and Ti diffusion has to take place for the growth of the nanostructure.

To detect and characterise nanofeatures, SEM (scanning electron microscopy) or AFM (atomic force microscopy) can be used. In particular with high-magnification SEM images, nanoparticles are easy to detect (Fig. 2.2). Evaluation of the most common sold implant brands reveals nanofeatures on many of them, such as SLActive (Straumann Institute, Basel, Switzerland), OsseoSpeed (Astra Tech Implant System, Dentsply, Germany), NanoTite (3i/Biomet, Florida, USA) and TiUnite (Nobel Biocare, Bern, Switzerland) surfaces. However, the density and appearance may vary as shown in Fig. 2.3.

Clinical results with implants including nanostructures are so far limited to about 10 years of follow-up. However the results are so far promising with cumulative survival rates for 10 years ranging from 95 to 100 % [11]. However, commercial oral implants would not display nanofeatures alone; in contrast such surfaces have combinations with microtopographical, chemical and/or physical characteristics, presenting with clear difficulties to single out one specific parameter such as nano-roughness to be behind good clinical results. Therefore, whether clinical results will be better with than without nanostructures is yet not known.

Chemical Properties

Various modifications of implant surfaces' chemical composition to allegedly promote bone healing have been frequently used over the years. An early modification was the hydroxyapatite (HA)

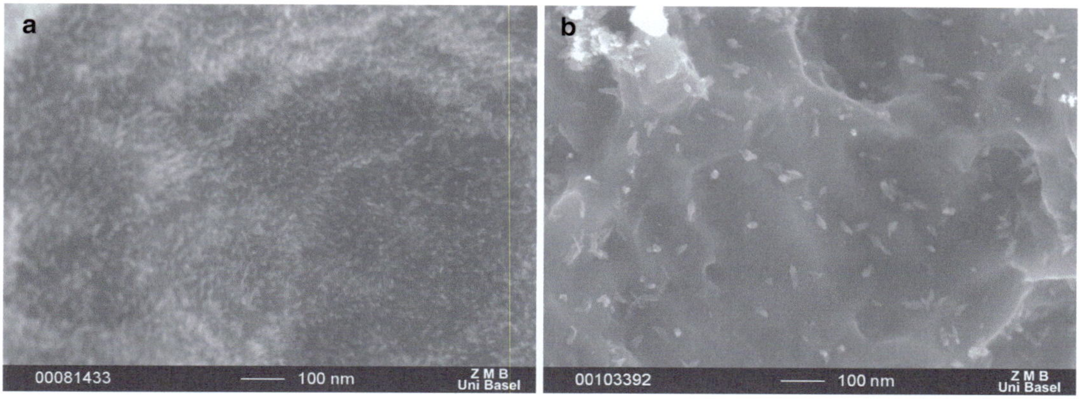

Fig. 2.3 SLActive surface and B TiZr surface both demonstrating the presence of nanostructures but (**a**) densely and (**b**) sparsely distributed

coat, introduced during the 1980s. HA coats allegedly having a similar chemical composition as the bone itself were hypothesised to promote chemical bonds between the implant surface and the bone tissue; thus, an immediate primary stability would occur, and the bone healing would be faster and firmer. Early experimental studies did show an enhanced bone healing compared to similar non-coated implants, but clinically HA-coated implants commonly demonstrated substantial bone resorption and, with time, very high implant failure rates, possibly associated with loss of the rather thick coats from the core metal. The loose coats created an inflammation, bone resorption and eventually implant failure. The HA coating not only changed the chemistry but the surface topography was considerably enlarged as well.

Today HA is again used as a coating but now in very thin layers of a thickness in the nanometre level. These coats seem to have better stability, but long-term clinical studies are still lacking.

Other chemical modifications of the implant surface include implementation of various ions with potentially bioactive properties. Calcium, magnesium and fluoride are some examples. These chemical modifications seldom influence the microtopography, but they often alter the nanotopography. In comparative experimental studies, impressive effects have been displayed with chemically altered surfaces, but their clinical effectiveness is yet to be demonstrated.

Physical Properties

In relation to implant surfaces, in particular the charge and the wettability have been hypothesised to have an impact on bone healing. Surface charge influences the surface energy which is a measure of the extent to which bonds are unsatisfied at the surface [12]. Thus various techniques to create very clean surfaces may increase the surface energy and ability to attach proteins. Such techniques include cleaning under argon or nitrogen protection and UV (ultraviolet) illumination. A high surface energy may result in a high degree of wettability; thus, when an implant is exposed to blood, the entire surface will almost immediately be covered by the liquid, again stimulating the blood proteins to attach to the surface to start the bone-healing process. However, from a clinical point of view, a recent overview failed to find convincing evidence of the effectiveness of increasing surface energies [13].

Mechanical Properties

The hardness of the implant surface may influence the wear, both of the implant itself and of the bone tissue during installation. Plastic deformation may cause residual stresses in the implant surface which may increase the corrosion rate. However, mechanical properties of the implant surface are very scarcely evaluated, and knowledge about their importance is very limited.

References

1. Lee DW, Choi YS, Park KH, Kim CS, Moon IS. Effect of microthread on the maintenance of marginal bone level: a 3-year prospective study. Clin Oral Implants Res. 2007;18:465–70.
2. Palmer RN, Palmer PJ, Smith BJ. A prospective study of a Astra single tooth implants. Clin Oral Implants Res. 2000;11(2):179–82.
3. Mertens C, Steveling HG, Stucke K, Pretzl B, Meyer-Baumer A. Fixed implant-retained rehabilitation of the edentulous maxilla: 11-years results of a prospective study. Clin Implant Dent Relat Res. 2012;14(6):816–27.
4. Hansson S. A conical implant-abutment interface at the level of the marginal bone improves the distribution of stresses in the supporting bone. Clin Oral Implants Res. 2003;14:286–93.
5. Chowdhary R, Halldin A, Jimbo R, Wennerberg A. Influence of micro threads alteration on osseointegration and primary stability of implants: an FEA and in vivo analysis in rabbits. Clin Implant Dent Relat Res. 2013. EPub ahead of print.
6. Albrektsson T, Wennerberg A. Oral implant surfaces. Part 1. A review focussing on topographical and chemical properties of different surfaces and in vivo responses to them. Int J Prosthodont. 2004;17:536–43.
7. Jimbo R, Albrektsson T. A comparison of marginal bone loss and clinical outcome between older, turned and newer, moderately rough implants. Implant Dentistry, accepted for publication 2014.
8. Webster TJ, Ahn ES. Nanostructured biomaterials for tissue engineering bone. Tissue Engineering II. Berlin: Springer; 2007. p. 275–308.
9. Wennerberg A, Svanborg Melin L, Berner S, Andersson M. Spontaneously formed nanostructures on titanium surfaces. Clin Oral Implants Res. 2013;24(2):203–9.
10. Szmukler-Moncler S, Bischof M, Nedir R, Ermrich M. Titanium hydride and hydrogen concentration in acid-etched commercially pure titanium and titanium alloy implants: a comparative analysis of five implant systems. Clin Oral Implants Res. 2010;21:944–50.
11. Albrektsson T, Buser D, Sennerby L. Crestal bone loss and oral implants. Clin Implant Dent Relat Res. 2012;14:783–91.
12. Hench LL, Ethridge EC. Biomaterials. An interfacial approach. New York: Academic; 1982.
13. Wennerberg A, Galli S, Albrektsson T. Current knowledge of the SLActive surface. Clin Cosmet Investig Dent (Dove Press). 2011;3:59–67.

Experimental and Clinical Knowledge of Surface Micro-topography

3

Ryo Jimbo, Ann Wennerberg, and Tomas Albrektsson

Abstract

Implant surface micro-topography has been of great interest for many years. Scientific evidence indicates that the micro-roughness of the implant is one of the regulatory factors for osseointegration, and roughness within a certain range has been proven to present the strongest bone responses. The so-called moderately rough micro-topography has been applied to most of the commercially available implants of today and has shown high clinical success rates, especially in compromised bone quality sites. This chapter will focus on the importance of micro-topography on implant osseointegration by exploring the experimental and clinical evidence available. Furthermore, the recent topics regarding micro-topography in relation to marginal bone maintenance will be briefly discussed.

Introduction

The reliability of the implant treatment as a clinical alternative for edentulism has significantly increased over the past 50 years owing to the advancements in numerous fields. Albrektsson et al. have suggested that implant success is an exquisite balance of six different factors consisting from implant material, implant design, implant finish, status of the bone, surgical technique, and implant loading conditions [1]. From an implant surface topography (finish) viewpoint, the experimental and clinical evidence concerning implant surface micro-topography and its biologic responses has led to the development of the so-called moderately rough implant surfaces [2]. As a result, most of the commercially available implants today possess a moderately rough micro-topography, which can be considered as one of the major features contributing to the clinical success of the implant [3], and furthermore, the implants of today possess a nano-topography within the micro-topography, which will be

R. Jimbo, DDS, PhD (✉)
Department of Prosthodontics, Malmo University, Malmo, Sweden
e-mail: ryo.jimbo@mah.se

A. Wennerberg, DDS, PhD
Oral Prosthodontics, Malmo University, Carl Gustavs Vag 34, Malmo 205 06, Sweden
e-mail: ann.wennerberg@mah.se

T. Albrektsson, MD, PhD, Odhc, RCPSG
Department of Prosthodontics, Malmo University, Malmo, Sweden

Dental School, Smedjegatan Malmo, Sweden
e-mail: tomas.albrektsson@biomaterials.gu.se

A. Wennerberg et al. (eds.), *Implant Surfaces and their Biological and Clinical Impact*,
DOI 10.1007/978-3-662-45379-7_3,

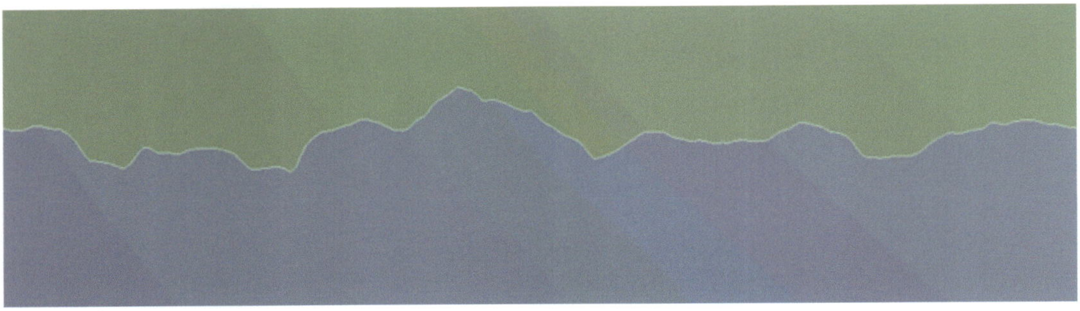

Fig. 3.1 Schematic image of the increased surface area generated by the micro-roughening procedure

discussed in a later chapter by Coelho et al. Although the manufacturing process can differ depending on implant systems, there is a general consensus today that implant micro-topography possessing Sa value of approximately 1.0–2.0 μm and Sdr of approximately 50 % presents the strongest bone responses [4].

Although the clinical documentation of the moderately rough implant surfaces is not as long as the traditional turned implant surfaces, it can be said that the addition of the moderately rough micro-topography has significant benefits especially when they are placed in sites with lower bone quality with thin cortical bone [5, 6]. This phenomenon can possibly be explained from biomechanical and biological aspects.

From a biomechanical viewpoint, the expanded surface area of the moderately rough implant surface, which is in contact with the surrounding bone tissue, increases the friction coefficiency and the kinetic friction during implant insertion (Fig. 3.1).

Along with implant macro-geometry, the increased kinetic friction naturally provides higher implant primary stability [7], which is equivalent to the lower micro-motion of the implant in the bone. The high primary stability of the implant provides a stable host bed, which allows growth factors and cells to successfully adhere to the implant surface.

From a biological viewpoint, the moderately roughened surface micro-topography seems to modulate the cellular events towards a more osteogenic atmosphere [8]. It has been reported that the surface micro-roughness is a regulatory factor for the production of growth factors, cell attachment, proliferation, differentiation, and mineralization [9, 10]. Interestingly, the scientific evidence from in vitro studies suggests that osteogenic cells possess a topography cognitive mechanism to micron or to sub-micron structures [11–13]. Ismail et al. have shown that the viability and attachment of osteoblasts to commercially available implant surfaces had altered depending on the micro-topography (in this case, different size microgrooves) [11]. What is more interesting is that these cells seem to follow the microgrooves created, which provided further stability of the cell attachment and improved osteogenesis [14]. The so-called contact guidance is a typical example of a micro-topography influencing the biological outcomes of osteogenic cells, which also strongly indicates the importance of micro-topography on biomaterial surfaces.

Thus, this chapter focuses on the effect of micro-topography on osseointegration from both experimental and clinical aspects. Furthermore, the different surface modification methodologies will be introduced to deepen the knowledge of implant surface topography, which should help the readers to better understand the following chapters on this topic.

Turned Implant Surfaces

The osseointegration implants initially utilized by the Swedish and the Swiss groups were the turned (or the so-called machined) implants, which in reality has the longest clinical documentation. The term 'machined' should be avoided as much as possible in this book since it is well known that implants are manufactured by a turning process in a turning machine. The term 'machined' could be any surface finish, since as long as a 'machine' is involved in the manufacturing process, the surface could be called 'machined'; thus, it is clear that the terminology is not suitable especially for a book focusing on implant surfaces. For example, implants that have a mechanically polished surface finish are often rightfully called 'machined' and compared with turned 'machined' surfaces. However, these polished implants possess a much smoother surface topography in the micro-level compared to the traditional Brånemark turned implant surfaces; thus, the comparison is not correct from a topographical point of view. Turned surface implants have indeed a long clinical history. Until the mid-1990s the turned implants dominated the market. One of the first long-term documentation concerning the survival of the turned osseointegrated implants stated that 81 % of the maxillary implants and 91 % of the mandibular fixtures remained stable after a 15-year period [15]. Attard and Zarb had replicated the studies performed in Sweden and reported in their prospective study that over a 20-year period (range 18–23 years), the implant success rate with fixed prosthesis in edentulous patients was 87 % [16]. These studies clearly highlight that the turned implants present good prognosis over a long period. According to Wennerberg and Albrektsson [4], these once commercially available turned Brånemark implants had a surface topographical value of Sa of 0.9 μm and an Sdr of 34 % [4]. Thus, it can be said that the effect of surface micro-topography may have contributed in the long-term clinical success of the turned commercially available implants. However naturally, their definitive role during functional loading over a long period is difficult to distinguish since implant success is a complex blend of multiple factors.

Rough Implant Surfaces

In general, the traditional Brånemark turned implants placed in the mandible, or the maxilla, followed a 2-stage protocol, which allowed the implants to heal (osseointegrate) [17]. Clinically, it has been suggested that the turned implants required a healing period of 3 months in the mandible and 6 months in the maxilla. This was probably one of the reasons why the so-called rough implant surfaces appeared on the market in order to provide higher grip between the implant surface and the bone. It can be said that back in the days when the development of these surfaces took place, there was little evidence on what is the optimal roughness. Although in general, from a mechanical viewpoint, the rougher surfaces have been known to provide higher stability, the clinical performance of these surfaces was without proper evidence. More on the optimal roughness, namely, the moderately roughened surface, will be introduced later in this chapter.

In this section, the two major surface-roughening procedures, i.e. evidence with regard to the titanium plasma spraying technique and hydroxyapatite coating technique, will be briefly introduced.

Titanium Plasma-Sprayed Rough Implant Surfaces

The plasma spray technique, which yields a bumpy surface configuration [3], was introduced to roughen the titanium outermost layer so that the implants allegedly would osseointegrate faster than the turned implants [18]. Wennerberg and Albrektsson [3] have summarized different implant surface topographies in their review and have stated that the surface roughness of the plasma-sprayed implants possess a surface roughness of approximately Ra 4–5 μm [3]. Although the Ra as we know is a two-dimensional parameter and cannot be directly correlated to the three-dimensional Sa, it is evident that the surface topography of the plasma-sprayed implant surfaces possesses quite a rough topography compared to the turned implant surfaces.

The rougher surface generated by the titanium plasma spray (TPS) technique seemed to accelerate osseointegration in some animal studies [18–20]; on the contrary, some studies including a clinical 5-year randomized, control clinical study by Roccuzzo et al. indicated no major benefits of the TPS surfaces [21–23]. Moreover, numerous studies indicated that there were more complications with these rough implant surfaces compared to the less rough or turned surfaces and caused more marginal bone loss [19, 24–28]. Especially with periodontally susceptible patients, De Boever et al. indicated that the survival of the TPS implants significantly decreased compared to the less rough implant surfaces [29]. This trend further worsens with periodontally susceptible patients with a smoking habit. Aglietta et al. have reported that patients in this group after 10 years showed an average marginal bone loss of 2.5 mm [30]. Although the cumulative survival rate (CSR) was 100 %, one can question the success of the implant, and this can be regarded as one of the drawbacks of presenting survival rates.

Rough and Thick Hydroxyapatite Coatings

Another type of implant surface that will be introduced in this section is the thick hydroxyapatite-coated implant with a rough microsurface, most of which are no longer commercially available. These surfaces have been well described by Wennerberg et al. [31], in their study observing the design and topographical characteristics of 13 different implant systems [31]. The authors found that the hydroxyapatite implant surface presented the highest surface roughness compared to the other textured surfaces.

Experimentally, this surface has proven to be bioactive and promotes osteogenesis especially in the short term [32–36]. On the contrary, Gottlander et al. have suggested that at relatively longer healing periods in the animal study, the outermost layer of the hydroxyapatite and the bone in proximity to the surface were affected by a macrophage-induced resorption [37]. Moreover, Registad et al. have reported a time course coat flaking and delamination of the hydroxyapatite with multinucleated giant cell activity and bone resorption [38]. This phenomenon is further evident with the clinical performance of these implants as it seems that the clinical success in the long term was less favourable with many of them resulting in marginal bone loss [39].

Albrektsson et al. have reported the existence of loose hydroxyapatite particles in the tissue around clinically failed hydroxyapatite implants [40]. As indicated by the same author, the surface roughness of these implants are normally Sa = 2.0 μm or higher, and the coat thickness is between 80 and 100 μm; thus, the initial stability and fit may seemingly be excellent [41]. However, it is also suggested that these features may actually act against their clinical prognosis. Insertion protocols and functional loading may promote loosening or breakage of the particles, which induces the foreign body reaction. Furthermore, hydroxyapatite rough surfaces may be a host bed for numerous microorganisms, which may be one of the reasons for implant complications.

Moderately Roughened Implant Surfaces

As of 2014, a majority of the implant surfaces have textured micro-topographies. In principle, the turned implants as a substrate are treated with different roughening procedures such as sand blasting [42–44], acid etching [45–47], anodic oxidation [48–50], and laser etching [51–53]. More importantly, a majority of the commercially available implants of today are strategically roughened in the micro-level to present the optimal bone responses. The moderately roughened micro-roughness, as mentioned in the introduction, is the major key to the success of the implant from a surface topography viewpoint.

This success stands on the knowledge that bone responds in a different manner to different surface topographies. Wennerberg et al. have shown that implant surfaces blasted with titania particles of 25 μm and alumina particles of 75 μm presented higher bone-to-implant contact than the turned implants. For the roughness parameters, especially the average height deviation, the Ra presented differences between the turned and the blasted surfaces, with the blasted surface presenting two to three times higher topographical values (Ra = 0.4 μm, and Ra = 0.9–1.3 μm, respectively) [54]. It was suggested in another study from Wennerberg et al. that the mode of roughening, in other words, the material used to roughen, did not play a significant role on the biological outcome and the alterations in surface topography were the influential factors with regard to osseointegration (direct bone-to-implant contact) [55, 56]. Although these experimental results suggested a linear relation between the surface roughness and osseointegration, another report from Wennerberg et al. has suggested that highly increased surface roughness presents lower bone-to-implant interactions. In brief, the implants blasted with 250 μm particles (average surface height deviation Sa = 1.88 μm) presented significantly lower bone-to-implant contact than the implants blasted with 25 μm particles (average surface height deviation Sa = 1.16 μm). Interestingly, the removal torque values and the bone area presented no significant differences, which combined with the bone-to-implant contact suggests a non-linear relation between surface roughness and osseointegration [57]. As shown in Fig. 3.2, which is a summary of the series of articles presented with regard to this topic by Wennerberg et al., there seems to be a range of surface roughness that presents the strongest bone responses, and as stated in the introduction, many of the commercially available implants of today possess a moderately roughened micro-topography.

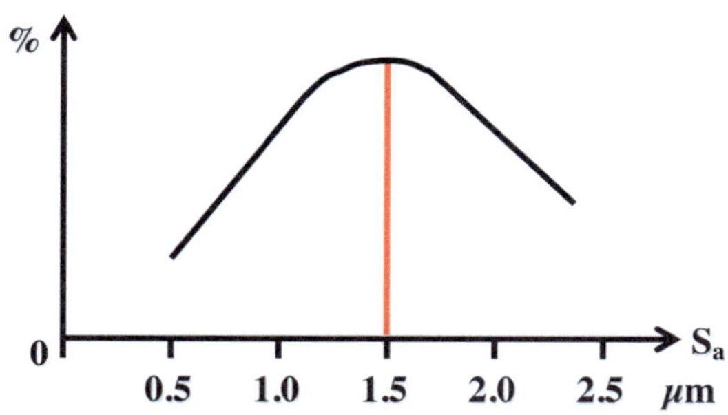

Fig. 3.2 Summary of the thesis work presented by Ann Wennerberg suggesting that the degree of osseointegration can vary depending on the surface micro-topography. It has been suggested that the moderately roughened implant micro-topography presents the strongest bone responses

Clinically, we know from experience that the moderately roughened implant surfaces osseointegrate faster and the time to functionally load has significantly reduced compared to the turned implant surfaces. Although it is difficult to prove that the implants are osseointegrating faster in the patients' bone, the alterations in loading protocols (from delayed to early or immediate) and their success clearly suggest the effects and benefits of the moderately roughened implants [58].

With regard to the clinical outcomes of the implants possessing moderately roughened surface topography after a 5-year period, the prognosis has been reported to present good outcomes. Gotfredsen and Karlsson have reported that commercially available implants with a moderately roughened surface topography presented 100 % survival after 5 years with low levels of marginal bone loss with a fixed partial prostheses as superstructures [59]. Akogulu et al. reported that three implants from different manufactures all possessing moderately roughened surfaces presented no differences in survival rates after 5 years (100 %) with marginal bone loss less than 0.4 mm with an overdenture reconstruction in the mandible.

When compared to the turned implants, the long-term implant survival of the moderately roughened implants presented no significant differences, if the implants are placed in sites such as fully healed sites or sites with good bone quality [60–62]. Thus, it seems that the moderately roughened implant surfaces do not present significant differences compared to the turned surfaces in normal situations; however, in compromised situations such as in poor quality bone, or in irradiated bone, the moderately roughened implants present their benefits. Khang et al. conducted a multicentre study testing the success of turned and dual acid-etched surfaces and reported that the success rates were notably higher for the dual acid-etched surfaces compared to the turned surfaces in poor bone quality conditions [63]. Pinholt has reported that in grafted maxillary bone, the moderately roughened implant surfaces outperformed the turned implant surfaces in terms of implant survival [64]. Buddula et al. investigated the differences in implant survival after 5 years using turned or moderately roughened implant surfaces in sites where radiation of at least 50 Gy was irradiated [65]. The results presented significantly higher survival rates for the moderately roughened implants both in the mandible and maxilla. In addition, a recent paper summarized 10 different non-controlled studies of moderately rough implant and found those to present a combined failure and peri-implantitis frequency within 5 % if followed up for 10 years or longer [66].

Concluding Remarks

This chapter focused on the importance of implant micro-topography on osseointegration and the clinical success of the osseointegrated oral implants. It is quite evident that the treatment modalities have changed due to the advancements in the surface micro-topography of the implant and there is a tendency to shorten the total treatment period. However, it is also important to understand and respect the biological phenomena since the bone cannot be formed in short healing periods or the bone can easily be damaged by coarse surgical or prosthetic procedures. Moderately roughened implant surfaces have been proven to present the most optimal clinical outcomes. To date, there is no evidence that these rough surfaces act negatively against bacterial infection and reducing the surface roughness of the implants could cause negative biologic reactions; thus, this trend should be cautiously observed.

References

1. Albrektsson T, Branemark PI, Hansson HA, Lindstrom J. Osseointegrated titanium implants. Requirements for ensuring a long-lasting, direct bone-to-implant anchorage in man. Acta Orthop Scand. 1981;52:155–70.
2. Albrektsson T, Wennerberg A. Oral implant surfaces: part 1–review focusing on topographic and chemical properties of different surfaces and in vivo responses to them. Int J Prosthodont. 2004;17:536–43.
3. Wennerberg A, Albrektsson T. Effects of titanium surface topography on bone integration: a systematic review. Clin Oral Implants Res. 2009;20:172–84.
4. Wennerberg A, Albrektsson T. On implant surfaces: a review of current knowledge and opinions. Int J Oral Maxillofac Implants. 2010;25:63–74.
5. Albrektsson T, Wennerberg A. Oral implant surfaces: part 2–review focusing on clinical knowledge of different surfaces. Int J Prosthodont. 2004;17:544–64.
6. Tabassum A, Meijer GJ, Wolke JGC, Jansen JA. Influence of surgical technique and surface roughness on the primary stability of an implant in artificial bone with different cortical thickness: a laboratory study. Clin Oral Implants Res. 2010;21:213–20.
7. dos Santos MV, Elias CN, Cavalcanti Lima JH. The effects of superficial roughness and design on the primary stability of dental implants. Clin Implant Dent Relat Res. 2011;13:215–23.
8. Lossdorfer S, Schwartz Z, Wang L, Lohmann CH, Turner JD, Wieland M, et al. Microrough implant surface topographies increase osteogenesis by reducing osteoclast formation and activity. J Biomed Mater Res A. 2004;70:361–9.
9. Martin JY, Schwartz Z, Hummert TW, Schraub DM, Simpson J, Lankford Jr J, et al. Effect of titanium surface roughness on proliferation, differentiation, and protein synthesis of human osteoblast-like cells (MG63). J Biomed Mater Res. 1995;29:389–401.
10. Mustafa K, Wennerberg A, Wroblewski J, Hultenby K, Lopez BS, Arvidson K. Determining optimal surface roughness of TiO (2) blasted titanium implant material for attachment, proliferation and differentiation of cells derived from human mandibular alveolar bone. Clin Oral Implants Res. 2001;12:515–25.
11. Ismail FS, Rohanizadeh R, Atwa S, Mason RS, Ruys AJ, Martin PJ, et al. The influence of surface chemistry and topography on the contact guidance of MG63 osteoblast cells. J Mater Sci Mater Med. 2007;18:705–14.
12. Im BJ, Lee SW, Oh N, Lee MH, Kang JH, Leesungbok R, et al. Texture direction of combined microgrooves and submicroscale topographies of titanium substrata influence adhesion, proliferation, and differentiation in human primary cells. Arch Oral Biol. 2012;57:898–905.
13. Birch MA, Johnson-Lynn S, Nouraei S, Wu QB, Ngalim S, Lu WJ, et al. Effect of electrochemical structuring of Ti6Al4V on osteoblast behaviour in vitro. Biomed Mater. 2012;7:035016.
14. Ricci JL, Grew JC, Alexander H. Connective-tissue responses to defined biomaterial surfaces. I. Growth of rat fibroblast and bone marrow cell colonies on microgrooved substrates. J Biomed Mater Res A. 2008;85:313–25.
15. Adell R, Lekholm U, Rockler B, Branemark PI. A 15-year study of osseointegrated implants in the treatment of the edentulous jaw. Int J Oral Surg. 1981;10:387–416.
16. Attard NJ, Zarb GA. Long-term treatment outcomes in edentulous patients with implant-fixed prostheses: the Toronto study. Int J Prosthodont. 2004;17:417–24.
17. Branemark PI, Adell R, Breine U, Hansson BO, Lindstrom J, Ohlsson A. Intra-osseous anchorage of

dental prostheses. I. Experimental studies. Scand J Plast Reconstr Surg. 1969;3:81–100.
18. Schroeder A, Pohler O, Sutter F. [Tissue reaction to an implant of a titanium hollow cylinder with a titanium surface spray layer]. Schweizerische Monatsschrift fur Zahnheilkunde =Revue mensuelle suisse d'odonto-stomatologie/SSO. 1976;86:713–27.
19. Simmons CA, Valiquette N, Pilliar RM. Osseointegration of sintered porous-surfaced and plasma spray-coated implants: an animal model study of early postimplantation healing response and mechanical stability. J Biomed Mater Res. 1999;47:127–38.
20. Gotfredsen K, Berglundh T, Lindhe J. Anchorage of titanium implants with different surface characteristics: an experimental study in rabbits. Clin Implant Dent Relat Res. 2000;2:120–8.
21. Vercaigne S, Wolke JG, Naert I, Jansen JA. The effect of titanium plasma-sprayed implants on trabecular bone healing in the goat. Biomaterials. 1998;19:1093–9.
22. Vercaigne S, Wolke JG, Naert I, Jansen JA. Histomorphometrical and mechanical evaluation of titanium plasma-spray-coated implants placed in the cortical bone of goats. J Biomed Mater Res. 1998;41:41–8.
23. Roccuzzo M, Aglietta M, Bunino M, Bonino L. Early loading of sandblasted and acid-etched implants: a randomized-controlled double-blind split-mouth study. Five-year results. Clin Oral Implants Res. 2008;19:148–52.
24. Mau J, Behneke A, Behneke N, Fritzemeier CU, Gomez-Roman G, d'Hoedt B, et al. Randomized multicenter comparison of 2 IMZ and 4 TPS screw implants supporting bar-retained overdentures in 425 edentulous mandibles. Int J Oral Maxillofac Implants. 2003;18:835–47.
25. Roynesdal AK, Ambjornsen E, Haanaes HR. A comparison of 3 different endosseous nonsubmerged implants in edentulous mandibles: a clinical report. Int J Oral Maxillofac Implants. 1999;14:543–8.
26. Roynesdal AK, Ambjornsen E, Stovne S, Haanaes HR. A comparative clinical study of three different endosseous implants in edentulous mandibles. Int J Oral Maxillofac Implants. 1998;13:500–5.
27. Astrand P, Anzen B, Karlsson U, Sahlholm S, Svardstrom P, Hellem S. Nonsubmerged implants in the treatment of the edentulous upper jaw: a prospective clinical and radiographic study of ITI implants–results after 1 year. Clin Implant Dent Relat Res. 2000;2:166–74.
28. Becker W, Becker BE, Ricci A, Bahat O, Rosenberg E, Rose LF, et al. A prospective multicenter clinical trial comparing one- and two-stage titanium screw-shaped fixtures with one-stage plasma-sprayed solid-screw fixtures. Clin Implant Dent Relat Res. 2000;2:159–65.
29. De Boever AL, Quirynen M, Coucke W, Theuniers G, De Boever JA. Clinical and radiographic study of implant treatment outcome in periodontally susceptible and non-susceptible patients: a prospective long-term study. Clin Oral Implants Res. 2009;20:1341–50.
30. Aglietta M, Siciliano VI, Rasperini G, Cafiero C, Lang NP, Salvi GE. A 10-year retrospective analysis of marginal bone-level changes around implants in periodontally healthy and periodontally compromised tobacco smokers. Clin Oral Implants Res. 2011;22:47–53.
31. Wennerberg A, Albrektsson T, Andersson B. Design and surface characteristics of 13 commercially available oral implant systems. Int J Oral Maxillofac Implants. 1993;8:622–33.
32. Massaro C, Baker MA, Cosentino F, Ramires PA, Klose S, Milella E. Surface and biological evaluation of hydroxyapatite-based coatings on titanium deposited by different techniques. J Biomed Mater Res. 2001;58:651–7.
33. Weng J, Wang M, Chen J. Plasma-sprayed calcium phosphate particles with high bioactivity and their use in bioactive scaffolds. Biomaterials. 2002;23:2623–9.
34. Heimann RB, Schurmann N, Muller RT. In vitro and in vivo performance of Ti6Al4V implants with plasma-sprayed osteoconductive hydroxylapatite-bioinert titania bond coat "duplex" systems: an experimental study in sheep. J Mater Sci Mater Med. 2004;15:1045–52.
35. Vercaigne S, Wolke JG, Naert I, Jansen JA. Bone healing capacity of titanium plasma-sprayed and hydroxylapatite-coated oral implants. Clin Oral Implants Res. 1998;9:261–71.
36. Gottlander M, Albrektsson T, Carlsson LV. A histomorphometric study of unthreaded hydroxyapatite-coated and titanium-coated implants in rabbit bone. Int J Oral Maxillofac Implants. 1992;7:485–90.
37. Gottlander M, Johansson CB, Albrektsson T. Short- and long-term animal studies with a plasma-sprayed calcium phosphate-coated implant. Clin Oral Implants Res. 1997;8:345–51.
38. Reigstad O, Johansson C, Stenport V, Wennerberg A, Reigstad A, Rokkum M. Different patterns of bone fixation with hydroxyapatite and resorbable CaP coatings in the rabbit tibia at 6, 12, and 52 weeks. J Biomed Mater Res B Appl Biomater. 2011;99:14–20.
39. Johnson BW. HA-coated dental implants: long-term consequences. J Calif Dent Assoc. 1992;20:33–41.
40. Albrektsson T, Åstrand P, Becker W, Eriksson AR, Lekholm U, Malmquist J, et al. Histologic studies of failed dental implants: a retrieval analysis of four different oral implant designs. Clin Mater. 1992;10:225–32.
41. Albrektsson T. Hydroxyapatite-coated implants: a case against their use. J Oral Maxillofac Surg. 1998;56:1312–26.
42. Masaki C, Schneider GB, Zaharias R, Seabold D, Stanford C. Effects of implant surface microtopography on osteoblast gene expression. Clin Oral Implants Res. 2005;16:650–6.
43. Coelho PG, Bonfante EA, Pessoa RS, Marin C, Granato R, Giro G, et al. Characterization of five different implant surfaces and their effect on osseointegration: a study in dogs. J Periodontol. 2011;82:742–50.

44. Ronold HJ, Ellingsen JE. Effect of micro-roughness produced by TiO2 blasting–tensile testing of bone attachment by using coin-shaped implants. Biomaterials. 2002;23:4211–9.
45. Klokkevold PR, Johnson P, Dadgostari S, Caputo A, Davies JE, Nishimura RD. Early endosseous integration enhanced by dual acid etching of titanium: a torque removal study in the rabbit. Clin Oral Implants Res. 2001;12:350–7.
46. Abrahamsson I, Zitzmann NU, Berglundh T, Wennerberg A, Lindhe J. Bone and soft tissue integration to titanium implants with different surface topography: an experimental study in the dog. Int J Oral Maxillofac Implants. 2001;16:323–32.
47. Cochran DL, Schenk RK, Lussi A, Higginbottom FL, Buser D. Bone response to unloaded and loaded titanium implants with a sandblasted and acid-etched surface: a histometric study in the canine mandible. J Biomed Mater Res. 1998;40:1–11.
48. Schupbach P, Glauser R, Rocci A, Martignoni M, Sennerby L, Lundgren A, et al. The human bone-oxidized titanium implant interface: a light microscopic, scanning electron microscopic, back-scatter scanning electron microscopic, and energy-dispersive x-ray study of clinically retrieved dental implants. Clin Implant Dent Relat Res. 2005;7 Suppl 1:S36–43.
49. Burgos PM, Rasmusson L, Meirelles L, Sennerby L. Early bone tissue responses to turned and oxidized implants in the rabbit tibia. Clin Implant Dent Relat Res. 2008;10:181–90.
50. Sawase T, Jimbo R, Wennerberg A, Suketa N, Tanaka Y, Atsuta M. A novel characteristic of porous titanium oxide implants. Clin Oral Implants Res. 2007;18:680–5.
51. Jimbo R, Tovar N, Yoo DY, Janal MN, Anchieta RB, Coelho PG. The effect of different surgical drilling procedures on full laser-etched microgrooves surface-treated implants: an experimental study in sheep. Clin Oral Implants Res. 2014;25(9):1072–7.
52. Cei S, Legitimo A, Barachini S, Consolini R, Sammartino G, Mattii L, et al. Effect of laser micromachining of titanium on viability and responsiveness of osteoblast-like cells. Implant Dent. 2011;20:285–91.
53. Kang SH, Cho SA. Comparison of removal torques for laser-treated titanium implants with anodized implants. J Craniofac Surg. 2011;22:1491–5.
54. Wennerberg A, Albrektsson T, Andersson B, Krol JJ. A histomorphometric and removal torque study of screw-shaped titanium implants with three different surface topographies. Clin Oral Implants Res. 1995;6:24–30.
55. Wennerberg A, Albrektsson T, Johansson C, Andersson B. Experimental study of turned and grit-blasted screw-shaped implants with special emphasis on effects of blasting material and surface topography. Biomaterials. 1996;17:15–22.
56. Wennerberg A, Albrektsson T, Lausmaa J. Torque and histomorphometric evaluation of c.p. titanium screws blasted with 25- and 75-microns-sized particles of Al2O3. J Biomed Mater Res. 1996;30:251–60.
57. Wennerberg A, Albrektsson T, Andersson B. Bone tissue response to commercially pure titanium implants blasted with fine and coarse particles of aluminum oxide. Int J Oral Maxillofac Implants. 1996;11:38–45.
58. Mertens C, Steveling HG. Early and immediate loading of titanium implants with fluoride-modified surfaces: results of 5-year prospective study. Clin Oral Implants Res. 2011;22:1354–60.
59. Gotfredsen K, Karlsson U. A prospective 5-year study of fixed partial prostheses supported by implants with machined and TiO2-blasted surface. J Prosthodont. 2001;10:2–7.
60. Eliasson A, Blomqvist F, Wennerberg A, Johansson A. A retrospective analysis of early and delayed loading of full-arch mandibular prostheses using three different implant systems: clinical results with up to 5 years of loading. Clin Implant Dent Relat Res. 2009;11:134–48.
61. Chang M, Wennstrom JL. Longitudinal changes in tooth/single-implant relationship and bone topography: an 8-year retrospective analysis. Clin Implant Dent Relat Res. 2012;14:388–94.
62. Friberg B, Jemt T. Clinical experience of TiUnite implants: a 5-year cross-sectional, retrospective follow-up study. Clin Implant Dent Relat Res. 2010;12 Suppl 1:e95–103.
63. Khang W, Feldman S, Hawley CE, Gunsolley J. A multi-center study comparing dual acid-etched and machined-surfaced implants in various bone qualities. J Periodontol. 2001;72:1384–90.
64. Pinholt EM. Branemark and ITI dental implants in the human bone-grafted maxilla: a comparative evaluation. Clin Oral Implants Res. 2003;14:584–92.
65. Buddula A, Assad DA, Salinas TJ, Garces YI, Volz JE, Weaver AL. Survival of turned and roughened dental implants in irradiated head and neck cancer patients: a retrospective analysis. J Prosthet Dent. 2011;106:290–6.
66. Albrektsson T, Buser D, Sennerby L. Crestal bone loss and oral implants. Clin Implant Dent Relat Res. 2012;14:783–91.

Experimental Evaluation of Implant Surface Chemistry

4

Martin Andersson

Abstract

The clinical outcome of implants is highly dependent on the surface properties of the implant material. Therefore, it is of outermost importance to accurately perform and interpret surface analyses. Different analytical tools give distinctive information about the surface at different depths and spatial resolutions. Knowledge about the working principles and strengths and weaknesses of the techniques is important to understand. Since it is the surface atoms of the implant that are in direct contact with the tissue, it is crucial that the proper techniques are chosen, which have the desired surface sensitivity. In this chapter, the most important and most frequently used surface analytical techniques of today's implant research are briefly reviewed. The modus operandi, the used notation, and the information that is acquired for the following techniques are included: X-ray photoelectron spectroscopy (XPS), Auger electron spectroscopy (AES), secondary ion mass spectroscopy (SIMS), energy-dispersive X-ray spectroscopy (EDX or EDS), and contact angle (CA).

The chemical composition of implant materials has a high impact on the clinical success. Different compounds give rise to different host tissue responses resulting in desired or undesired outcomes. Accordingly, it is necessary to understand the connection between surface properties and the performance of the implant. In this context surface characterization plays an important role. Since it is the outermost atoms on the surface of the implant that are in direct contact with the tissue, it is crucial that the proper techniques are chosen, which have the desired surface sensitivity. A wide range of available techniques are used to quantitatively and qualitatively analyze the chemical composition of implants, and it is therefore important to grasp the different strengths and weaknesses of the techniques to properly review and compare different implants.

The surface of an implant is inherently different from the bulk material. For titanium implants this is evident by the always-present native oxide layer that however is not uniform at different depths of the layer. The degree of crystallinity, chemical

M. Andersson, PhD
Chemical and Biological Engineering, Chalmers University of Technology,
Kemivagen 10, Goteborg 412 96, Sweden
e-mail: martin.andersson@chalmers.se

A. Wennerberg et al. (eds.), *Implant Surfaces and their Biological and Clinical Impact*,
DOI 10.1007/978-3-662-45379-7_4, © Springer-Verlag Berlin Heidelberg 2015

composition, and presence of desired or undesired elements are properties that frequently are different, comparing the surface with its bulk. The concept of surface energy is an important property that is a true surface feature directly linked to the properties of the outermost atoms. A high surface energy material, which includes most metals, is hydrophilic and is easily wet by aqueous body fluids, such as blood, and allows for protein adsorption with relatively low remodeling of the protein conformation. Whether the metal surface is intentionally through surface modification or unintentionally through contamination covered with a molecular monolayer having, for example, methyl end groups, the surface energy is dramatically decreased resulting in low or no wettability, which would induce high conformational changes of adsorbed proteins. If relatively short polar polymers, such as polyethylene glycol (PEG), are attached to the implant surface, protein adsorption can be more or less totally inhibited, which affects the immune response of the foreign material. Hence, a few nm-thick layer on the implant could have a high impact on the clinical outcome. Moreover, the presence of nano-sized features also contributes to the surface character, thus further changing the implant surface properties from the bulk. For example, if the nano-sized feature contains fewer atoms than needed to reach the bulk concentration of a certain element, it is inevitable that the chemical composition is different than the bulk. More specifically, if a material is doped with 5 ppm of a certain element, it is not possible to know what the composition of the surface would be if it exists as nano-sized features containing less than one million atoms. Also, if the size of the implant surface features is in the order of 5 nm or less, there are generally more surface atoms than bulk atoms resulting in a highly surface-active material. Such a material is more prone to interact with the surroundings compared to surfaces without such small structures, which makes them easily functionalized, however, sensitive to undesired surface contaminations.

In this chapter, the five most frequently used surface-sensitive methods being utilized in today's implant research are briefly introduced and discussed with emphasis on their functionality, what is being measured, what information can be extracted, and with what resolution this can be obtained. The techniques are X-ray photoelectron spectroscopy (XPS), Auger electron spectroscopy (AES), secondary ion mass spectroscopy (SIMS), energy-dispersive X-ray spectroscopy (EDX or EDS), and contact angle (CA). This is not intended to be a full review of the techniques but rather to present the most important concepts needed to grasp the essence of the surface analyses and to acquire the needed nomenclature and notations to read and understand presented data.

XPS

X-ray photoelectron spectroscopy (XPS) also known as electron spectroscopy for chemical analysis (ESCA) is a surface-sensitive spectroscopy technique that can be used to answer the following key questions [1]:

- Which elements are present on a surface, within the top 3–10 nm (except hydrogen and helium)?
- What is the chemical composition in atomic percent (down to ppm in detection limit)?
- What is the chemical state of the elements?
- Is there a thin film present on the surface and if so how thick is it?

The modus operandi of the instrument is based on photoemission, that is, ejection of electrons by the use of X-ray photons, as is illustrated in Fig. 4.1.

The kinetic energy (KE) of the emitted electrons is measured using a spectrometer. From the kinetic energy, the element-specific binding energy (BE) is obtained, which is easily calculated by subtracting the KE and spectrometer working function (φ) from the incoming X-ray energy ($h\nu$), a calculation most often performed directly by the instrument software. The resulting data is presented as a graph where the electron binding energy (eV) is plotted as a function of intensity (counts), i.e., the XPS spectrum. Two examples of XPS spectra are presented in Fig. 4.2 for commercially pure titanium (a) and titanium coated with a thin layer of hydroxyapatite, HA (b).

The peaks in the XPS spectra represent the different types of photoelectrons ejected from the

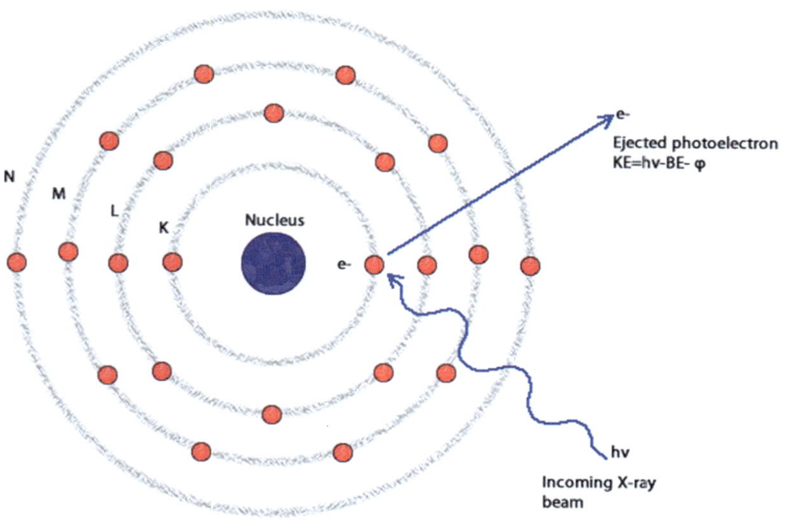

Fig. 4.1 The principle behind XPS: an incoming X-ray excites the atoms and as result emits a photoelectron (Courtesy of Jose J. Chavez, Ph.D. Candidate – Department of Electrical Engineering, The University of Texas at El Paso)

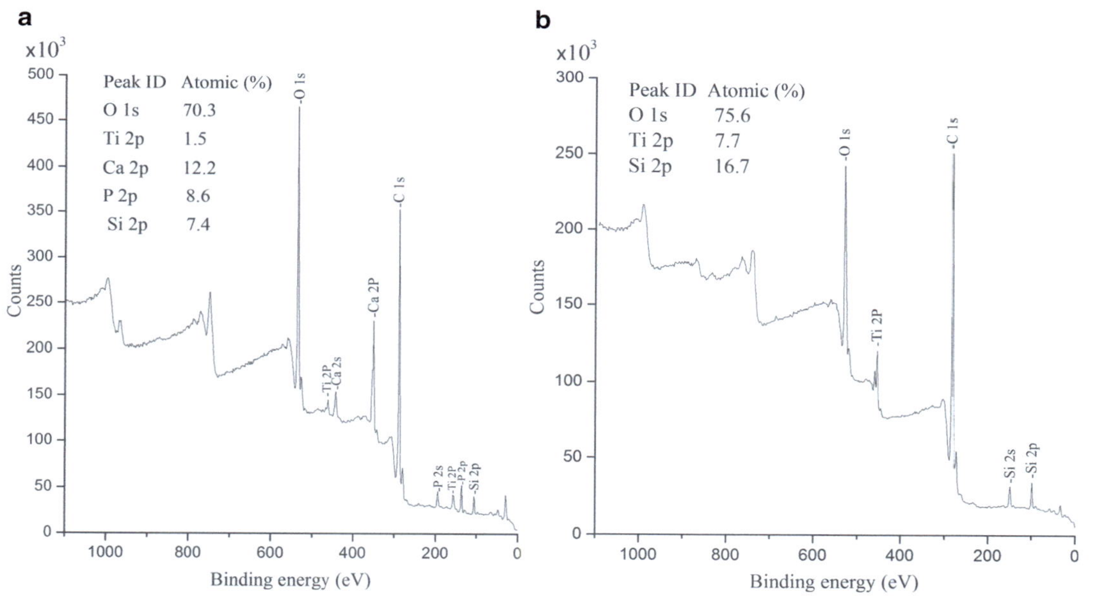

Fig. 4.2 Typical XPS survey spectra for a titanium implant (**a**) and a hydroxyapatite (HA)-coated titanium implant (**b**)

sample and are labeled according to their quantum numbers. The labeling is usually following the scheme *xyz*, where *x* is the principal quantum number (1, 2, 3…), *y* is the orbital (s, p, d, f, etc.), and *z* describes the differences in spin angular momentum, which results in some peaks that are split into two. For example, values of *z* for p orbitals are 1/2 and 3/2, while for d orbitals they are 3/2 and 5/2. XPS is a surface-sensitive technique; however, there is always a penetration depth of the signal, which is dependent on the kinetic energy of the photoelectrons. The depth of analysis is determined by the attenuation length of the electrons and is dependent on the element being analyzed and is in the range of 3–10 nm. The spatial resolution is, however, much less and often in the order of 3 μm^2. All XPS analyses are performed under ultrahigh vacuum (UHV) range of 10^{-8} to 10^{-10} mbar. The low pressure is needed to reduce scattering of the photoelectrons and to avoid surface contamination from the surrounding air. The samples analyzed need to be carefully handled to prevent contamination, and storage in, for example, plastic bags should be avoided. With the exception for careful handling, most dry solid samples can be directly analyzed without any other pretreatments. Besides for direct surface compositional measurements, XPS can also be used for depth profiling. If the emitted electrons are detected at some angle to the normal, the information depth is decreased, something often related to as angle resolved XPS (ARXPS). In addition to ARXPS, surface material can be removed from the sample within the spectrometer by the use of ion sputtering; hence, deeper depths can be analyzed.

Implant materials are often characterized by XPS since it gives details including:

- Chemical composition of the surface
- Presence of undesired contaminants
- The thickness of possibly present layers such as oxides or additional coatings, for example, hydroxyapatite coatings on titanium

It should be noted that carbon contaminants always are present when analyzing, for example, titanium implants due to adsorption from the surrounding air (see Fig. 4.2). Such detection can be avoided to some extent by the use of surface sputtering. XPS can be considered as the gold standard for chemical characterization of implants.

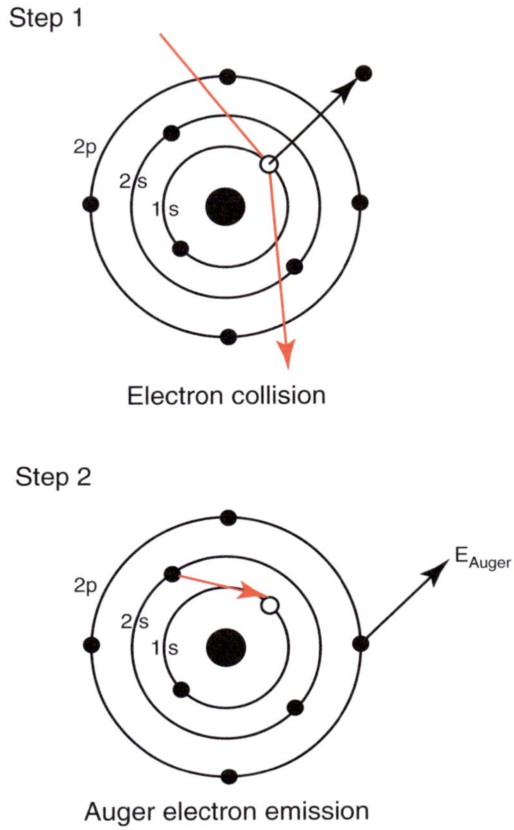

Fig. 4.3 An illustration of the sequences occurring in Auger spectroscopy. Step 1, an electron from the incoming beam kicks out an electron (secondary electron) from an atom in the sample leaving an electron hole. Step 2, an electron from a higher-energy shell fills the hole through an internal transition, and a second electron, named Auger electron, is emitted and detected (Source: http://commons.wikimedia.org/wiki/File:Auger_Process.svg)

AES

Auger electron spectroscopy (AES) shares many similarities with XPS when it comes to the actual material properties that can be measured; however, the working principle is somewhat different (see Fig. 4.3) [1].

In AES, incoming electrons are used to eject core electrons from the sample, often referred to as secondary electrons. When the secondary electrons are replaced within the material, through an internal transition by another electron positioned in a higher energy level, another electron is emitted from the sample due to the first law of thermodynamics, i.e., the conservation of energy. This second emitted electron is termed an Auger electron. The kinetic energy of the Auger electron is element specific and is plotted as a function of intensity. The notation used in AES is different from the XPS. In AES three electrons need to be accounted for, and an Auger electron can, for example, be written as $L_2M_5M_5$, which means that a secondary electron from the L_2 energy level (sometimes also referred to as an energy shell) is kicked out and replaced by an electron from the M_5 energy level. A second electron from the M_5 energy is emitted, which is the one being measured. Sometimes, the subscripts are excluded leaving LMM as a common notation for an Auger electron. AES bares many similarities to XPS, both being surface-sensitive techniques; however, there are strengths and weaknesses of each technique. Both techniques require the presence of UHV, which to some extent limits the flexibility regarding sample preparations. In AES, difficulties arising from charging effects are more cumbersome, resulting in difficulties in analyzing nonconducting samples, including implants made of ceramics and polymers. The quantification, i.e., surface composition determinations, is less accurate using AES. The lower sensitivity in AES is due to the coexistence of several different internal processes within the atoms resulting in competitive signals. The Auger electrons carry less information about the chemical nature of the samples compared to the photoelectrons analyzed in XPS. It is, for example, not possible to detect the oxidation state of the atoms using AES. The big advantage with AES lies in the high spatial resolution, being less than 10 nm in today's instruments. Through the combination with scanning electron microscopy (SEM) in the same instrument, it is possible to both visualize surface features down to a few nm as well as have them surface analyzed, a technique coined scanning Auger microscopy (SAM). This possibility is of advantage, for example, when samples are inhomogeneous. For standard characterization of implants, AES is not as frequently used as XPS, which is a combination of availability and the acquired information that is desired. Most often, an implant is chemically homogeneous throughout its surface, and information about what elements that are present, in what concentration, and to some extent their chemical nature is desired; hence, XPS is the preferred choice over AES. However, the ongoing developments implementing nanostructured implant surfaces should cause higher attention toward AES.

SIMS

Secondary ion mass spectroscopy (SIMS) is the most surface-sensitive spectroscopy technique with the ability to measure depths of 1–2 nm with

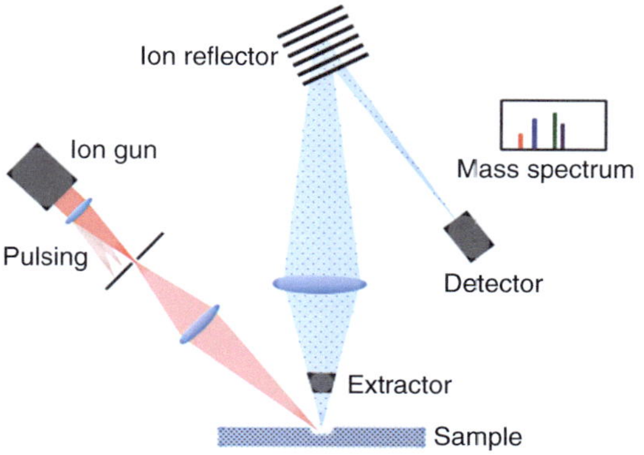

Fig. 4.4 The working principle of SIMS. Here illustrated with a time-of-flight (TOF) mass detector

a sensitivity of parts per billion (ppb) [2]. There are two modes of operation: static SIMS and dynamic SIMS. For surface analysis, static SIMS is the preferred mode and involves only the outer atomic layer of the surface in contrast to dynamic SIMS, which is used for more bulk analysis. The working principle of SIMS is that ions (usually Ar, Ga, O, and Cs) are hurled toward the sample surface, which is etched resulting in the formation of secondary ions. The secondary ions are identified and quantified using a mass spectrometer (sector, quadrupole, or time-of-flight) where the mass per charge is measured. The working principle of a TOF-SIMS is shown in Fig. 4.4.

Typical mass spectra contain large numbers of peaks, which can be identified as molecular ions, molecular fragment of ions, or element ions of the sample. Accurate quantification of samples is not as straightforward as with, for example, XPS due to large variation in ionization ability between different materials (matrix effects), and standards of known compositions are needed. Since the sample surface is etched with the incoming ions, depth profiling is possible to achieve, and there is a direct correlation between the exposure time and etching depth. Depth profiling should, however, be performed with care when rough surfaces, such as implants, are analyzed. As an example, undercuts could erroneously be taken for being at a certain depth instead of at the outer surface. As a consequence, control samples should be used to receive accurate depth profiles. A strong advantage with SIMS compared to XPS and AES is the possibility to receive molecular recognition of, for example, polymers, where fragment ions of characteristic side chains and backbones can be identified. With SIMS it is also possible to detect hydrogen, which makes it an interesting technique when, for example, the hydrogenation degree of metal implants is desired. The SIMS measurements are performed in vacuum or in ultrahigh vacuum. As with all surface analysis, care needs to be taken when it comes to sample handling; however, due to the etching principle of SIMS, surface contaminants are naturally removed during the measurements. The lateral resolution can be relatively high, less than 100 nm if a highly focused primary ion beam is used, placing it in between XPS and AES. Hence, SIMS can be used to produce elemental maps.

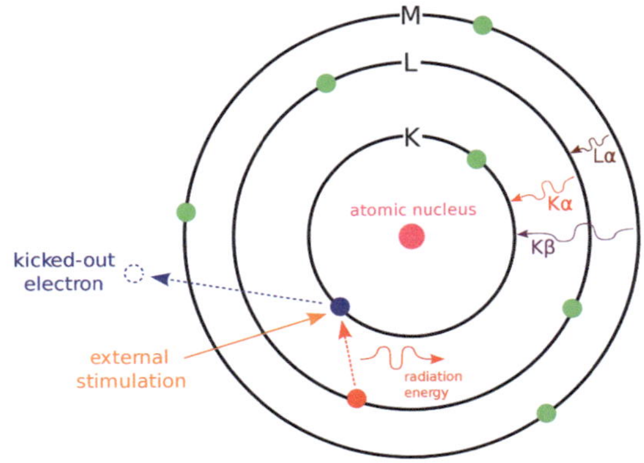

Fig. 4.5 An illustration of the principle events occurring in EDS (Source: http://commons.wikimedia.org/wiki/File:EDX-scheme.svg, author Muso)

EDS/EDX

Energy-dispersive X-ray spectroscopy (EDX or EDS) is an analytical spectroscopy technique often coexisting with electron microscopy, SEM and TEM [3]. It can be used to identify and quantify the present elements in a sample (beryllium and heavier). The principle behind the technique is to measure the energy of X-rays emitted from the sample when it is being bombarded with a focused beam of electrons (see Fig. 4.5). The useful X-rays, often referred to as the characteristic X-rays, result from inner transitions within the atoms. An inner shell electron is kicked out by the incoming electron and is replaced by an electron from an outer shell of higher energy. The energy difference between the two electrons is element specific and hence is used for elemental identification.

The characteristic X-rays are identified by Roman letters associated with the energy shell from where the electron was kicked out (K, L, M, N…). These letters are combined with a Greek letter depending on the origin of the electron "falling" down and a number denoting the intensity within the shell. For example, $K\alpha_1$ means the characteristic X-ray is associated with an electron hole being filled in the K shell with an electron originating from the most intense line in the L shell. Even though the measurement is being performed on the surface, at least in the SEM, the relative high penetrability and spreading of the incoming electrons in combination with the low absorption of the emitted X-rays result in low nominal resolution and low surface sensibility. The resolution increases with decreasing accelerating voltage of the incoming electron beam; however, typical surface penetrability is of the size of about 1 μm. The sensitivity of the technique is about 1,000 ppm and the analytical precision is on the order of 1–2 atomic %. It is possible to perform mapping using the EDS signal, which is useful when the uniformity of a surface is investigated. The strength with the EDS technique is due to the fact that it is often present together with SEM and is relatively easy and fast to use. When analyzing implants, it provides a good estimate of the bulk material chemical composition, and most often the elemental compositions of surface coatings can be measured, given a thickness of at least about 10 nm. If nonconducting samples are analyzed using a conventional SEM/EDS instrument, precautions are needed to be performed, hindering charging of the sample, such as surface sputtering. However, care needs to be taken regarding the sputtered thickness as well as choice of sputtering source to hinder unwanted artifacts in the analysis. Preferably, carbon sputtering should be applied. EDS cannot replace XPS, AES, or SIMS due to its relatively low surface sensibility but should be used as a complement.

Contact Angle

Contact angle (CA) is a very surface-sensitive technique that measures surface energy/wettability of the outermost layer of atoms, below 1 nm in depth. No chemical quantification can be made of the actual elements on the surface; however, since CA is very sensitive to changes in surface chemistry, it is often used to give a first estimate of the surface properties, for example, the effect of different surface treatments of implants. The technique is simple and straightforward to use; a liquid droplet (often water) is placed on the material, and its angle with the surface, the contact angle, is measured either manually or automatically using a camera in an instrument called a goniometer. Another less accurate but easy to use method, without the need of instruments, is to measure the diameter of a droplet of known volume seen from the above. The Young's equation, Eq. 4.1, which is valid only for ideal totally flat surfaces, correlates the interfacial tension between the solid and the liquid (γ_{SL}) and the horizontal component of the surface tension between the liquid and gas ($\gamma_{LG} \cos \theta_c$) with the opposite interfacial tension between the solid and gas (γ_{SG}):

$$\gamma_{SG} = \gamma_{SL} + \gamma_{LG} \cos \theta_c \qquad (4.1)$$

where θ_c is defined as the contact angle.

The involved interfacial surface tensions and contact angle are illustrated in Fig. 4.6.

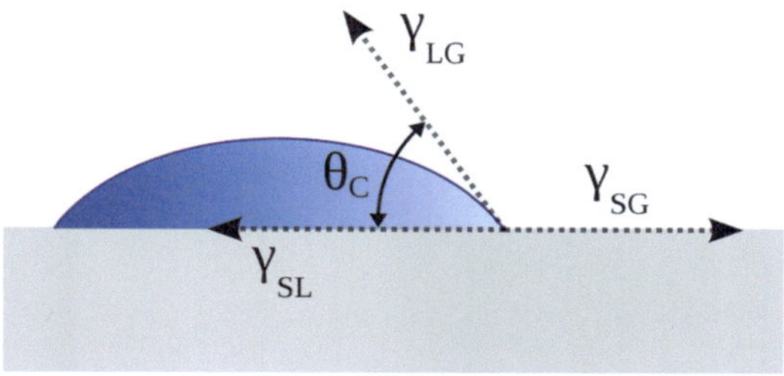

Fig. 4.6 An illustration showing the relationship between the interfacial tensions between solid and liquid (γ_{SL}), liquid and gas (γ_{LG}), solid and gas (γ_{SG}), and the contact angle (θ_c) (Source: http://commons.wikimedia.org/wiki/File:Contact_angle.svg)

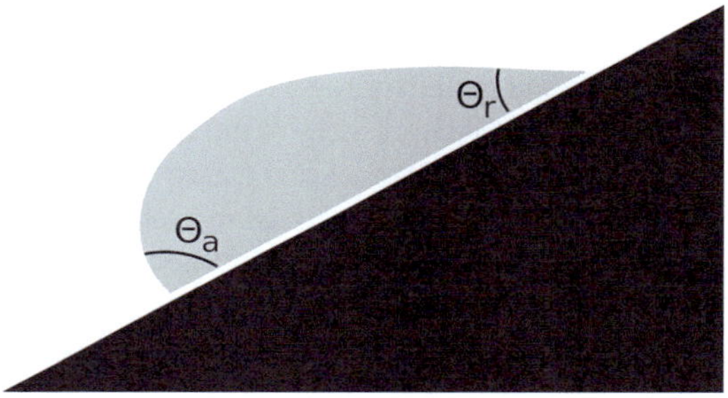

Fig. 4.7 The definition of the advancing angle (θ_a) and receding angle (θ_r) on a tilted plane (Source: http://commons.wikimedia.org/wiki/File:Hysteresis.svg author Emmanuelle rio slr)

By definition, surfaces having contact angles of water above 90° are termed hydrophobic whereas those below 90° are termed hydrophilic. Not only surface chemistry affects the contact angle; also the surface roughness plays an important role [4]. Interestingly, an increased surface roughness of an already hydrophobic surface renders it even more hydrophobic, and an increased surface roughness of a hydrophilic surface makes it even more hydrophilic. This dependence on roughness is commonly the main reason for why, for example, titanium surfaces, having very similar surface chemistry, may have significantly different wettability. When the surface is nonideal, for example, due to surface roughness, the contact angles will show hysteresis, for example, decrease with time after the drop has been placed on the surface. The difference between the highest measured angle, the advancing angle, and the lowest measured angle, the receding angle, is called the contact angle hysteresis. The contact angle hysteresis can, for example, be used to investigate differences in surface roughnesses between different implants. It can be obtained either by dynamic contact angle measurements, where the contact angle is measured as a function of time when being added and removed (sucked up) from the surface, or by measuring the angles that the droplet forms when the surface is tilted just until it starts to move. In this latter technique, the angle being formed in the front of the tilted drop is the advancing angle (θ_a), and the one being formed at the rear is the receding angle (θ_r) (see Fig. 4.7).

Table 4.1 Features of the different techniques described in the text

Technique	Incident radiation	What is measured	Elements detectable	Quantification	Depth of analysis	Spatial resolution
XPS	X-rays	Energy, e^-	He>	Good	3–10 nm	3 μm
AES	e^-	Energy, e^-	Li>	Good	3–10 nm	<10 nm
SIMS	Ions	Mass, ions	All	Poor	1–2 nm	1 μm
EDX/EDS	e^-	X-ray	Be>	Reasonable	1 μm	1 μm
CA	–	Angle	–	–	1 nm	–

As seen from Young's equation (Eq. 4.1), the contact angle is directly coupled to the surface energies/interfacial tensions of the system. A surface having a high surface energy has a low contact angle and is easily wetted by water in contrast to a low-energy surface with a high contact angle. Since the contact angle is dependent on the used liquid, the surface and gas environment, it is sometimes of interest to calculate the energy of the surface. There are several different theories that can be used to calculate the surface energy, and the most straightforward one is to use the so-called Zisman plot. In this technique, the static contact angle is measured using different liquids with known surface tensions (often alkanes with varying lengths), and the highest surface tension needed to totally wet the surface is extrapolated. This surface tension at $\theta_c=0$ is then equal to the surface energy of the material.

As mentioned before, the CA is dependent on both surface chemistry and surface roughness and gives a number on the wettability of a surface. For implant studies this is an important measure, which has been shown to directly affect the biological response. Yet, another strength (or sometimes a weakness) with the technique is that it is very sensitive toward surface contaminants, which affects both the static contact angle as well as the hysteresis between the advancing and receding angle. Hence, contact angle measurements can be used, for example, to study how the storage of implants is affecting the surface and to give a hint on the reproducibility of implant production.

Availability and key questions related to an implant's surface chemistry dictate the characterization techniques being used. The techniques described in this chapter all have their strengths and weaknesses and are often used in combination as complement to give a better understanding of the surface. It is important to stress that even though the different techniques are defined as being surface sensitive (except for EDS), they all measure at different depths of the material. In many cases this has a strong impact and care needs to be taken when comparing data when measurements have been performed with different analytical techniques. In Table 4.1, a short summary of the described techniques is presented with emphasis on the type of information that can be extracted and from what depths and spatial resolution it can be obtained.

References

1. Watts JF, Wolstenholme J. An introduction to surface analysis by XPS and AES. West Sussex: Wiley; 2003. ISBN 978-0-470-84712-1.
2. Belu AM, Graham DJ, Castner DG. Time-of-flight secondary ion mass spectrometry: techniques and applications for the characterization of biomaterial surfaces. Biomaterials. 2004;24:3635–53.
3. Goldstein JL, et al. Scanning electron microscopy and x-ray microanalysis. 3rd ed. New York: Plenum Press; 2003. ISBN 978-1-4613-4969-3.
4. Quere D. Wetting and roughness. In: Annual Reviews, Annual review of materials research, vol. 38. Palo Alto; 2008. p. 71–99.

Experimental and Clinical Knowledge of Nanometer Scale Designing on Endosteal Implants

5

Paulo G. Coelho, Ryo Jimbo, and Estevam A. Bonfante

Abstract

Recent advances in engineering methods and characterization have rendered the addition of nanometer scale features on endosteal implant surfaces. Such modifications usually occur hierarchically in tandem with modifications at the micrometer scale level, and its main objective is to support the bone response through enhanced interaction between the immediate and intermediate implant and host after surgical placement. This chapter describes the increasing basic science experimental basis for surface nanotopographical alterations and the limited clinical evidence of nanometer scale surface modifications.

Introduction

Historically, implant surfaces in their majority transitioned from turned (machined) to textured [1]. Such transition has occurred since multiple studies have unequivocally demonstrated that surface topographical modifications have a dramatic effect on early osseointegration, significantly reducing the amount of time needed for the establishment of the implant–bone system biomechanical competence for functional load bearing [2].

It is currently a general consensus that the mechanism, which surface modifications at any scale strengthen the bone response, is through enhancing the initial interaction between the implantable device and the host biofluids [3–5]. Of special interest is the effect that surface modifications have on maintaining a more intimate interaction between the blood clot and the surface immediately after placement. Such intimate interaction between the blood clot and implant surface permits the development of a continuous biological pathway between instrumented healing bone and implant [6]. Through this continuous pathway,

P.G. Coelho, DDS, PhD (✉)
Department of Biomaterials and Biomimetics, Department of Periodontology and Implant Dentistry, New York University, 345 East 24th street room 804s, New York, NY 10010, USA

Division of Engineering, New York University Abu Dhabi, New York, NY, USA
e-mail: pgcoelho@nyu.edu

R. Jimbo, DDS, PhD
Department of Prosthodontics, Malmo University, Carl Gustavs Vag 34, Malmo 205 06, Sweden
e-mail: ryo.jimbo@mah.se

E.A. Bonfante, DDS, PhD
Department of Prosthodontics, University of São Paulo – Bauru College of Dentistry, Bauru, SP, Brazil
e-mail: estevam.bonfante@fob.usp.br

A. Wennerberg et al. (eds.), *Implant Surfaces and their Biological and Clinical Impact*,
DOI 10.1007/978-3-662-45379-7_5, © Springer-Verlag Berlin Heidelberg 2015

osteogenic cells more easily migrate towards the proximity of the implant to form bone that will establish osseointegration [7]. Thus, through the appropriate combination of implant hardware configuration (implant macrogeometry and surgical instrumentation dimensional interplay) and surface engineering at multiple scales, bone response may be maximized [8].

After Albrektsson et al. pioneered the concept of the importance of surface treatment at the micrometer-level length scale on the biological response to an implant [9], materials science engineering has enabled the fabrication of implant surfaces presenting intended nanometer scale components [10]. From a theoretical perspective, the presence of intended nanometer scale features in the implant surface would further support the bone-to-implant response by enhancing the implant–biofluid interaction immediately after placement due to alteration in properties inherent to the nanometer length scale [11–13]. It is speculated that otherwise, the non-intended nanotopography would have no controlled biologic effects, since heterogeneous nanostructures can be formed by native oxidation of the base titanium substrate. For better understanding of the potential effects of nanometer scale features on implant surfaces, this chapter describes the importance of reduced scale engineering in the field of materials science before presenting the preclinical and clinical evidence of nanometer scale inclusions on implant surfaces.

The Nanometer Size Scale and Its Importance in Materials Science and Engineering: Quantum Confinement

The building blocks of atoms (protons, neutrons, and electrons) and their electromagnetic relationship occur at the Angstrom scale (10^{-10} m) and rapidly build up to the nanometer scale (10^{-9} to 10^{-6} m, namely, from 1 to 1,000 nm) to the micrometer and to the macrometer scale. While it is obvious that the nanometer scale can be utilized for multiple engineering purposes due to its reduced physical dimensions, the quantized (as a function of size) effects that originate due to the reduced dimensions (especially from 1 to 100 nm, which defines the grain size of materials fabricated with nanotechnology) have been responsible for the significant interest currently devoted to this material class. From a physical standpoint, the size of nanoparticles is small enough to interact even with the DNA (approximately 2 nm diameter) [14].

The physical principles governing materials science in the macro- and micrometer scale have been developed over the past centuries through the development of quantum mechanical relationships that led physical sciences into developing the fields of condensed matter physics (especially solid-state physics) along with statistical mechanics and thermodynamics. While these relationships have been experimentally validated by materials scientists, modern manufacturing techniques that allow precise atomic buildup at the nanometer scale have shown that materials presenting reduced length scale in at least one of the three dimensions exhibited substantial departures in their electronic configuration relative to their larger-scale counterparts. Such phenomenon has been described as quantum confinement and is dependent on the number of dimensions presenting reduced length scale (typically below 100 nm) in the *xy*, *xz*, and *yz* planes. In short, alteration in electronic configuration that is tailorable based on the number of atoms that build up the reduced scale domains has been well received by the materials science community as it allowed substantial advances in the understanding of matter that are currently being made useful for a variety of applications [15].

The Hierarchical Placement of Nanometer Scale Features on Dental Implants: Targeting Cells

Concerning implant surfaces and nanomaterials, the possibilities are limitless as nanometer scale fabrication methods are becoming widely available. Nanotechnology manufacturing processes may easily alter the texture length scale and patterning of implant surfaces while at the same time altering the chemical properties of the substrate due to dimensional confinement [13].

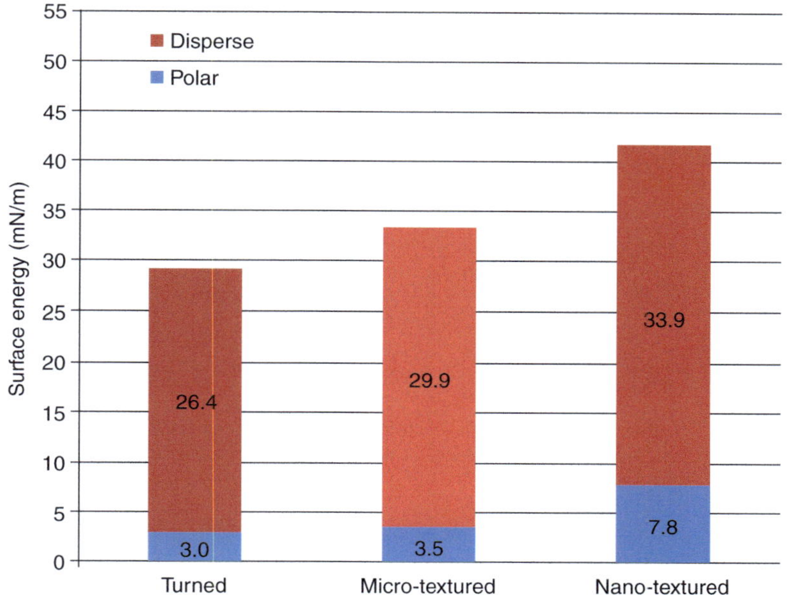

Fig. 5.1 Surface energy measured by the OWRK method of turned, micro-textured, and nano-textured Ti-6Al-4V substrates (Source: Paulo G. Coelho's laboratory archives)

From a general perspective, recent research strongly supports that alterations in surface topography also lead to changes in surface chemistry, and such phenomenon may be exacerbated further when nanometer scale features are considered. Not surprisingly, nanometer scale features presenting both short- and long-range ordering have been shown to alter various aspects of cell behavior and are the subject of active research [16].

For instance, if one considers nanotopographical texturing of any surface, an exponential gain in surface area is expected along with alterations in surface electronic properties due to the two-dimensional confinement that exists due to the formation of nanometer scale peaks. Thus, it is expected that the surface energy resulting from nanotopographical texturing will deviate from both smooth and micrometer scale texturing. Such panorama is depicted in Fig. 5.1 for Ti-6Al-4V with different degrees of texture (turned, micro-textured, and nano-textured, Fig. 5.2), where an increase, rendered by nanotopography, arises not only due to alterations in surface roughness (represented by the disperse component contribution to surface energy) but also due to alterations in surface chemistry due to the reduced scale (represented by the polar component contribution to surface energy). Other studies considering nanometer scale and micrometer scale topographies demonstrated improved wettability for the nanometer scale surface [17]. This may be attributed to the fact that the surface area significantly increases with the nanolevel surface modification, and at many occasions, the surface is negatively charged [17]. Thus, due to both physical and chemical features inherent to the nanometer length scale, such surfaces have been widely described to affect cell behavior.

The positive effect of surfaces presenting nanometer scale features on the adhesion, spreading, motility, proliferation, adhesion selectivity, and differentiation of osteoblasts has been previously compiled [18–22]. Thus, there is unequivocal evidence that cells can be triggered through nanometer length scale modifications and that such modifications should be incorporated into dental implant designing to support the bone response.

From a hierarchical implant design perspective, the implant hardware and microgeometric/topographical role is to not only provide the device primary stability through mechanical engagement and an increase in friction between implant and bone, respectively, but also to allow adequate bone healing conditions where substantial interaction between blood clot and implant surface exists immediately after placement [23]. While implant

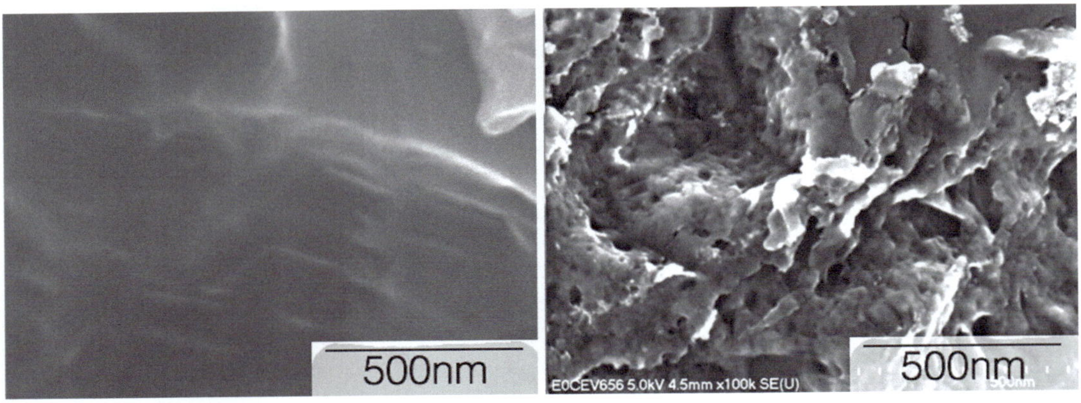

Fig. 5.2 High-resolution FE-SEM micrograph of a (*left*) micrometer scale textured surface and (*right*) a nanometer scale textured surface (Source: Paulo G. Coelho's laboratory archives)

hardware and micrometer scale modifications will dictate tissue-level interaction and healing pathway cascade around the implant [6, 8, 23, 24], nanometer scale features present potential in boosting osteoblastic behavior and thus supporting the bone response. However, while in vitro cell culture studies demonstrated positive effects of nanometer scale features on osteoblastic cells [25–27], direct translation of nanometer scale features to implants, without considering implant hardware features and micrometer scale design parameters, may not relate with laboratory in vivo findings. Such contradiction led to the rationale for the hierarchical placement of nanometer scale features within micrometer scale texturing when designing dental implant surfaces. Such strategy attempts to assure adequate intimate interaction between blood clot and the implant surface so osteogenic cells may travel through a seamless pathway towards the device surface to be further altered in phenotype by nanometer scale features. Under this design guideline, implant surfaces presenting nanometer scale texture and chemistry alteration have been manufactured.

Commercially Available Implant Surfaces Presenting Nanometer Scale Features

Reduced scale manufacturing techniques have been compiled in the engineering literature and are beyond the scope of this chapter. From a manufacturing perspective, many if not all of the available techniques may be utilized for patterning implant surfaces with nanometer scale features [14]. However, since high throughput is necessary for economically viable implant surface manufacturing, industrial methods for nanometer scale surface modification are restricted to a reduced number of additive and subtractive methods. To date, four representative implant surfaces presenting nanometer scale features have been made commercially available. Out of these four, two comprise surface modifications presenting calcium-and-phosphate bioactive components manufactured through initially subtractive methods followed by additive methods, and the other two are manufactured mainly through subtractive processes.

The nanometer scale surfaces presenting bioactive ceramic components were both named NanoTite™ by their respective manufacturers (Bicon LLC, Boston, USA; Biomet 3i, Palm Beach Gardens, USA). While their final physicochemical configuration is distinctively different, both surfaces are manufactured by an initial subtractive method prior to the additive methods that are distinct. For the Bicon surface, a 20–50 nm-thickness ion beam-assisted deposition (IBAD) of calcium phosphate results in the coating of a moderately rough micro-textured substrate obtained by alumina blasting/acid etching (AB/AE) [28]. For the Biomet 3i surface, a sol–gel process is performed for the deposition of calcium phosphate nanometer-sized (called discrete crystalline deposition, DCD) particles onto their textured acid-etched surface. Previous work has demonstrated that the particle component covered approximately 50 % of the surface [29]. While both surfaces presented bioactive components on their surfaces, the rationale for their presence and intended coating kinetics in vivo substantially differed.

The rationale for the IBAD of 20–50 nm mainly amorphous coating thickness onto the AB/AE micro-textured surface was to take advantage of the highly osteoconductive properties of the calcium phosphate coating properties while avoiding long-term issues presented by thick plasma-sprayed hydroxyapatite coatings in which long-term performance is highly dependent on implant hardware configuration [30]. In short, the basis was to provide the healing site with the known osteogenic properties of bioactive calcium phosphate elements, and due to the IBAD coating amorphous configuration, the coating would be entirely dissolved/resorbed from the surface and an intimate contact between bone and the AB/AE micro-textured surface would result. Different from the IBAD coating, the DCD method for nanometer scale feature incorporation intended to increase the substrate osteoconductivity due to the multiscale texture levels (micro- and nano-texturing) and chemical composition rendered by the DCD method.

The two other surfaces presenting nanometer scale features are both manufactured by subtractive methods [31]. The first surface, OsseoSpeed™ (Astra Tech, AB, Mölndal, Sweden), from here on referred by the OSP acronym, initially utilizes a titanium oxide blasting procedure that renders the surface with micrometer-level texture, followed by a hydrofluoric acid etching procedure that results in nanometer scale texturing within the micrometer scale texturing. The second one, OSSEAN™ (Intra-Lock International, Boca Raton, FL, USA), from hereon referred to by the OSS acronym, is fabricated by robotic micro-blasting of a resorbable blasting media powder that simultaneously results in nanometer scale topography within the larger-scale micro-topography. Regardless of fabrication method, no long-range ordering of the nanometer scale features is obtained [31, 32].

Despite the substantially different fabrication methods, from a topographical standpoint, all four surfaces present nano-texture within micro-textured surface features. From a surface chemistry standpoint, the IBAD fabricated surface presents primarily Ca, P, and O in its surface since it is a uniform coating at the nanometer length scale thickness, whereas the DCD surface presents elements from both bioactive ceramic and substrate components [29, 33]. Along with the substrate alloy components, fluoride presence at minute quantities has been detected on OSP [34], whereas bioactive ceramic along with substrate alloy elements is present on the OSS surface [35].

It must be stated here that some of the implant surfaces other than the abovementioned were discovered afterwards by scientific reports to possess nanoscale features. For example, TiUnite (Nobel Biocare, Zurich, Switzerland), SLActive (Institut Straumann, Basel, Switzerland), and OsseoSpeed (DENTSPLY IH, Mölndal, Sweden), all of them, which were originally not claiming of possessing nanoscale features, were discovered to have distinctive nano-patterns [2, 36, 37]. Whether intended or not intended, these features may be one of the reasons for the enhanced bone apposition observed when compared to their respective predecessors.

Biological Response to Nanotextured Implant Surfaces Made Commercially Available

Despite the recent introduction of the nanometer scale onto implant surfaces, a substantial body of work has been developed. The early studies investigating the biological response to nanometer scale surfaces were funded by manufacturers and often utilized their predecessor surfaces as control groups. A series of studies followed and at times different nanometer scale surfaces were compared within studies.

Cell Culture Studies

The IBAD surface was evaluated in three different cell culture studies, where the IBAD surface was compared to its AB/AE uncoated substrate and as-machined surfaces [38–40]. The first study, carried out with primary human osteoblasts, presented mixed results between the IBAD and AB/AE surfaces regarding events related to osteogenesis [38]. The second study aimed to evaluate the same three surfaces under human osteogenic cells, peripheral blood mononuclear cells (PBMC), and osteogenic cells cocultured with PBMC without exogenous stimuli. In general, relative differences in results were observed between surfaces for three different cultures (always favoring the IBAD and AB/AE surfaces relative to the as-machined control); however, the "multicell type" interactions played a more remarkable role than the surface texture or chemistry on the in vitro cellular events related to initial stages of bone formation [40]. Finally, the same three surfaces were evaluated in human polymorphonuclear neutrophil (PMN) culture. The results showed that the addition of a thin CaP coating to the AB/AE surface influenced the secretion profile of proinflammatory cytokines [39]. Altogether, cell culture studies including the IBAD surface presented mixed results that demonstrated substantial disagreement with the in vivo preclinical results between IBAD, AB/AE, and turned surfaces as subsequently discussed.

The DCD surface has been evaluated in primary mouse alveolar bone cells relative to Astra OsseoSpeed, Nobel Biocare TiUnite, and Straumann SLA surfaces [41]. The results following a 48-h culture, Astra and Straumann systems displayed the highest degrees of cell adhesion. Specific to the DCD surface, it presented significantly lower degrees of cell confluence relative to the other surfaces [41].

The OSP surface has been compared to its titanium oxide blasted predecessor in a mouse preosteoblast MC3T3-E1 cell culture model [42]. The study results showed no differences in cell viability and proliferation but more branched cell morphology was observed for OSP relative to the control at 48 h. At 14 days, increased degrees of IGF-I, BSP, and osterix gene expression were observed for the OSP surface, concluding that osteoblast differentiation and mineralization were affected by the nanometer scale surface [42]. A more comprehensive real-time PCR study considering bone-specific gene expression in the same two surfaces plus a turned control in a MC3T3-E1 cell culture model and in implant adherent cells from a rabbit tibia model depicted that OSP surface outperformed the control surface in osteogenic gene expression events [43]. Another study evaluating adherent mesenchymal stem cells on OSP and its predecessor presented favorable osteoinductivity and osteogenesis of these cells for the OSP surface [44]. As previously mentioned, when OSP was compared to the DCD surface in a primary mouse alveolar bone cell culture model, favorable results were observed for the OSP surface relative to the DCD surface [41]. Masaki et al. also demonstrated that OSP altered cell behavior relative to other surfaces [45].

Cell culture studies considering the OSS surface also compared it to its micrometer scale textured predecessor [38]. In this study, cell adhesion, proliferation, and alkaline phosphatase activity were assessed with human SaOS-2 17 osteoblasts and bone mesenchymal stem cells in nonosteogenic culture conditions. The results demonstrated higher osteoblastic differentiation for the nanometer scale surface relative to its micrometer scale counterpart [38].

In general, cell culture studies depicted favorable results for nanometer scale surfaces relative to their micrometer scale predecessors. To date, no such study has been performed for the DCD surface, and the mixed results observed for the IBAD surface relative to the uncoated AB/AE substrate were possibly related to the amorphous coating dissolution. Specific to the OSP and OSS surfaces, where similar micrometer-level textured surfaces were used as controls against nanometer scale within micrometer scale topography surfaces, it is unequivocal that the nanometer scale features substantially altered cell behavior favoring osteogenic cellular events.

Preclinical In Vivo Models

Unlike the mixed results obtained in cell culture assays for the IBAD surface, a series of studies demonstrated its superiority to uncoated surfaces in both biomechanical and histometric outcomes

[46–48]. When cylindrical implants were utilized with the IBAD surface versus its uncoated counterpart, higher degrees of osteoconductivity were observed along with higher degrees of biomechanical fixation at early implantation times [46–48]. Furthermore, it has been demonstrated that the coating thickness played a role on biomechanical results [47]. When commercially available implants were utilized in larger preclinical in vivo models, significantly higher levels of bone-to-implant contact (BIC) and biomechanical fixation were observed [28, 33, 49–51]. While significant improvements were consistently obtained relative to its uncoated counterpart, studies that considered the IBAD- versus PSHA-coated implants demonstrated that the PSHA-coated implants outperformed the IBAD-coated groups, especially when biomechanical competence at early implantation time is concerned [33, 47, 50, 52].

The DCD surface showed promising results in rodent models relative to its micrometer scale textured counterpart [53–55]. In a bone healing chamber design in a rat model, higher degrees of bone ingrowth were observed [54], as well as higher degrees of bone adhesion were detected when bone pullout from DCD-coated implants was compared to the predecessor control (regarded as bone bonding due to the presence of nanometer scale features on the implant surface) [53]. However, different than observed in rodent models, no differences in bone response to both DCD and its predecessor surface in a beagle dog model were detected [56–59]. When the DCD surface was compared to other moderately rough surfaces in the challenging immediate extraction socket scenarios, it did present significantly lower BIC levels relative to a dual acid-etched surface, an SLA surface, and an anodized surface. When socket architecture was considered, no difference was detected between the four different implant groups [60].

The OSP surface has also been well documented in laboratory preclinical animal models versus its moderately rough micrometer scale textured predecessor and against other surfaces. Ellingsen et al. [61] demonstrated higher biomechanical competence and BIC levels for the OSP relative to its micrometer scale predecessor (TiOblast, Astra Tech AB, Mölndal, Sweden) in a rabbit tibia model. Through modification in the relationship between implant macrogeometry and surgical instrumentation (forming healing chambers between threads [6, 7, 24]), Berglundh et al. [34] demonstrated superior results for the OSP surface relative to its predecessor when the amount of bone formation within healing chambers was concerned.

The OSP surface has also been compared to other micrometer scale surfaces in numerous preclinical laboratory animal models. In a rabbit model, at 2 weeks in vivo, OSP surface presented significantly higher bone response when compared to an anodized surface presenting micrometer-level texturing [62]. In a crestal bone maintenance study conducted in minipigs by Heitz-Mayfield et al. [63], the OSP along with SLA implants presented higher degrees of crestal bone maintenance relative to an implant presenting an anodized surface with micrometer-level texturing [63].

The OSP has also been evaluated against other micrometer scale textured surfaces with enhanced surface wettability in fresh extraction sockets in beagle dogs [64], and after 4 and 12 weeks, no differences in host-to-implant response were detected. Another study comparing OSP versus other surfaces in fresh extraction sockets failed to demonstrate differences between groups in all parameters evaluated [65]. It should be noted that this particular study primarily comprised the evaluation of soft tissue measurement outcomes and not osseointegration measurements. However, bone maintenance around implants immediately placed in extraction sockets has been shown to influence soft tissue measurements [66, 67].

The OSP surface has also been compared to other nanometer scale surfaces in numerous preclinical laboratory animal models. These studies are described subsequently in the text.

The OSS has also been well documented versus its AB/AE predecessor in a series of preclinical in vivo studies. The first was conducted by Marin et al. [68], where OSS and AB/AE surfaces were histometrically and biomechanically evaluated in a beagle model. The group reported that while no significant differences were observed in BIC between surfaces at both 2 and 4 weeks, an approximately 100 % increase in removal torque was observed for the OSS surface relative to its predecessor counterpart, strongly suggesting that bone around the OSS surface presented higher mechanical properties [23]. Similar results were obtained by Marin et al. [69] when the OSS surface was compared to a dual acid-etched moderately rough surface presenting micrometer-level texture.

In a protocol similar to Mendes et al. [53], who reported bone bonding between the DCD nanometer scale modified surface and bone, Coelho et al. observed the same bone bonding phenomenon when the OSS surface was compared to its AB/AE micrometer scale textured counterpart, suggesting that bone bonding can also be achieved by the lower levels of Ca and P on the OSS implant surface (note that crystalline HA particles are present at much higher amounts for the DCD surface) [70]. Alternatively, the authors speculated that bone bonding to the OSS surface was possibly due to the nanometer scale texture rather than due to the low levels of Ca and P on the OSS surface relative to the DCD process. To address the question of whether nanometer scale texture or the surface chemistry was responsible for the high osteoconductive properties of the OSS surface, a nanometer scale presenting texture similar to the OSS surface was produced through silica blasting and thus no Ca and P content was present in its surface chemistry [71]. When these were compared in vivo in a beagle model, no differences in bone response (torque and BIC) were detected between surfaces, suggesting a stronger nano-texture contribution in the OSS surface osseointegration relative to its low level of Ca and P presence on its surface [71]. These results strongly suggest that the bone bonding achieved in Coelho et al. was likely due to the nanotopographical component of the OSS surface and experimental studies should be conducted to further address the nanometer scale texture and chemistry's contribution to bone bonding to implant surfaces [70]. Another histometric, nanomechanical, and gene-expression study conducted in a rodent model unequivocally showed higher BIC, bone mechanical properties (hardness and modulus of elasticity), and osteogenic gene expression for the OSS surface versus its predecessor, indicating that the nanometer scale surface indeed modulates osteoblastic cell response, leading to faster osseointegration and bone mechanical property achievement [72]. Finally, the OSS surface when evaluated in a more challenging scenario such as immediate placement in extraction sockets was able to maintain higher levels of bone attachment at the buccal flange relative to implants presenting a smooth cervical region [73].

When compared to other micrometer scale surfaces, the OSS presented favorable biomechanical and histometric results. For instance, a study comparing the OSS surface relative to several other micrometer scale textured surfaces obtained through AB/AE and resorbable blasting media (RBM) alone, plasma-treated micrometer textured surfaces, and RBM acid-etched surfaces depicted significantly higher torque levels for the OSS surface relative to others [74]. Another study comprising the histometric and nanomechanical assessment of bone mechanical property of OSS versus OSP, SLA, anodized, and RBM surfaces demonstrated higher BIC for the OSS at the earliest time point in vivo and that bone mechanical properties slightly differed between surfaces but not to a significant extent [35].

Relative to other nanometer scale surfaces, the OSS surface was compared to the DCD surface and other micrometer scale textured surfaces in a canine model at 10 and 30 days postimplantation [29]. Worth noting is that in this study, all implant macrogeometries and surgical instrumentation were the same, minimizing osseointegration confounding factors due to implant hardware. This study showed that the OSS surface presented significantly higher biomechanical competence (assessed by removal torque) than the other groups at 30 days in vivo [29].

One study directly comparing the biomechanical performance of the OSS, OSP, and DCD implants is available in the literature. The implants were placed in the beagle dog mandible at 1 and 3 weeks in vivo prior to euthanasia.

When torqued out, the OSS implant system presented significantly higher removal torque values compared to the OSP and DCD surfaces. At 3 weeks, both OSS and OSP implants presented similar results and both were significantly higher than the DCD surface [75]. While insightful, the results of this particular study must be interpreted with care, as it did not compare the performance of the three different surfaces but the performance of three different implant systems with nanometer scale surfaces. Specific to the removal torque results, it must be noted that the significant differences between groups may have been exacerbated by differences in implant hardware that possibly mitigated the effect of the nanometer scale in osseointegration.

Human Implant Retrieval Studies

Cell culturing and preclinical laboratory animal model studies are remarkable methods for initial evaluation of the effect of multiple scale design features in osseointegration. Even though slightly contradictory, the literature presented thus far regarding cell cultures and animal models in nanometer scale textured implants has shown the merit of such features in achieving favorable results in cell modulation, osseointegration, biomechanical fixation, and bone mechanical properties relative to micrometer scale surface texturing. While all laboratory preclinical work is valid to determine whether there is potential clinical application for novel design features, careful experimental work conducted in humans under appropriate IRB approval provides one of the most valuable tools for evaluation of both implant success and failures [76–78]. Once the removal of the implantable device is completed, this specimen contains important information regarding the biological reaction from the host and the effects of the implant presence in bone modeling/remodeling. Human implant retrieval studies have been conducted for some of the nanometer scale surfaces that have been made commercially available about the IBAD surface.

Orsini et al. [79] histologically and histomorphometrically evaluated the DCD surface versus its acid-etched predecessor in a study where both implant surfaces were placed in the posterior maxilla of 15 patients in a nested within subject study design. Following implant retrieval after 2 months healing, they evaluated the implants under a confocal microscope and concluded that the DCD presented significantly higher degrees of osseointegration relative to its predecessor [79].

Rocci et al. [80] compared OSP implants versus its micrometer scale textured predecessor placed in the mandible in a nested within subject design. Eight weeks after placement, the implants were retrieved and histometrically evaluated. Despite the small number of samples, the overall results of all histometric outcomes favored OSP relative to its control. In a study that evaluated the early temporal-wide genome transcription regulation by the surface topography at the bone–implant interface between OSP and its predecessor, paired samples collected at 3 and 7 days after placement from 11 healthy patients demonstrated that collagen fibrillogenesis, extracellular matrix organization, and the inflammatory/immune responses were observed in implant adherent cells early (3–7 days) after implantation [81]. The same study also reported different gene expression between surfaces at 3 and 7 days, further reinforcing that surface modifications do have strong potential for modulating cell behavior [81].

The OSS surface was also evaluated against its predecessor in a study where implants were placed in pairs in the posterior maxilla of ten subjects [82]. Implants were retrieved following a period of 8 weeks. The histometric results showed significantly higher BIC and osteocyte density within the newly formed bone for the OSS versus the control [82].

Clinical Research

Outcomes of a few published clinical trials regarding some implant surfaces with nanotopography will be described in this section and summarized in Table 5.1. The DCD surface has been evaluated in a prospective 1-year clinical study with tapered implants placed in 42 patients, with

Table 5.1 Clinical outcomes of prospective studies of implant surfaces presenting nanotopography

Author/implant surface	Prostheses design	Survival rate (%)	Observation period (study design)	Immediate occlusal loading	Control group (non nano-enabled surface)
Östman et al. [83]/DCD	20 SC, 30 FDP, 7 FA	99.4 % (one implant failure)	1 year (prospective)	Yes	No
Östman et al. [84]/DCD	14 SC, 26 FDP, 4 FA	99.2 % (one implant failure)	1 year (prospective)	Yes	No
Cecchinato et al. [85]/OSP	91 SC	Not described	3 years (prospective)	Yes	No
Collaert et al. [86]/OSP	25 FA	100 %	2 years (prospective)	Yes	No
De Bruyn et al. [87]/OSP	132 SC	94–98 %	3 years (prospective)	No	No
Mertens and Steveling [88]/OSP	31 SC, 4 FDP, 1 FA	97 %	5 years (prospective)	Yes/early loading included	No
Mertens et al. [89]/OSP	Fixed and removable	97.85 %	28 months (prospective)	No	No
Noelken et al. [90]/OSP	SC and FDP	100 %	2 years (prospective)	No	No
Raes et al. [91]/OSP	SC	98 %	1 year (prospective)	Yes	No

DCD Discrete Crystalline Deposition™, *OSP* OsseoSpeed™, *SC* single crown, *FDP* fixed dental prostheses, *FA* full arch

55 % located in the posterior region (20 single-tooth, 30 fixed dental prostheses, and 7 full-arch maxillary reconstructions). Survival rate at 1 year was 99.4 % [83]. The same surface was evaluated in an immediate-loading prospective 1-year clinical study but on a different macrogeometry (Prevail®). Thirty-five patients received 102 implants (65 % in the posterior region), to support 14 single crowns (SC), 26 fixed dental prostheses (FDP), and 4 full-arch reconstructions. The survival rate was 99.2 % (one implant failure) [84].

The OSP implant surface has been evaluated in several studies including: (1) immediate loading for soft tissue long-term (3 years) evaluation, where 93 patients were treated with 93 implants [85]; (2) immediate loading of 125 implants placed to support full-arch rehabilitations, followed up prospectively for 2 years with a survival rate of 100 % [86]; (3) immediate provisionalization (no centric or eccentric occlusal contact) of 132 implants supporting single crowns in the anterior maxilla (62 placed in extraction sockets and 70 in healed sites), with survival rates of 94.5 and 98.3 % [87]; (4) 17 patients received 33 implants in the maxilla and 16 in the mandible to support single crowns, fixed dental prostheses, or full-arch restoration [88]; (5) 15 patients received 99 implants at 19 different intraoral recipient sites (15 in the maxilla and 4 in the mandible), previously grafted with calvarial split grafts, and loaded after 3 months with fixed and removable prostheses. The 28 months follow-up showed an implant survival rate of 97.85 % [89]; (6) 37 implants immediately placed and provisionalized, without occlusal contact, with single crowns and FDP where 17 replaced central incisors, 9 lateral incisors, 6 canines, and 5 premolars, presenting a 2-year survival rate of 100 % [90]; (7) 48 patients received single implants to be immediately loaded after either conventional implant placement, immediate placement, or grafted sites. After 1 year of function, the prospective follow-up indicated a 98 % survival rate [91].

From the studies described above and included in the table, it is observed that a combination of treatment concepts even within the same study is commonplace with some involving: immediate and early loading, placement into grafted and non-grafted sites, different prosthesis designs including single crowns, FDP, removable, and full-arch prostheses sometimes screw- or cement-retained, varied implant diameters and lengths, implant placement in different areas in the mouth (anterior or posterior, maxilla or mandible). It becomes clear that comparative efforts even within the same implant surface among studies become a heuristic task. Of remarkable interest is that none of the studies that investigated the clinical outcomes of implants with nanosurface alterations have included a control (same implant macrodesign without the nano-enabled features) for sound observation of the real impact of nanofeatures in immediate, early, and long-term clinical results.

In the lack of controlled studies, it must be regarded as unknown whether nanometer surface alterations really have a clinical impact. Furthermore, even if controlled studies will be presented in the future, the fact that modern oral implant surfaces share a mix of a number of different surface characteristics including nanometer indentations, it would seem most difficult to prove a clinical support from nanometer scale texture/modifications alone.

Final Considerations

A report on the market share of nanotechnology-enabled products has early emphasized that nanotechnology represents a value chain and not an industry or sector per se. In this report, revenue projections for 2014 were that nanotechnology would represent 4 % of general manufactured goods, 50 % of electronics and information technology products, and 16 % of goods in healthcare. Ten years ago, the revenues for products incorporating nanotechnology were about US $ 13 billion, where US $ 8.5 billion came from the automotive and aerospace applications. Revenue rise for 2014 was projected to US $ 2.6 trillion, a period when nanotechnology in healthcare and life sciences would become significant in pharmaceutics and for medical devices, considering that lengthy, well-designed randomized controlled clinical trials (RCT) would have been able to demonstrate that nano-enabled materials substantially altered the nature of a product and its host response [92]. Obviously, this does not seem to be the case in implant dentistry, not only because RCTs comprise a substantially large patient pool and standardized prostheses design, in patients receiving implants with and without nano-intended features, are not available, but also because the multifaceted success criteria in implant dentistry are commonly not acknowledged [93]. To date, a large gap between the promise of nanotechnology and its integration into a new generation of nano-enabled products is remarkably evident [94]. It must also be emphasized that this chapter primarily concerned what has been made commercially available and that a plethora of nanometer scale surface modifications for bone healing modulation is currently under development and showing remarkable improvement such as increasing bone healing velocity while also resulting in higher bone mechanical properties [95], features of utmost importance if challenging loading protocols are to be common practice and not solely utilized in selected cases.

It is unequivocal that implant hardware does shift bone healing modes and that such healing mode shifting may increase the contribution of micrometer- and nanometer-scale level contribution to osseointegration. There is also an immense number of published work unequivocally demonstrating that micrometer level surface modifications support the bone response through facilitating early host-to-implant response through tissue healing that facilitates cell migration and also shifts cell phenotype. Moreover, not yet mentioned in this chapter, would be the biomolecular tagging ad hocs to implant surfaces that may potentially be better engineered due to nanometer scale properties and fabrication methods [96].

Since it has been experimentally determined that all length scale implant design levels have a substantial contribution to the science of osseointegration, a continued experimental and clinical testing of novel implant surface innovations would be of a challenge. Thus, given the inconsistencies encountered in the implant literature, a substantial amount of work is warranted for adequate collection of data that will enable enhanced osseointegration. Upon completion of such germane series of studies, it is anticipated that an optimal combination in the macrometer, micrometer, nanometer, and biomolecular scale design will be identified.

Acknowledgments The authors would like to express their gratitude to all their collaborators and students, who are the body and soul of the work presented in this chapter.

References

1. Wennerberg A, Albrektsson T. Effects of titanium surface topography on bone integration: a systematic review. Clin Oral Implants Res. 2009;20 Suppl 4:172–84.
2. Wennerberg A, Albrektsson T. On implant surfaces: a review of current knowledge and opinions. Int J Oral Maxillofac Implants. 2010;25(1):63–74.
3. Gittens RA, Scheideler L, Rupp F, Hyzy SL, Geis-Gerstorfer J, Schwartz Z, et al. A review on the wettability of dental implant surfaces II: biological and clinical aspects. Acta Biomater. 2014;10:2907–18.
4. Zambuzzi WF, Coelho PG, Alves GG, Granjeiro JM. Intracellular signal transduction as a factor in the development of "smart" biomaterials for bone tissue engineering. Biotechnol Bioeng. 2011;108(6):1246–50.
5. Kieswetter K, Schwartz Z, Dean DD, Boyan BD. The role of implant surface characteristics in the healing of bone. Crit Rev Oral Biol Med. 1996;7(4):329–45.
6. Leonard G, Coelho P, Polyzois I, Stassen L, Claffey N. A study of the bone healing kinetics of plateau versus screw root design titanium dental implants. Clin Oral Implants Res. 2009;20(3):232–9.
7. Berglundh T, Abrahamsson I, Lang NP, Lindhe J. De novo alveolar bone formation adjacent to endosseous implants. Clin Oral Implants Res. 2003;14(3):251–62.
8. Coelho PG, Granato R, Marin C, Teixeira HS, Suzuki M, Valverde GB, et al. The effect of different implant macrogeometries and surface treatment in early biomechanical fixation: an experimental study in dogs. J Mech Behav Biomed Mater. 2011;4(8):1974–81.
9. Albrektsson T, Branemark PI, Hansson HA, Lindstrom J. Osseointegrated titanium implants. Requirements for ensuring a long-lasting, direct bone-to-implant anchorage in man. Acta Orthop Scand. 1981;52(2):155–70.
10. Jimbo R, Andersson M, Vandeweghe S. Nano in implant dentistry. Int J Dent. 2014;2014:1–2.
11. Gittens RA, Olivares-Navarrete R, McLachlan T, Cai Y, Hyzy SL, Schneider JM, et al. Differential responses of osteoblast lineage cells to nanotopographically-modified, microroughened titanium-aluminum-vanadium alloy surfaces. Biomaterials. 2012;33(35):8986–94.
12. Hayashi M, Jimbo R, Lindh L, Sotres J, Sawase T, Mustafa K, et al. In vitro characterization and osteoblast responses to nanostructured photocatalytic TiO2 coated surfaces. Acta Biomater. 2012;8(6):2411–6.
13. Tomsia AP, Lee JS, Wegst UG, Saiz E. Nanotechnology for dental implants. Int J Oral Maxillofac Implants. 2013;28(6):e535–46.
14. Suri S, Ruan G, Winter J, Schmidt C. Microparticles and nanoparticles. In: Ratner B, Hoffman A, Schoen F, Lemons J, editors. Biomaterials science: an introduction to materials in medicine. Elsevier: San Diego; 2013. p. 360–88.
15. Cahay M, editor. Quantum confinement VI: nanostructured materials and devices. Proceedings of the International Symposium 2001: the electrochemical society, San Francisco, CA, USA.
16. Elias CN, Meirelles L. Improving osseointegration of dental implants. Expert Rev Med Devices. 2010;7(2):241–56.
17. Rupp F, Scheideler L, Eichler M, Geis-Gerstorfer J. Wetting behavior of dental implants. Int J Oral Maxillofac Implants. 2011;26(6):1256–66.
18. Gittens RA, McLachlan T, Olivares-Navarrete R, Cai Y, Berner S, Tannenbaum R, et al. The effects of combined micron-/submicron-scale surface roughness and nanoscale features on cell proliferation and differentiation. Biomaterials. 2011;32(13):3395–403.
19. Biggs MJ, Richards RG, Gadegaard N, McMurray RJ, Affrossman S, Wilkinson CD, et al. Interactions with nanoscale topography: adhesion quantification and signal transduction in cells of osteogenic and multipotent lineage. J Biomed Mater Res A. 2009;91(1):195–208.
20. Dalby MJ, McCloy D, Robertson M, Wilkinson CD, Oreffo RO. Osteoprogenitor response to defined topographies with nanoscale depths. Biomaterials. 2006;27(8):1306–15.
21. Palin E, Liu H, Webster TJ. Mimicking the nanofeatures of bone increases bone-forming cell adhesion and proliferation. Nanotechnology. 2005;16(9):1828.
22. Mendonca G, Mendonca DB, Aragao FJ, Cooper LF. Advancing dental implant surface technology–from micron- to nanotopography. Biomaterials. 2008;29(28):3822–35.
23. Coelho PG, Suzuki M, Guimaraes MV, Marin C, Granato R, Gil JN, et al. Early bone healing around different implant bulk designs and surgical techniques: a study in dogs. Clin Implant Dent Relat Res. 2010;12(3):202–8.
24. Marin C, Granato R, Suzuki M, Gil JN, Janal MN, Coelho PG. Histomorphologic and histomorphometric evaluation of various endosseous implant healing chamber configurations at early implanta-

tion times: a study in dogs. Clin Oral Implants Res. 2010;21(6):577–83.
25. Webster TJ, Siegel RW, Bizios R. Osteoblast adhesion on nanophase ceramics. Biomaterials. 1999;20(13):1221–7.
26. Webster TJ, Ejiofor JU. Increased osteoblast adhesion on nanophase metals: Ti, Ti6Al4V, and CoCrMo. Biomaterials. 2004;25(19):4731–9.
27. Webster TJ, Ergun C, Doremus RH, Siegel RW, Bizios R. Enhanced functions of osteoblasts on nanophase ceramics. Biomaterials. 2000;21(17):1803–10.
28. Granato R, Marin C, Suzuki M, Gil JN, Janal MN, Coelho PG. Biomechanical and histomorphometric evaluation of a thin ion beam bioceramic deposition on plateau root form implants: an experimental study in dogs. J Biomed Mater Res B Appl Biomater. 2009;90(1):396–403.
29. Bonfante EA, Granato R, Marin C, Jimbo R, Giro G, Suzuki M, et al. Biomechanical testing of microblasted, acid-etched/microblasted, anodized, and discrete crystalline deposition surfaces: an experimental study in beagle dogs. Int J Oral Maxillofac Implants. 2013;28(1):136–42.
30. Albrektsson T. Hydroxyapatite-coated implants: a case against their use. J Oral Maxillofac Surg. 1998;56(11):1312–26.
31. Coelho PG, Granjeiro JM, Romanos GE, Suzuki M, Silva NR, Cardaropoli G, et al. Basic research methods and current trends of dental implant surfaces. J Biomed Mater Res B Appl Biomater. 2009;88(2):579–96.
32. Dohan Ehrenfest DM, Coelho PG, Kang BS, Sul YT, Albrektsson T. Classification of osseointegrated implant surfaces: materials, chemistry and topography. Trends Biotechnol. 2010;28(4):198–206.
33. Coelho PG, Granato R, Marin C, Bonfante EA, Janal MN, Suzuki M. Biomechanical and bone histomorphologic evaluation of four surfaces on plateau root form implants: an experimental study in dogs. Oral Surg Oral Med Oral Pathol Oral Radiol Endod. 2010;109(5):e39–45.
34. Berglundh T, Abrahamsson I, Albouy JP, Lindhe J. Bone healing at implants with a fluoride-modified surface: an experimental study in dogs. Clin Oral Implants Res. 2007;18(2):147–52.
35. Jimbo R, Anchieta R, Baldassarri M, Granato R, Marin C, Teixeira HS, et al. Histomorphometry and bone mechanical property evolution around different implant systems at early healing stages: an experimental study in dogs. Implant Dent. 2013;22(6):596–603.
36. Meirelles L, Currie F, Jacobsson M, Albrektsson T, Wennerberg A. The effect of chemical and nanotopographical modifications on the early stages of osseointegration. Int J Oral Maxillofac Implants. 2008;23(4):641–7.
37. Wennerberg A, Galli S, Albrektsson T. Current knowledge about the hydrophilic and nanostructured SLActive surface. Clin Cosmet Investig Dent. 2011;3:59.
38. Bucci-Sabattini V, Cassinelli C, Coelho PG, Minnici A, Trani A, Dohan Ehrenfest DM. Effect of titanium implant surface nanoroughness and calcium phosphate low impregnation on bone cell activity in vitro. Oral Surg Oral Med Oral Pathol Oral Radiol Endod. 2010;109(2):217–24.
39. Moura CC, Machado JR, Silva MV, Rodrigues DB, Zanetta-Barbosa D, Jimbo R, et al. Evaluation of human polymorphonuclear behavior on textured titanium and calcium-phosphate coated surfaces. Biomed Mater. 2013;8(3):035010.
40. Moura CG, Souza MA, Kohal RJ, Dechichi P, Zanetta-Barbosa D, Jimbo R, et al. Evaluation of osteogenic cell culture and osteogenic/peripheral blood mononuclear human cell co-culture on modified titanium surfaces. Biomed Mater. 2013;8(3):035002.
41. Liu R, Lei T, Dusevich V, Yao X, Liu Y, Walker MP, et al. Surface characteristics and cell adhesion: a comparative study of four commercial dental implants. J Prosthodont. 2013;22(8):641–51.
42. Monjo M, Petzold C, Ramis JM, Lyngstadaas SP, Ellingsen JE. In vitro osteogenic properties of two dental implant surfaces. Int J Biomater. 2012;2012:181024.
43. Guo J, Padilla RJ, Ambrose W, De Kok IJ, Cooper LF. The effect of hydrofluoric acid treatment of TiO2 grit blasted titanium implants on adherent osteoblast gene expression in vitro and in vivo. Biomaterials. 2007;28(36):5418–25.
44. Valencia S, Gretzer C, Cooper LF. Surface nanofeature effects on titanium-adherent human mesenchymal stem cells. Int J Oral Maxillofac Implants. 2009;24(1):38–46.
45. Masaki C, Schneider GB, Zaharias R, Seabold D, Stanford C. Effects of implant surface microtopography on osteoblast gene expression. Clin Oral Implants Res. 2005;16(6):650–6.
46. Coelho PG, Cardaropoli G, Suzuki M, Lemons JE. Early healing of nanothickness bioceramic coatings on dental implants. An experimental study in dogs. J Biomed Mater Res B Appl Biomater. 2009;88(2):387–93.
47. Coelho PG, Lemons JE. Physico/chemical characterization and in vivo evaluation of nanothickness bioceramic depositions on alumina-blasted/acid-etched Ti-6Al-4V implant surfaces. J Biomed Mater Res A. 2009;90(2):351–61.
48. Coelho PG, Suzuki M. Evaluation of an IBAD thin-film process as an alternative method for surface incorporation of bioceramics on dental implants: a study in dogs. J Appl Oral Sci. 2005;13(1):87–92.
49. Granato R, Marin C, Gil JN, Chuang SK, Dodson TB, Suzuki M, et al. Thin bioactive ceramic-coated alumina-blasted/acid-etched implant surface enhances biomechanical fixation of implants: an experimental study in dogs. Clin Implant Dent Relat Res. 2011;13(2):87–94.
50. Suzuki M, Calasans-Maia MD, Marin C, Granato R, Gil JN, Granjeiro JM, et al. Effect of surface modi-

fications on early bone healing around plateau root form implants: an experimental study in rabbits. J Oral Maxillofac Surg. 2010;68(7):1631–8.
51. Suzuki M, Guimaraes MV, Marin C, Granato R, Gil JN, Coelho PG. Histomorphometric evaluation of alumina-blasted/acid-etched and thin ion beam-deposited bioceramic surfaces: an experimental study in dogs. J Oral Maxillofac Surg. 2009;67(3):602–7.
52. Quaranta A, Iezzi G, Scarano A, Coelho PG, Vozza I, Marincola M, et al. A histomorphometric study of nanothickness and plasma-sprayed calcium-phosphorous-coated implant surfaces in rabbit bone. J Periodontol. 2010;81(4):556–61.
53. Mendes VC, Moineddin R, Davies JE. The effect of discrete calcium phosphate nanocrystals on bone-bonding to titanium surfaces. Biomaterials. 2007;28(32):4748–55.
54. Mendes VC, Moineddin R, Davies JE. Discrete calcium phosphate nanocrystalline deposition enhances osteoconduction on titanium-based implant surfaces. J Biomed Mater Res A. 2009;90(2):577–85.
55. Lin A, Wang CJ, Kelly J, Gubbi P, Nishimura I. The role of titanium implant surface modification with hydroxyapatite nanoparticles in progressive early bone-implant fixation in vivo. Inter J Oral Maxillofac Implants. 2009;24(5):808–16.
56. Calvo-Guirado JL, Satorres-Nieto M, Aguilar-Salvatierra A, Delgado-Ruiz RA, Mate-Sanchez de Val JE, Gargallo-Albiol J, et al. Influence of surface treatment on osseointegration of dental implants: histological, histomorphometric and radiological analysis in vivo. Clin Oral Investig. 2014. doi: 10.1007/s00784-014-1241-2. [Epub ahead of print]
57. Calvo-Guirado JL, Satorres M, Negri B, Ramirez-Fernandez P, Mate-Sanchez JE, Delgado-Ruiz R, et al. Biomechanical and histological evaluation of four different titanium implant surface modifications: an experimental study in the rabbit tibia. Clin Oral Inv. 2014;18(5):1495–505.
58. Abrahamsson I, Linder E, Larsson L, Berglundh T. Deposition of nanometer scaled calcium-phosphate crystals to implants with a dual acid-etched surface does not improve early tissue integration. Clin Oral Implants Res. 2013;24(1):57–62.
59. Vignoletti F, Johansson C, Albrektsson T, De Sanctis M, San Roman F, Sanz M. Early healing of implants placed into fresh extraction sockets: an experimental study in the beagle dog. De novo bone formation. J Clin Periodontol. 2009;36(3):265–77.
60. Bonfante EA, Janal MN, Granato R, Marin C, Suzuki M, Tovar N, et al. Buccal and lingual bone level alterations after immediate implantation of four implant surfaces: a study in dogs. Clin Oral Implants Res. 2013;24(12):1375–80.
61. Ellingsen JE, Johansson CB, Wennerberg A, Holmen A. Improved retention and bone-to-implant contact with fluoride-modified titanium implants. Int J Oral Maxillofac Implants. 2004;19(5):659–66.
62. Choi JY, Lee HJ, Jang JU, Yeo IS. Comparison between bioactive fluoride modified and bioinert anodically oxidized implant surfaces in early bone response using rabbit tibia model. Implant Dent. 2012;21(2):124–8.
63. Heitz-Mayfield LJ, Darby I, Heitz F, Chen S. Preservation of crestal bone by implant design. A comparative study in minipigs. Clin Oral Implants Res. 2013;24(3):243–9.
64. Alharbi HM, Babay N, Alzoman H, Basudan S, Anil S, Jansen JA. Bone morphology changes around two types of bone-level implants installed in fresh extraction sockets – a histomorphometric study in Beagle dogs. Clin Oral Implants Res. 2014. doi: 10.1111/clr.12388. [Epub ahead of print]
65. de Sanctis M, Vignoletti F, Discepoli N, Munoz F, Sanz M. Immediate implants at fresh extraction sockets: an experimental study in the beagle dog comparing four different implant systems. Soft tissue findings. J Clin Periodontol. 2010;37(8):769–76.
66. Araujo MG, Sukekava F, Wennstrom JL, Lindhe J. Tissue modeling following implant placement in fresh extraction sockets. Clin Oral Implants Res. 2006;17(6):615–24.
67. Araujo MG, Wennstrom JL, Lindhe J. Modeling of the buccal and lingual bone walls of fresh extraction sites following implant installation. Clin Oral Implants Res. 2006;17(6):606–14.
68. Marin C, Granato R, Suzuki M, Gil JN, Piattelli A, Coelho PG. Removal torque and histomorphometric evaluation of bioceramic grit-blasted/acid-etched and dual acid-etched implant surfaces: an experimental study in dogs. J Periodontol. 2008;79(10):1942–9.
69. Marin C, Granato R, Bonfante EA, Suzuki M, Janal MN, Coelho PG. Evaluation of a nanometer roughness scale resorbable media-processed surface: a study in dogs. Clin Oral Implants Res. 2012;23(1):119–24.
70. Coelho PG, Zavanelli RA, Salles MB, Yeniyol S, Tovar N, Jimbo R. Enhanced bone bonding to nanotextured implant surfaces. Biomech Tensile Test Rat Femur. Submitted. 2014.
71. Coelho PG, Granato R, Marin C, Jimbo R, Lin S, Witek L, et al. Effect of Si addition on Ca- and P-impregnated implant surfaces with nanometer-scale roughness: an experimental study in dogs. Clin Oral Implants Res. 2012;23(3):373–8.
72. Coelho PG, Takayama T, Yoo D, Jimbo R, Karunagaran S, Tovar N, et al. Nanometer-scale features on micrometer-scale surface texturing: a bone histological, gene expression, and nanomechanical study. Bone. 2014;65C:25–32.
73. Coelho PG, Marin C, Granato R, Bonfante EA, Lima CP, Suzuki M. Surface treatment at the cervical region and its effect on bone maintenance after immediate

implantation: an experimental study in dogs. Oral Surg Oral Med Oral Pathol Oral Radiol Endod. 2010;110(2):182–7.
74. Coelho PG, Bonfante EA, Pessoa RS, Marin C, Granato R, Giro G, et al. Characterization of five different implant surfaces and their effect on osseointegration: a study in dogs. J Periodontol. 2011;82(5):742–50.
75. Coelho PG, Granato R, Marin C, Bonfante EA, Freire JN, Janal MN, et al. Biomechanical evaluation of endosseous implants at early implantation times: a study in dogs. J Oral Maxillofac Surg. 2010;68(7):1667–75.
76. Coelho PG, Bonfante EA, Marin C, Granato R, Giro G, Suzuki M. A human retrieval study of plasma-sprayed hydroxyapatite-coated plateau root form implants after 2 months to 13 years in function. J Long-Term Eff Med Implants. 2010;20(4):335–42.
77. Coelho PG, Marin C, Granato R, Suzuki M. Histomorphologic analysis of 30 plateau root form implants retrieved after 8 to 13 years in function. A human retrieval study. J Biomed Mater Res B Appl Biomater. 2009;91(2):975–9.
78. Baldassarri M, Bonfante E, Suzuki M, Marin C, Granato R, Tovar N, et al. Mechanical properties of human bone surrounding plateau root form implants retrieved after 0.3–24 years of function. J Biomed Mater Res B Appl Biomater. 2012;100(7):2015–21.
79. Orsini G, Piattelli M, Scarano A, Petrone G, Kenealy J, Piattelli A, et al. Randomized, controlled histologic and histomorphometric evaluation of implants with nanometer-scale calcium phosphate added to the dual acid-etched surface in the human posterior maxilla. J Periodontol. 2007;78(2):209–18.
80. Rocci M, Rocci A, Martignoni M, Albrektsson T, Barlattani A, Gargari M. Comparing the tioblast and osseospeed surfaces. Histomorphometric and histological analysis in humans. Oral Implantol. 2008;1(1):34–42.
81. Thalji GN, Nares S, Cooper LF. Early molecular assessment of osseointegration in humans. Clin Oral Implants Res. 2014;25:1273–85.
82. Shibli JA, Grassi S, Piattelli A, Pecora GE, Ferrari DS, Onuma T, et al. Histomorphometric evaluation of bioceramic molecular impregnated and dual acid-etched implant surfaces in the human posterior maxilla. Clin Implant Dent Relat Res. 2010;12(4):281–8.
83. Ostman PO, Wennerberg A, Ekestubbe A, Albrektsson T. Immediate occlusal loading of NanoTite tapered implants: a prospective 1-year clinical and radiographic study. Clin Implant Dent Relat Res. 2013;15(6):809–18.
84. Ostman PO, Wennerberg A, Albrektsson T. Immediate occlusal loading of NanoTite PREVAIL implants: a prospective 1-year clinical and radiographic study. Clin Implant Dent Relat Res. 2010;12(1):39–47.
85. Cecchinato D, Lops D, Salvi GE, Sanz M. A prospective, randomized, controlled study using osseospeed implants placed in maxillary fresh extraction socket: soft tissues response. Clin Oral Implants Res. 2013. doi: 10.1111/clr.12295. [Epub ahead of print]
86. Collaert B, Wijnen L, De Bruyn H. A 2-year prospective study on immediate loading with fluoride-modified implants in the edentulous mandible. Clin Oral Implants Res. 2011;22(10):1111–6.
87. De Bruyn H, Raes F, Cooper LF, Reside G, Garriga JS, Tarrida LG, et al. Three-years clinical outcome of immediate provisionalization of single osseospeed() implants in extraction sockets and healed ridges. Clin Oral Implants Res. 2013;24(2):217–23.
88. Mertens C, Steveling HG. Early and immediate loading of titanium implants with fluoride-modified surfaces: results of 5-year prospective study. Clin Oral Implants Res. 2011;22(12):1354–60.
89. Mertens C, Steveling HG, Seeberger R, Hoffmann J, Freier K. Reconstruction of severely atrophied alveolar ridges with calvarial onlay bone grafts and dental implants. Clin Implant Dent Relat Res. 2013;15(5): 673–83.
90. Noelken R, Neffe BA, Kunkel M, Wagner W. Maintenance of marginal bone support and soft tissue esthetics at immediately provisionalized osseospeed implants placed into extraction sites: 2-year results. Clin Oral Implants Res. 2014;25(2): 214–20.
91. Raes F, Cosyn J, De Bruyn H. Clinical, aesthetic, and patient-related outcome of immediately loaded single implants in the anterior maxilla: a prospective study in extraction sockets, healed ridges, and grafted sites. Clin Implant Dent Relat Res. 2013;15(6): 819–35.
92. PRNewswire. Revenue from nanotechnology-enabled products to equal IT and Telecom by 2014, exceed biotech by 10 times. http://www.prnewswire.com/news-releases/revenue-from-nanotechnology-enabled-products-to-equal-it-and-telecom-by-2014-exceed-biotech-by-10-times-74956547.html. Source: Lux Research; 2014.
93. Papaspyridakos P, Chen CJ, Singh M, Weber HP, Gallucci GO. Success criteria in implant dentistry: a systematic review. J Dent Res. 2012;91(3):242–8.
94. Manoharan M. Research on the frontiers of materials science: the impact of nanotechnology on new material development. Technol Soc. 2008;30(3):401–4.
95. Jimbo R, Coelho PG, Bryington M, Baldassarri M, Tovar N, Currie F, et al. Nano hydroxyapatite-coated implants improve bone nanomechanical properties. J Dent Res. 2012;91(12):1172–7.
96. Coelho PG, Teixeira HS, Marin C, Witek L, Tovar N, Janal MN, et al. The in vivo effect of P-15 coating on early osseointegration. J Biomed Mater Res B Appl Biomater. 2014;102:430–40.

Development of a Novel Fluoride-Modified Implant Surface for Clinical Use

6

Jan Eirik Ellingsen, Marta Monjo, and Joana Maria Ramis

Abstract

The OssseoSpeed™ implant is the first bone-anchored dental implant with a chemical surface modification of titanium to improve bone healing after implantation. Fluoride modification of titanium alters the surface oxide layer and creates a fluoride containing titanium oxide layer with a characteristic nanostructural surface topography. These small changes in surface chemistry and topography improve the properties of titanium as an implant material with increased bone-to-implant contact at an earlier stage after implantation as one important feature with clinical impact. This book chapter reviews the development of the fluoride-modified titanium implants and summarizes in vitro and in vivo scientific studies documenting and describing the physicochemical properties and biological responses that are experienced with this implant surface. Finally, the clinical studies of the commercial implant (OsseoSpeed™) are presented and discussed.

Development of a Novel Fluoride-Modified Implant Surface

The introduction of the principle of osseointegration and titanium (Ti) as material for dental implants changed oral implantology from a non-predictable mode of treatment with number of failures and in some cases serious trauma for the patients to a well-accepted treatment with good predictability [1–4].

The established treatment protocol recommended, however, long healing time between insertion of the implants and loading, 6 months healing in the maxillae and 3–4 months healing following implantation in the mandible [1, 5–7]. This guideline was based on the acquired knowledge and experience of the bone healing and regeneration process to establish a tight and sound connection between alveolar bone and the implants, the osseointegration.

Histological studies showed that the bone growth occurred from the cut surface of old bone

J.E. Ellingsen, DDS, Dr.odont (✉)
Department of Prosthodontics, Institute of Clinical Dentistry, University of Oslo, Geitmyrsveien 71, 1109, Blindern, Oslo 0317, Norway
e-mail: j.e.ellingsen@odont.uio.no

M. Monjo, PhD • J.M. Ramis, PhD
Department of Fundamental Biology and Health Sciences, Research Institute on Health Sciences (IUNICS), Instituto de Investigación Santaria de Palma (IdISPa), Palma de Mallorca, Spain

A. Wennerberg et al. (eds.), *Implant Surfaces and their Biological and Clinical Impact*,
DOI 10.1007/978-3-662-45379-7_6, © Springer-Verlag Berlin Heidelberg 2015

towards the implant surface to finally establish a tight connection between the newly formed bone and the implant surface [8]. Since the process of establishing this tight connection between the bone and the implant material was slow, the speed of the healing process was regarded as a limitation for the use of implants and thus the acceptance among patients and dentists. The slow bone healing and regeneration had thus also consequences in limiting the load-bearing capacity of the implants during this initial period.

Persistence and maintenance of the marginal alveolar bone surrounding implants is essential for the long-lasting survival of the implant-retained prosthetic construction, but minor changes of the marginal bone level will also influence treatment success with increased frequencies of deep pockets or retraction of the supporting soft tissue followed by exposure of marginal parts of the implants [9]. From clinical studies, it was reported an initial general marginal resorption progressing to the first thread during the first 1–2 years after implantation and thereafter reaching a steady state with a slow loss of marginal bone [4, 10, 11]. A mean marginal bone loss on patient level of 1.5 mm during the first year in function and 0.2 mm annually thereafter was accepted as a natural response of the alveolar bone and an expected consequence of a successful implant installation [12–15]. A successful treatment with dental implants thus included some major limitations: long healing time, limited load-bearing capacity in the early phase due to limited bone-to-implant contact (BIC), and marginal bone resorption.

A project was then started in 1990 addressing those identified limitations in dental implant treatment with the aim of trying to optimize the implant qualities for an improved regenerative process with bone-to-implant integration as well as the speed of the osseointegration process.

During the process of bone regeneration, a number of biological factors have influence due to their activity in stimulating or inhibiting the different steps in the healing cascade. The approach in the project was not to add synthetically produced bone-promoting factors like bone morphogenetic proteins to improve the bone regeneration but rather modify the implant surface to trigger the bone tissue regenerative activity and possibly guide the mesenchymal stem cell (MSC) differentiation towards the osteoblastic line and thus bone formation.

The goal was to identify a chemical modification of the superficial titanium dioxide (TiO_2) layer that through ion incorporation and nanostructural modification could induce improved bone regeneration. This effect could add on to already established positive bone regenerative responses to Ti/TiO_2 and microstructures with an improved regenerative potential as result [6, 16–22].

The element fluoride was selected as a surface modification agent due to its specific qualities both in contact with calcified tissues and also in contact with Ti. Fluoride was known to have a particular affinity for calcified tissues and had proven an effect as a prophylactic agent against dental caries by binding to calcium forming calcium fluoride and also fluorapatite, leading to an increased stability of the hydroxyl apatite structure and resistance against acid attach [23–25].

The calcium-binding capacity of fluoride has also been successfully used in the treatment of systemic bone diseases such as osteoporosis [26]. Systemic treatment with fluoride was reported to give an increased trabecular density and further an induced calcification of bone, leading to a stronger bone with improved load-bearing capacities and improved fracture resistance [27–30]. There were indications in the literature that fluoride acted primarily on osteoprogenitor cells or undifferentiated osteoblasts and thus had an effect at the cellular level in addition to a physicochemical effect [31–34]. It was reported in studies that fluoride treatment of bone triggered acute increases of intrinsic calcium levels, further indicating a cellular effect of fluoride [35]. A surface modification of Ti implants with fluoride incorporated into the superficial TiO_2 layer could thus lead to an implant with an improved bone response compared to non-modified titanium implants. Studies were therefore initiated to establish a method for modifying titanium with the use of fluoride to create an implant intended to have improved biological properties. This project resulted in the Astra Tech OsseoSpeed™ implant.

Physicochemical Surface Characteristics of Fluoride-Modified Titanium Implants

Natural Ti is highly reactive and will instantly be covered by an oxide layer after exposure to oxygen in air [36–39]. This oxide layer, a few nanometers thick, is considered to be very stable and makes the surface corrosion resistant with excellent repassivation ability [40]. This corrosion-resistant Ti surface is, however, reactive to fluoride.

The OsseoSpeed™ dental implant is made of grade 4 Ti and blasted with TiO_2 particles to a rough surface and thereafter treated with diluted HF. The blasting procedure is an invasive technique that removes parts of the surface on the microlevel, makes it irregular and increases the surface area significantly, and thus creates an isotropic surface regarded as medium rough. Since the surface is blasted with TiO_2 particles, no additional undesired elements will contaminate the biological exposed surface. The developed rough surface has a natural potential for mechanical retention, but with its increased surface area, it has also improved potential for biological reaction after implant installation [41]. When this blasted titanium surface is treated with diluted HF, small but significant changes occur on the surface. The roughness parameter Sa is slightly reduced (Table 6.1), and through scanning electron microscopy (SEM) investigation, a more rounded structure can be observed with less sharp edges giving a coral-like impression of the surface structure [42]. At high magnification, a new feature can be observed present on the surface: small, nanoscale structures evenly distributed on the surface both in the valleys and on the peaks (Fig. 6.1). This nanoscale topography is not present on the blasted-only surfaces but only on surfaces treated with fluoride [43]. Although the nanoscale topography can easily be observed by 3D-SEM at high magnification, atomic force microscope is needed to quantify and describe the created texture.

Chemical analyses of these surfaces by the use of X-ray photoelectron spectroscopy (XPS) spectra has revealed binding energies corresponding to oxygen, titanium, carbon, fluoride, and traces of nitrogen [42]. Fluoride was in this study present at a level of 1.0 %, a similar level also reported by Petersson et al. [44], but lower fluoride values of the OsseoSpeed™ surface, 0.4 %, are reported in the literature also using XPS analysis [45]. Exact analysis of fluoride on this level is technique sensitive, and these differences may be due to variations between the analytical protocols. By treating titanium with fluoride, the fluoride ions will exchange with hydroxyl groups at the surface. The fluoride content that remain on the TiO_2 surface of dental implants after a rinsing process are calculated to occupy approximately 5 % of all active sites equaling that every 20th site is occupied by an exchanged fluoride ion. This change in the surface TiO_2 composition increases the conductivity and lowers the surface charge of the implant that may have biological consequences [44]. It is further hypothesized that the fluoride ion as such may contribute directly to the calcification process through ion exchange and binding to phosphate molecules in the bone structure [46, 47]. The nanoscale roughness created by the fluoride modification may add further bone-promoting effect to the already seen by the

Table 6.1 Summary of surface characterization studies of fluoride-modified titanium implants

Parameter measured	Result	Reference
SEM characterization	Fluoride treatment reduces roughness at the micrometer scale but produces nanostructures	[42, 45, 66, 67, 69, 88, 133–135]
Roughness (average surface roughness/S_a, μm)	1.32–1.82	[44, 69, 71, 75, 79, 88, 93, 134, 135]
XPS (F atomic %)	0.3–1.0	[42, 44, 45, 69, 93]
Contact angle (°)	138	[136]

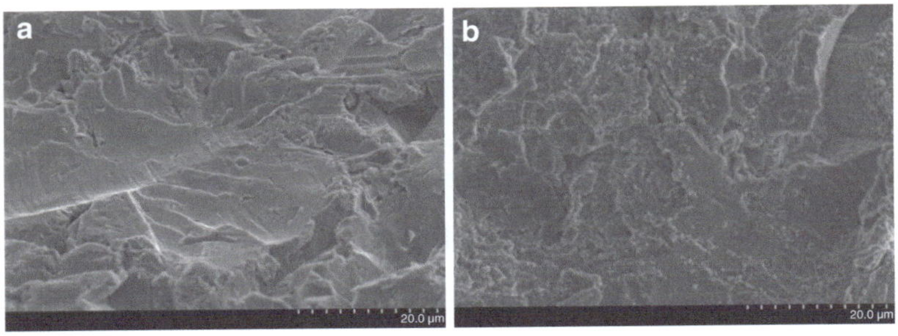

Fig. 6.1 SEM images of blasted titanium implant surfaces before (**a**) and after (**b**) fluoride treatment, obtained at 10 kV and ×2,000 magnification

microstructure due to the blasting. A unique nucleating effect is demonstrated by fluoride-modified Ti in that when the implant is immersed into a liquid saturated with respect to calcium and phosphate, it attracts these ions to the surface and crystals of calcium phosphate start to grow [48]. Based on physicochemical evaluation, this designed implant surface had potential for improving bone integration and regeneration.

Molecular and Cellular In Vitro Response to Fluoride-Modified Titanium Implants

The formation of mineralized bone at the bone-to-implant interface requires the recruitment of osteoprogenitor cells, its proliferation, and differentiation to mature osteoblasts followed by the production and mineralization of extracellular matrix at the surface [49]. Osteoblast cell culture in vitro models provide a useful tool to study the cellular and molecular events of osteoblasts in response to different implant surfaces [50].

Osteoblast maturation in vitro has been divided into three major developmental stages, a period of growth and proliferation, a period of extracellular matrix development and maturation, and a mineralization stage (Fig. 6.2), with characteristic changes in gene expression at each stage [51–54]. The analysis of cell attachment, proliferation, gene expression, and mineralization in cells cultured onto different implant surfaces are valuable data to define the effect of the different surfaces at the implant interface.

The main sources of osteoprogenitor cells are MSC, multipotent cells that can differentiate along a variety of cell lineages [55]. During the commitment towards a specific lineage, a master gene, such as a transcription factor, is induced and starts a cascade that leads to the sequential expression of other transcription factors and of phenotype-specific genes [56]. Runt-related transcription factor 2 (RUNX2 or formerly called Cbfa1), a member of the runt homology domain transcription factor family, is the master gene necessary for the osteoblast lineage commitment [57], also influences on the signaling pathways and transcriptional factors which regulate osteoblastogenesis [58], and modulates the expression of bone extracellular matrix protein genes [59]. Downstream of RUNX2 is Osterix (OSX), a specific osteogenic zinc finger transcription factor that is required for the ongoing differentiation within the osteogenic pathway [60], and is involved in the differentiation step from pre-osteoblast to fully functional osteoblast [61].

During osteoblast differentiation, type I collagen (COLL-I) is expressed in high levels in the early synthetic stage, supporting cell proliferation [54], and its expression is gradually decreased as the cell matures. Alkaline phosphatase (ALP), a membrane-bound enzyme contained in matrix vesicles that contributes to rendering the extracellular matrix competent for mineralization [54], is considered an early marker of osteoblast differentiation; hence, its expression increases during extracellular matrix maturation and decreases when mineralization is well progressed [62]. Bone sialoprotein (BSP) is transiently expressed very early and then upregulated again in differentiated osteoblasts at the onset of mineralization. Osteopontin (OPN) is a sialoprotein that mediates hydroxyapatite binding, being produced early in the differentiation of bone cells with higher expression levels after mineralization has been

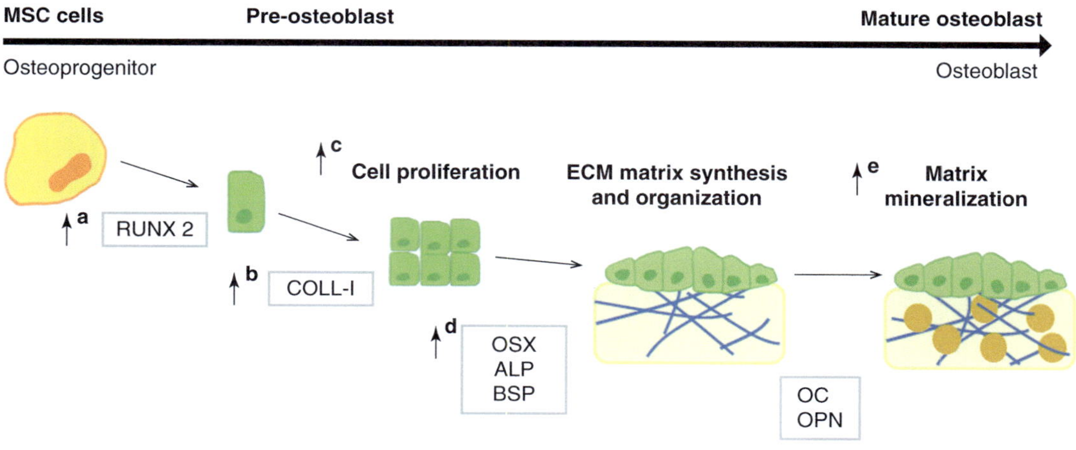

Fig. 6.2 In vitro effects of fluoride-modified implants during osteoblast differentiation. Drawing of the different stages of osteoblast differentiation and the reported effects of fluoride-modified implants. (*a*) [67–69, 74]; (*b*) [66]; (*c*) [43, 65, 66]; (*d*) [65, 68, 73–75]; (*e*) [75]

initiated [63, 64]. Finally, osteocalcin (OC) appears with mineralization, being only expressed by fully differentiated osteoblasts [51, 54].

The cellular response to fluoride-modified Ti implants has been assessed in different osteoblast cellular models (Table 6.2) using MSCs from different origin [65–69], primary cultures of osteoblasts [70–73], nontransformed clonal cell lines (MC3T3-E1) [43, 74, 75], or osteosarcoma cell lines (MG63) [76]. The different cellular models, time-point of the analysis, or implant production might explain the differences in the reported results. Thus, while some studies have reported increased proliferation on fluoride-modified titanium implants [43, 65, 66], others failed [67, 75]. In solution, fluoride has been proved to stimulate bone cell proliferation [77], but its effect varies according to the stage of differentiation of the cells; thus, the fluoride ion acts primarily on osteoprogenitor cells or undifferentiated osteoblasts rather on more differentiated osteoblasts [78]. In addition, some studies find higher cell adhesion [71] in fluoride-modified titanium implants compared to control; other studies found no differences [65, 66, 68, 73]. In this regard, it is important to include the importance of the surface topography when discussing the number of cells attached on the surfaces since the modification of titanium surface with HF is influenced by HF concentration, the exposure time, and the initial surface topography [43]. In the same line, differences in the results of gene expression analysis (Table 6.2) might also be explained by differences in the roughness or chemical composition of the surfaces used in the different studies. However, fluoride-modified Ti implants (Fig. 6.2) stimulate osteoblast differentiation and expression of bone-specific mRNA [43, 74], as does fluoride in monolayer bone cell cultures [78]. Thus, fluoride-modified Ti implants increase the expression of RUNX2 [67–69, 74], OSX [68, 74, 75], COLL-I [66], and BSP [65, 75] and increases ALP activity [73]. In addition, fluoride modification augments the thrombogenic properties of titanium, promoting fibrinogen activation and rapid coagulation, resulting in a less dense fibrin clot that could promote osteoblast migration to the implant surface in vivo [79].

Bone Healing Around Fluoride-Modified Titanium Implants in In Vivo Models

In general, Ti implants are classified as bioinert [80], characterized by contact osteogenesis, in which the osteogenic cells migrate directly to the surface where they will establish de novo bone formation [81]. In the very first animal study performed with fluoride-modified Ti, it was observed

Table 6.2 Summary of in vitro studies investigating the cellular response to fluoride-modified titanium implants

Reference	Cell type	Cell culture time	Type of surface	Type of analysis	Cell response
[76]	Human osteoblast-like cells (MG-63)	<45 min	TiOblast/OsseoSpeed/machined Ti	Cytodetachment	Higher cytodetachment in OsseoSpeed than in TiOblast, but not statistically significant. Machined Ti significantly lower cytodetachment than rough surfaces
[65]	hMSC	1 h–28 days	GB/GB-HF	Cell adhesion, proliferation, and gene expression analysis	No differences in cell adhesion Greater proliferation and increased BSP and BMP-2 expression in GB-HF than GB
[70]	Primary human mandibular bone cells	12 h–10 days	Fluoride etched/Alkali-head treated/magnesium ion incorporated anodized/nano-HA coated and heat treated/GB	CaP formation in SBF	Earlier CaP formation in all modified surfaces than GB, but after 72 h, GB showed higher CaP formation than the modified surfaces
				Cell attachment, OC, and protein production	The fluoride-etched surface treated for 72 h with SB before cell culture showed similar or lower bone cell response than GB
[66]	Human bone marrow MSCs	3 h–14 days	GB/GB-HF	Cell adhesion, proliferation, and protein production and activity	No differences in cell adhesion Higher proliferation and increased COLL-I and OPG expression levels on GB-HF than GB
[74]	Mouse pre-osteoblasts (MC3T3-E1)	1–14 days	GB/GB-HF	Gene expression analysis	Higher levels of Runx-2 and Osterix in GB-HF than GB
[67]	Human embryonic palatal MSC	1, 3, 7 days	GB/GB-HF	Cell proliferation, ALP activity, gene expression analysis	No differences in proliferation Higher expression levels of Runx-2 in GB-HF
[43]	Mouse pre-osteoblasts (MC3T3-E1)	1–7 days	P/P-HF (treated for 40, 90, 120, and 150 s)	Cytotoxicity, cell number and gene expression analysis	Lower cytotoxicity in P-HF, being significant in Ti treated with HF for longer times (120 and 150 s) Higher cell number after 7 days in P-HF treated for 120 and 150 s No significant differences on gene expression
[71]	Primary mouse alveolar bone cells	48 h	Nanotite/OsseoSpeed/TiUnite/SLActive	Cell adhesion analysis	Higher cell adhesion rate in OsseoSpeed and SLActive than the other surfaces (being as well the two surfaces with higher roughness)
[68]	Human mesenchymal pre-osteoblasts (HEPM)	72 h	TiOblast/OsseoSpeed/SLA-1/SLA-2	Cell attachment and gene expression analysis	No differences in cell attachment Increased Runx-2 and Osterix expression levels in TiOblast and OsseoSpeed

[75]	Mouse pre-osteoblasts (MC3T3-E1)	2–14 days	TiOblast/OsseoSpeed	Cytotoxicity, cell morphology and proliferation, ALP activity, gene expression, and release of osteoblast markers	No differences on cell viability and cell proliferation Increased secretion of BMP-2 secretion after 2 days of culture in OsseoSpeed Increased IGF-I, BSP, and Osterix gene expression levels in OsseoSpeed after 14 days Increased mineralization in OsseoSpeed after 14 days
[72]	Human osteoblasts	1 day	P/P-HF/GB/GB-HF	Gene expression analysis by microarray and RT-PCR	Identification of novel genes involved in the early response of osteoblasts to rough and to fluoride-modified titanium implants
[73]	Primary mouse osteoblastic cells	21 days	sulfuric-hydrochloric acid/anodic oxidation with phosphoric acid/chemical attack plus thermal oxidation immersion NaF	Cell attachment, proliferation, and differentiation	No differences on cell attachment Higher ALP activity in the sulfuric-hydrochloric surface and in the chemical attack plus thermal oxidation immersion NaF
[79]	No cells: in vitro slide chamber model furnished with heparin in contact with blood, PRP, or PPP		Hydroxyapatite surface/machined Ti/TiOblast/OsseoSpeed	Generation of thrombin-antithrombin complexes	Higher thrombin-antithrombin complexes formation in OsseoSpeed compared to the other surfaces
[69]	Human MSCs	1–28 days	GB/GB-HF	Gene expression analysis	Osteoblast differentiation more rapid and to a greater extent in GB-HF Higher expression of Runx-2, Smads, insulin-like growth factor 2, BMPs, and bone matrix proteins

that non-threaded conically shaped Ti implants with a machined surface increased the retention three to four times as measured by a push-out test when the surface had been modified by fluoride; the push-out values were depending on the fluoride solution used [46]. It was further reported from this study that the test implants had bone firmly attached to the surface after the push-out as observed by SEM. This first observation clearly indicated that the bone had reacted differently to the fluoride-modified implants compared to the control Ti implants with a natural TiO_2 layer. The observation of an attachment between the implant and bone with increased implant retention was further evaluated by Ellingsen and co-workers who placed 80 threaded grit-blasted implants with or without fluoride-modified surface into the rabbit tibiae [82]. The functional attachment of the threaded implants to bone was evaluated by a removal torque test after 1 and 3 months healing time. In this study, there were no significant differences in removal torque values after 1 month healing time, but significant higher values were recorded in the fluoride-modified group compared to the blasted group, 85 Ncm versus 54 Ncm, after 3 months healing. In the histomorphometric analysis, significantly higher BIC for the fluoride-modified implants was observed already after 1 month healing time, and the difference between the groups was even more pronounced after 3 months healing. The lack of significance between the groups when evaluating functional attachment after 1 month healing time could be due to that the bone that was formed, with significant higher BIC, was not yet fully mature and calcified and thus not able to resist the removal torque forces. Later, Cooper and co-workers placed grit-blasted Ti implants into rat tibiae and compared these to implants with similar surface treatment, but with an additional fluoride modification. At day 21 after surgery, the rats were euthanized and the implants were prepared for histology and histomorphometric analysis [65]. In this study, the grit-blasted implant group had a mean direct BIC of 34.2 %, whereas the fluoride-modified group had a significantly higher direct BIC of 55.5 %. In the same study, significantly increased expression of genes related to bone regeneration was recorded in the fluoride-modified group as discussed in the previous section. Then, the early stage of osseointegration was investigated by placing grit-blasted implants with or without fluoride modification in the alveolar process of mongrel dogs [83]. The bone regeneration and growth in a chamber created between the cut surface of the old bone was studied, and the authors reported that the amount of new bone that formed in the chambers within the first 2 weeks of healing was larger at sites where the internal walls of the wound chamber were designed with a fluoride-modified surface (test) than with a control surface (TiOblast®). The BIC that had been established in the macro-threaded part of the implant was significantly larger at the fluoride-modified implants than the grit-blasted-only control implants. In another interesting study from the same group, the focus was on the healing of marginal bone when implants were placed without direct contact to the bone, imitating the clinical situation of implant placement into extraction sockets [84]. The marginal 50 % of the prepared canal for the implant was widened to give a free space of 1 mm around the implant, and the bone regeneration in this gap was evaluated. Abrahamsson and co-workers found that the quality of the contact between the implant and the newly formed bone differed between test and control implants. The % of BIC within the defect area was in the 2-week specimens 55.7 % at test sites and 33.7 % at control sites. After 6 weeks of healing, the % of BIC had increased to 63.7 and 45.2 % at test and control sites, respectively. The histological analysis in this study thus revealed a significantly larger area of osseointegration within the defect at fluoride-modified (OsseoSpeed™) implants than at implants with a grit-blasted-only (TiOblast™) surface after 6 weeks of healing. Another interesting fact of the fluoride-modified Ti implants was found by Thor and co-workers who demonstrated that Ti in whole blood activates the thrombogenic response to a higher degree than platelet-rich plasma (PRP) and that a fluoridated Ti surface augmented the effect compared with the control. This property was further evaluated by the same group in an implant defect model in dogs [79, 85]. The defects of 1.25 mm were made around the implant and the regeneration of bone was evaluated regarding the influence

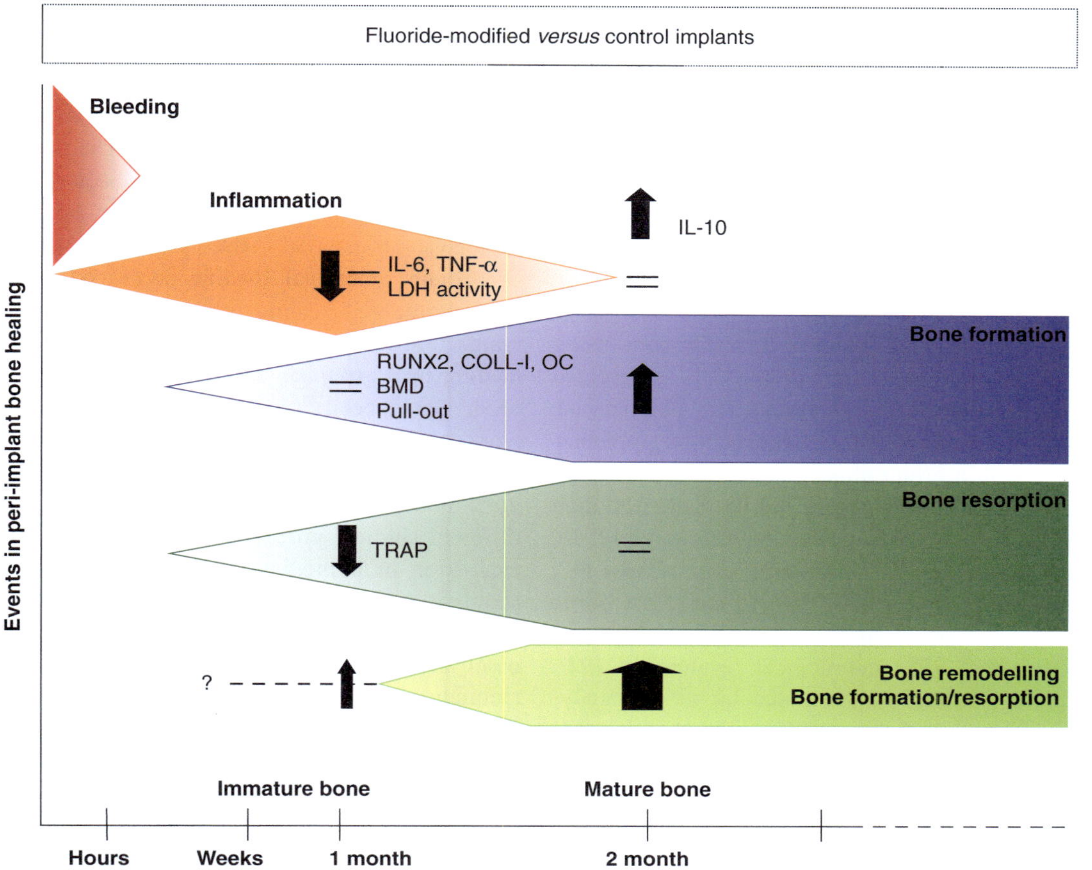

Fig. 6.3 Events in the peri-implant bone healing in fluoride versus control modified implants. Schematic representation of the events in the peri-implant bone healing and the reported effects of the fluoride-modified implants analyzed by enzymatic analyses, gene expression, biomechanical test, and micro-computed tomography (Results extracted from Monjo et al. [86])

of PRP, whole blood, grit-basted surface and grit-blasted surface, and fluoride modification. The authors confirmed the findings from the previous in vitro study that PRP does not improve bone regeneration in peri-implant tissue compared to whole blood and a statistically significant higher bone fill was recorded in the defects with OsseoSpeed™ implants compared to TiOblast™ implants. The most superior point of the bone envelope in marginal bone was attached at a shorter distance from a perpendicular point on the OsseoSpeed™ implants compared with the control, irrespective of defect-fill PRP or whole blood.

An even more detailed information about the regeneration process around the OsseoSpeed™ implants after their installation in vivo in rabbits was given by Monjo and co-workers who analyzed bone-implant retention in combination with gene expression of several inflammatory and osteogenic markers of the peri-implant bone after the tensile test was completed. In addition, enzymatic analyses of the wound fluid and micro-computed tomography (micro-CT) analysis of the intact bone were performed [86]. Implant placement elicits a sequence of healing events leading to osseointegration including bleeding, inflammation, and subsequent resorption of traumatized bone around the titanium implant concomitant with new bone formation and mineralization (Fig. 6.3). The present investigation demonstrated that in this sequence of events, necrosis and gene expression of inflammatory and resorption markers were reduced at the surface of fluoride-modified Ti implants after an early healing period of 4 weeks. This was followed after a longer healing period of 8 weeks by a significant increased bone-to-implant retention, gene expression of bone formation markers, and bone mineral density, reflecting an improved bone remodeling activity.

In conclusion, all these investigations using different animal models (Table 6.3) represented and demonstrated clearly that this new surface gave an improved bone response after implantation with a firmer attachment and higher degree of contact between bone and implant. Although most of the studies focused on histology [42, 46, 65, 82–85, 87–95] and biomechanical tests [42, 46, 82, 86, 89, 93, 94, 96] to study the bone-implant interface, also resonance frequency analysis [96, 97], radiological evaluation [92], micro-CT [86, 94], and molecular biology analysis [74, 86] were used, giving altogether valuable information of the osseointegration process mechanisms of fluoride-modified implants. In summary, the bone-implant interface with fluoride-modified implants was characterized by (1) high BIC in later healing, (2) improved biomechanical properties, (3) good primary stability and low radiological marginal bone loss, (4) increased bone mineral density and bone volume ratio, and (5) high gene expression of osteogenic markers.

Clinical Results

A number of clinical studies have been performed in evaluating the clinical performance of OsseoSpeed™ implants. The favorable biological responses that are demonstrated in cell studies and in in vivo animal models have indeed also been reported from clinical studies confirming an improved healing of the alveolar bone with clinical significance. Results with the OsseoSpeed™ implant show good functionality [98–107], high esthetics [108–112], and predictable and maintained marginal bone levels at OsseoSpeed™ implants. Based on the preclinical observations, studies have also focused on the possibility to reduce the time from implant installation to loading of the restoration without compromising the clinical outcome. The potential of the OsseoSpeed™ implant has been evaluated both in immediate and early loading protocols [105, 107, 109, 113–123]. When immediate functional loading were compared with submerged healing followed by abutment connection and functional loading after 3 months healing in a group of 151 patients with single tooth Osseospeed™ implants, Donati and coworkers could not find any significant differences between the groups when assessing marginal bone level after 12 months [118]. Two different surgical procedures were used for the evaluation of immediate loading in this study, standard preparation procedure and osteotome technique, but the authors were not able to document any significant differences between these techniques regarding marginal bone level. Twelve months after implant installation, a mean marginal bone level change was not significantly increased compared to the bone level after 3 months healing. Similar positive effects on the marginal bone level was also reported by Collaert et al. when studying healing of the marginal bone in 25 patients with totally edentulous mandibles receiving five Osseospeed™ implants each that were functionally loaded after 24 h and evaluated after 3, 6, 12, and 24 months [117]. All 125 implants survived over the 2-year observation period. The marginal bone level was observed to be stable with very little bone resorption. Mean marginal bone loss compared to baseline was reported to be 0.14, 0.13, 0.11, and 0.11 mm after 3, 6, 12, and 24 months, respectively, which demonstrated an initial loss followed by a stable bone level after the first 3 months of healing. A similar stable bone level was reported after 5-year follow-up in a prospective study including 49 implants placed in the maxilla or mandible [120]. The implants had a different loading protocol that varied from immediate loading of 14 implants; the remaining 35 implants were loaded after a mean healing period of 9.56 weeks. The radiographic

Table 6.3 Summary of in vivo animal studies investigating the tissue response to fluoride-modified titanium implants

Reference	Animal	Implant location	Healing time	Type of surface	Type of implant	Type of analysis	Tissue response
[84]	Mongrel dogs	Mandible	2 and 6 weeks	TiOblast/ OsseoSpeed	Screw: 3.5 × 8 mm	Histology	Higher % of BIC within the defect area at OsseoSpeed implants than at the TiOblast implants
[83]	Mongrel dogs	Mandible	2 and 6 weeks	TiOblast/ OsseoSpeed	Screw: 3.5 × 8 mm	Histology	Higher % BIC and amount of bone at OsseoSpeed implants fluoride-modified in the early phase of healing (2 weeks) following implant installation
[96]	Cows	Ribs	Cadaveric	OsseoSpeed/ Biohorizons	Screw: OsseoSpeed conical 11 × 4 mm/ cylindrical 11 × 3.5 mm Biohorizons tapered internal screw 12 × 3.8 mm/12 × 4.6 mm	Resonance frequency analysis and insertion torque	OsseoSpeed conical dental implants with a wide diameter show better primary stability
[87]	Labrador dogs	Mandible	4 months	OsseoSpeed	Screw: 4 × 6 mm, 4 × 11 mm	Histology	Shorter implants (6 mm) present with equal osseointegration than do longer implants (11 mm)
[88]	New Zealand white rabbits	Tibia	2 weeks	OsseoSpeed/TiUnite	Screw: 4 × 11 mm, 4 × 11.5 mm	Histology	No significant differences in % BIC and bone area between OsseoSpeed and TiUnite in early healing
[89]	Beagle dogs	Mandible	1 and 3 weeks	Nanotite/ OsseoSpeed/ Ossean	Screw: 4 × 10 mm, 4 × 11 mm, 4 × 10 mm	Torque test and histology	At 3 weeks, OsseoSpeed and Ossean implant presented comparable torque value and were higher than Nanotite. Histologically, no differences among the groups
[65]	Sprague-Dawley rats	Tibia	3 weeks	TiO_2 blasted (75 μm), TiO_2 blasted (75 μm) + HF	Screw: 1.5 × 2 mm	Histology	Higher % BIC in fluoride treated compared to control implants
[91]	Beagle dogs	Mandible	6 weeks	3i Osseotite/Astra OsseoSpeed/ Tommen SPI element/Straumann ITI-standard plus	Screw: 3.25 × 11 mm, 3.5 × 11 mm, 3.5 × 9.5 mm, 3.3 × 11 mm	Histology	No statistically significant difference was observed in the histomorphometry (% BIC) among the four-implant systems when used in fresh extraction sockets

(continued)

Table 6.3 (continued)

Reference	Animal	Implant location	Healing time	Type of surface	Type of implant	Type of analysis	Tissue response
[90]	Beagle dogs	Mandible	6 weeks	3i Osseotite/Astra OsseoSpeed/ Tommen SPI element/Straumann ITI-standard plus	Screw: 3.25×11 mm, 3.5×11 mm, 3.5×9.5 mm, 3.3×11 mm	Histology	No differences in the soft tissue healing outcome when placing four different implant systems into fresh extraction sockets
[92]	Minipigs	Mandible and maxilla	2 and 3 months	Sand-blasted and acid-etched OsseoSpeed	Screw: 3.5×8 mm	Radiological evaluation and histology	Higher radiological marginal bone loss with sand-blasted and acid-etched implants. Higher peri-implant bone fraction with OsseoSpeed implants
[46]	Chinchilla rabbits	Ulna	4 and 8 weeks	Control/0.5 % NaF, pH 3.5/4 % NaF, pH 3.5 /4 % NaF, pH 3.0	Screw: conical 2(3)×5 mm	Push-out and histology	Improved retention and bone formation in fluoride-treated implants
[82]	New Zealand white rabbits	Tibia	1 and 3 months	TiO2 blasted, TiO2 blasted+HF	Screw: 3.5×8 mm	Torque test and histology	Improved retention and bone formation in fluoride-treated implants
[74]	Sprague-Dawley rats	Tibia	1, 3, and 7 days	TiO2 blasted (75 µm), TiO2 blasted (75 µm) + HF	Screw: 1.5×1 mm	Gene expression analysis	Fluoride treatment increases gene expression of osteogenic markers in vivo
[93]	New Zealand white rabbits	Femur	6 weeks	OsseoSpeed/TiO2 blasted + oxalic/ TiO2 blasted + oxalic + HF	Screw: 3.5×8 mm	Torque test, fluorochrome labeling and histology	Greater bone tissue integration of implants treated with oxalic acid and HF both with biomechanical and with histomorphometrical tests
[97]	Cows	Ribs	Cadaveric	TiUnite/SLA/ OsseoSpeed	Screw: 4×8.5 mm, 4.1×8 mm, 4×9 mm	Resonance frequency analysis	In type II bone, ISQ values were not significantly different between implant types. In bone types III and IV, the ISQ value of the Straumann implant was significantly less than that of other implants
[94]	Ovariectomized Sprague-Dawley rats	Femur	12 weeks	Titanium blasted with 25 µm Al2O3 particles/titanium blasted with 25 µm Al2O3 particles + fluoride	Rods: 1.2×10 mm	Push-out test, micro-computed tomography, and histology	Improved retention and bone formation in fluoride-treated implants

[42]	New Zealand white rabbits	Tibia	4 weeks	TiO2 blasted, TiO2 blasted + HF, TiO2 blasted + nano-HA	Screw: 3.5 × 7.5 mm	Torque test and histology	Nanotopography produced in the TiO2 blasted + HF and TiO2 blasted + nano-HA might explain the improved retention after 4 weeks. No differences in the histology were observed among the groups
[86]	New Zealand white rabbits	Tibia	4 and 8 weeks	TiO2 blasted, TiO2 blasted + HF	Coin shaped: 6.25 × 1.95 mm	Pull-out test, wound fluid analysis, gene expression, and micro-computed tomography	Higher pull-out, gene expression of osteogenic markers and higher BMD in fluoride implants after 8 weeks
[85]	Labrador dogs	Mandible	5 weeks	TiOblast/ OsseoSpeed	Screw: 5 × 9 mm	Histology	Fluoride implants increased bone formation compared with control, regardless of using PRP or whole blood
[95]	Beagle dogs	Mandible	6 weeks	3i Osseotite/Astra OsseoSpeed/ Tommen SPI element/Straumann ITI-standard plus	Screw: 3.25 × 11 mm, 3.5 × 11 mm, 3.5 × 9.5 mm, 3.3 × 12 mm	Histology	Straumann implant demonstrated a higher absolute vertical bone resorption when compared to the adjacent control site, without implant

evaluation revealed that after 5 years, there were no differences in marginal bone level between the immediate loaded implants and the non-immediately loaded implants. The maximum bone loss was 1.7 mm and the maximum bone gain was 0.7 mm. The authors reported a mean bone loss of 0.1 mm and in 83 % of the implants there were no changes in the marginal bone level during the 5-year observation period. In another 5-year study, the marginal bone level was followed after placing 134 OsseoSpeed™ implants in the posterior mandible that were functionally loaded after 7 weeks [121]. In this study the resonance frequency were recorded at the time of implant placement, 2 and 6 weeks after and 1, 3, 6, and 12 months after loading. A significant reduction of the implant stability quotient (ISQ) values was reported 2 weeks after implant placement, a value that increased steadily during the rest of the observation period to a highly significantly higher value 12 months after onset of loading. In this study, the marginal bone level was reduced with 0.21 mm (mean value) from implant installation to loading after 7 weeks, but thereafter, only a nonsignificant marginal bone loss of −0.16 mm occurred during the 5-year observation period. The majority of the implants, 61 %, exhibited no bone loss, and no implants were lost during the study. These studies with immediate or early loading protocols confirm the observations from in vivo animal studies that a very high degree of preservation of the surrounding marginal bone can be expected when installing the OsseoSpeed™ implant with a microrough and fluoride-modified surface.

Cecchinato and co-workers evaluated the marginal bone healing and osseointegration in the posterior maxilla of periodontitis-susceptible patients by installing mini-implants that were retrieved with the surrounding bone after 3 months and analyzed by histomorphometry [124]. The study showed that there were no apparent difference between the periodontitis-susceptible patients and the control group with respect to BIC or percentage of mineralized bone within the implant threads. The authors concluded that this high percentage of BIC had already been established after 3 months of healing. Furthermore, they documented that the fluoride-modified surface of the micro-implants had excellent osteoconductive property. This osteoconductive property has further as well been documented clinically with high survival rates and low marginal bone resorption even when the implants are used in challenging clinical situations as in combination with sinus lift surgery, severely absorbed alveolar ridges, irradiated bone, and in smokers [125–132].

Concluding Remarks

Placement of an endosseous implant is followed by a sequence of peri-implant healing events that result in the establishment of osseointegration. The result of this healing process is determined by a number of factors including the patients' general condition, bone volume and quality, and soft tissue. The qualifications of the dentist and the methods used during the surgery will as well influence the outcome of the healing process. Finally, qualities of the implant, bulk material, macroscopic design and thread configuration, surface macro- and nanostructure, and the surface chemistry are as well essential for the clinical outcome. Depending on the implant characteristics, different biologic responses are elicited on the neighboring bone upon insertion. In the development of the OsseoSpeed™ implant surface, it was the intention to create a surface with qualities that gave a response in the living bone with increased regenerative activity. From early scientific reports in 1995 until present, OsseoSpeed™ implants have shown to stimulate osteoblast differentiation in vitro, to improve osseointegration and decrease marginal bone loss in animals and good functionality with maintained marginal bone levels clinically, even when used in immediate loading protocols in challenging clinical situations (Fig. 6.4).

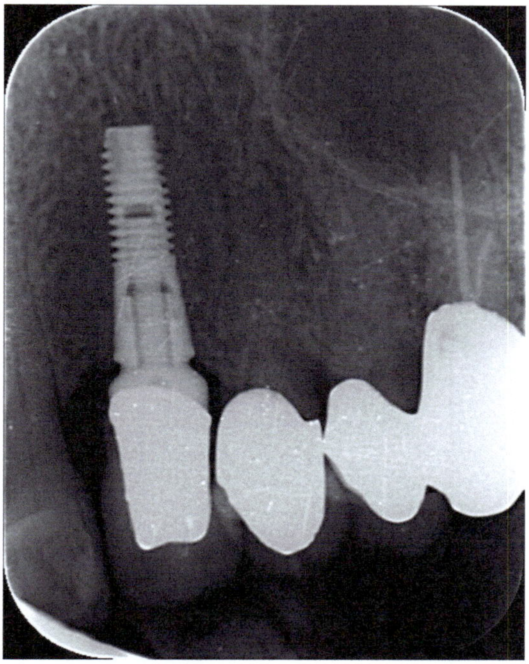

Fig. 6.4 Marginal bone level surrounding the first fluoride-modified implant placed in a human after 14 years in function

References

1. Branemark PI, Hansson BO, Adell R, Breine U, Lindstrom J, Hallen O, et al. Osseointegrated implants in the treatment of the edentulous jaw. Experience from a 10-year period. Scand J Plast Reconstr Surg Suppl. 1977;16:1–132.
2. Adell R, Lekholm U, Rockler B, Branemark PI. A 15-year study of osseointegrated implants in the treatment of the edentulous jaw. Int J Oral Surg. 1981;10(6):387–416.
3. Adell R, Eriksson B, Lekholm U, Branemark PI, Jemt T. Long-term follow-up study of osseointegrated implants in the treatment of totally edentulous jaws. Int J Oral Maxillofac Implants. 1990;5(4): 347–59.
4. Albrektsson T, Branemark PI, Hansson HA, Lindstrom J. Osseointegrated titanium implants – requirements for ensuring a long-lasting, direct bone-to-implant anchorage in man. Acta Orthop Scand. 1981;52(2):155–70.
5. Branemark PI, Adell R, Breine U, Hansson BO, Lindstrom J, Ohlsson A. Intra-osseous anchorage of dental prostheses. I. Experimental studies. Scand J Plast Reconstr Surg. 1969;3(2):81–100.
6. Buser D, Schenk RK, Steinemann S, Fiorellini JP, Fox CH, Stich H. Influence of surface characteristics on bone integration of titanium implants – a histomorphometric study in miniature pigs. J Biomed Mater Res. 1991;25(7):889–902.
7. Buser D, Weber HP, Bragger U, Balsiger C. Tissue integration of one-stage ITI implants: 3-year results of a longitudinal study with Hollow-Cylinder and Hollow-Screw implants. Int J Oral Maxillofac Implants. 1991;6(4):405–12.
8. Sennerby L. On the bone tissue response to titanium implants. Gothenburg: University of Gothenburg; 1991.
9. Lang NP, Pjetursson BE, Tan K, Bragger U, Egger M, Zwahlen M. A systematic review of the survival and complication rates of fixed partial dentures (FPDs) after an observation period of at least 5 years – II. Combined tooth-implant-supported FPDs. Clin Oral Implants Res. 2004;15(6):643–53.
10. Astrand P, Engquist B, Anzen B, Bergendal T, Hallman M, Karlsson U, et al. A three-year follow-up report of a comparative study of ITI Dental Implants and Branemark System implants in the treatment of the partially edentulous maxilla. Clin Implant Dent Relat Res. 2004;6(3):130–41.
11. Berglundh T, Abrahamsson I, Lindhe J. Bone reactions to longstanding functional load at implants: an experimental study in dogs. J Clin Periodontol. 2005;32(9):925–32.
12. Albrektsson T, Zarb G, Worthington P, Eriksson AR. The long-term efficacy of currently used dental implants: a review and proposed criteria of success. Int J Oral Maxillofac Implants. 1986;1(1):11–25.
13. Albrektsson T, Zarb GA. Current interpretations of the osseointegrated response: clinical significance. Int J Prosthodont. 1993;6(2):95–105.
14. Roos J, Sennerby L, Lekholm U, Jemt T, Grondahl K, Albrektsson T. A qualitative and quantitative method for evaluating implant success: a 5-year retrospective analysis of the Branemark implant. Int J Oral Maxillofac Implants. 1997;12(4):504–14.
15. Albrektsson T, Isidor F, editors. Consensus report of Session IV. 1st European workshop on periodontology. London: Quintessence Publishing; 1993.
16. Thomas KA, Cook SD. An evaluation of variables influencing implant fixation by direct bone apposition. J Biomed Mater Res. 1985;19(8):875–901.
17. Thomas KA, Kay JF, Cook SD, Jarcho M. The effect of surface macrotexture and hydroxyapatite coating on the mechanical strengths and histologic profiles of titanium implant materials. J Biomed Mater Res. 1987;21(12):1395–414.
18. Larsson C, Esposito M, Liao H, Thomsen P. The titanium-bone interface in vivo. Titanium in medicine. Berlin: Springer; 2001. p. 587–648.
19. Carlsson L, Rostlund T, Albrektsson B, Albrektsson T. Removal torques for polished and rough titanium implants. Int J Oral Maxillofac Implants. 1988;3(1): 21–4.

20. Gotfredsen K, Nimb L, Hjorting-Hansen E, Jensen JS, Holmen A. Histomorphometric and removal torque analysis for TiO2-blasted titanium implants. An experimental study on dogs. Clin Oral Implants Res. 1992;3(2):77–84.
21. Gotfredsen K, Wennerberg A, Johansson C, Skovgaard LT, Hjortinghansen E. Anchorage of TiO2-blasted, ha-coated, and machined implants – an experimental-study with rabbits. J Biomed Mater Res. 1995;29(10):1223–31.
22. Wieland M. Experimental determination and quantitative evaluation of the surface composition and topography of medical implant surfaces and their influence on osteoblastic cell-surface interactions. Zürich: ETH Zurich; 1999.
23. Cruz R, Rolla G, Ogaard B. Formation of fluoride on enamel in vitro after exposure to fluoridated mouthrinses. Acta Odontol Scand. 1991;49(6):329–34.
24. Rolla G, Ogaard B, Cruz RD. Topical application of fluorides on teeth – new concepts of mechanisms of interaction. J Clin Periodontol. 1993;20(2):105–8.
25. Saxegaard E, Rolla G. Kinetics of acquisition and loss of calcium-fluoride by enamel in vivo. Caries Res. 1989;23(6):406–11.
26. Pitt P, Berry H. Fluoride treatment in osteoporosis. Postgrad Med J. 1991;67(786):323–6.
27. Baud CA, Bang S, Very JM. Minor elements in bone mineral and their effects on its solubility. J Biol Buccale. 1977;5(3):195–202. Epub 1977/09/01.
28. Gedalia I, Zipkin I. The role of fluoride in bone structure. St. Louis: Warren H. Green Inc.; 1973.
29. Farley JR, Tarbaux N, Hall S, Baylink DJ. Mitogenic action(s) of fluoride on osteoblast line cells: determinants of the response in vitro. J Bone Miner Res. 1990;5 Suppl 1:S107–13. Epub 1990/03/01.
30. Resch H, Libanati C, Farley S, Bettica P, Schulz E, Baylink DJ. Evidence that fluoride therapy increases trabecular bone density in a peripheral skeletal site. J Clin Endocrinol Metab. 1993;76(6):1622–4. Epub 1993/06/01.
31. Lau KH, Farley JR, Freeman TK, Baylink DJ. A proposed mechanism of the mitogenic action of fluoride on bone cells: inhibition of the activity of an osteoblastic acid phosphatase. Metabolism. 1989;38(9):858–68. Epub 1989/09/01.
32. Bellows CG, Heersche JN, Aubin JE. The effects of fluoride on osteoblast progenitors in vitro. J Bone Miner Res. 1990;5 Suppl 1:S101–5. Epub 1990/03/01.
33. Kassem M, Mosekilde L, Eriksen EF. Effects of fluoride on human bone cells in vitro: differences in responsiveness between stromal osteoblast precursors and mature osteoblasts. Eur J Endocrinol. 1994;130(4):381–6. Epub 1994/04/01.
34. Kassem M, Mosekilde L, Eriksen EF. 1,25-dihydroxyvitamin D3 potentiates fluoride-stimulated collagen type I production in cultures of human bone marrow stromal osteoblast-like cells. J Bone Miner Res. 1993;8(12):1453–8. Epub 1993/12/01.
35. Kanagaraja S, Wennerberg A, Eriksson C, Nygren H. Cellular reactions and bone apposition to titanium surfaces with different surface roughness and oxide thickness cleaned by oxidation. Biomaterials. 2001;22(13):1809–18. Epub 2001/06/09.
36. Lausmaa J. Surface spectroscopic characterization of titanium implant materials. J Electron Spectrosc Relat Phenom. 1996;81(3):343–61.
37. McCafferty E, Wightman JP. An X-ray photoelectron spectroscopy sputter profile study of the native air-formed oxide film on titanium. Appl Surf Sci. 1999;143(1–4):92–100.
38. Pouilleau J, Devilliers D, Garrido F, Durand-Vidal S, Mahé E. Structure and composition of passive titanium oxide films. Mater Sci Eng B. 1997;47(3):235–43.
39. Sittig C, Textor M, Spencer ND, Wieland M, Vallotton PH. Surface characterization of implant materials c.p. Ti, Ti-6Al-7Nb and Ti-6Al-4V with different pretreatments. J Mater Sci Mater Med. 1999;10(1):35–46.
40. Tengvall P, Lundstrom I. Physico-chemical considerations of titanium as a biomaterial. Clin Mater. 1992;9(2):115–34. Epub 1991/12/10.
41. Ronold HJ, Ellingsen JE. Effect of micro-roughness produced by TiO2 blasting–tensile testing of bone attachment by using coin-shaped implants. Biomaterials. 2002;23(21):4211–9. Epub 2002/08/27.
42. Meirelles L, Currie F, Jacobsson M, Albrektsson T, Wennerberg A. The effect of chemical and nanotopographical modifications on the early stages of osseointegration. Int J Oral Maxillofac Implants. 2008;23(4):641–7. Epub 2008/09/24.
43. Lamolle SF, Monjo M, Rubert M, Haugen HJ, Lyngstadaas SP, Ellingsen JE. The effect of hydrofluoric acid treatment of titanium surface on nanostructural and chemical changes and the growth of MC3T3-E1 cells. Biomaterials. 2009;30(5):736–42. Epub 2008/11/22.
44. Petersson IU, Loberg JE, Fredriksson AS, Ahlberg EK. Semi-conducting properties of titanium dioxide surfaces on titanium implants. Biomaterials. 2009;30(27):4471–9. Epub 2009/06/16.
45. Kang BS, Sul YT, Oh SJ, Lee HJ, Albrektsson T. XPS, AES and SEM analysis of recent dental implants. Acta Biomater. 2009;5(6):2222–9. Epub 2009/03/06.
46. Ellingsen JE. Pre-treatment of titanium implants with fluoride improves their retention in bone. J Mater Sci Mater Med. 1995;6(12):749–53.
47. Ellingsen JE. Surface configurations of dental implants. Periodontol 2000. 1998;17:36–46. Epub 1999/05/25.
48. Ellingsen JE. On the properties of surface modified titanium. In: Davies JE, editor. Bone engineering. Toronto: E-squared ltd; 2000. p. 183–9.
49. Albrektsson T, Johansson C. Osteoinduction, osteoconduction and osseointegration. Eur Spine J. 2001;10 Suppl 2:S96–101.

50. Mendonca G, Mendonca DB, Aragao FJ, Cooper LF. Advancing dental implant surface technology–from micron- to nanotopography. Biomaterials. 2008;29(28):3822–35. Epub 2008/07/12.
51. Aubin JE. Advances in the osteoblast lineage. Biochem Cell Biol. 1998;76(6):899–910. Epub 1999/07/07.
52. Aubin JE. Regulation of osteoblast formation and function. Rev Endocr Metab Disord. 2001;2(1):81–94. Epub 2001/11/14.
53. Lian JB, Stein GS, Stein JL, van Wijnen AJ. Transcriptional control of osteoblast differentiation. Biochem Soc Trans. 1998;26(1):14–21. Epub 2000/07/18.
54. Stein GS, Lian JB, Stein JL, Van Wijnen AJ, Montecino M. Transcriptional control of osteoblast growth and differentiation. Physiol Rev. 1996;76(2):593–629.
55. Caplan AI. Mesenchymal stem cells. J Orthop Res. 1991;9(5):641–50. Epub 1991/09/01.
56. Berkes CA, Tapscott SJ. MyoD and the transcriptional control of myogenesis. Semin Cell Dev Biol. 2005;16(4–5):585–95. Epub 2005/08/16.
57. Ducy P, Zhang R, Geoffroy V, Ridall AL, Karsenty G. Osf2/Cbfa1: a transcriptional activator of osteoblast differentiation. Cell. 1997;89(5):747–54.
58. Jensen ED, Gopalakrishnan R, Westendorf JJ. Regulation of gene expression in osteoblasts. Biofactors. 2010;36(1):25–32. Epub 2010/01/21.
59. Komori T, Yagi H, Nomura S, Yamaguchi A, Sasaki K, Deguchi K, et al. Targeted disruption of Cbfa1 results in a complete lack of bone formation owing to maturational arrest of osteoblasts. Cell. 1997;89(5):755–64. Epub 1997/05/30.
60. Nakashima K, Zhou X, Kunkel G, Zhang Z, Deng JM, Behringer RR, et al. The novel zinc finger-containing transcription factor osterix is required for osteoblast differentiation and bone formation. Cell. 2002;108(1):17–29. Epub 2002/01/17.
61. Tu Q, Valverde P, Chen J. Osterix enhances proliferation and osteogenic potential of bone marrow stromal cells. Biochem Biophys Res Commun. 2006;341(4):1257–65. Epub 2006/02/10.
62. Guida L, Annunziata M, Carinci F, Di Feo A, Passaro I, Oliva A. In vitro biologic response of human bone marrow stromal cells to enamel matrix derivative. J Periodontol. 2007;78(11):2190–6.
63. McKee MD, Nanci A. Osteopontin and the bone remodeling sequence. Colloidal-gold immunocytochemistry of an interfacial extracellular matrix protein. Ann N Y Acad Sci. 1995;760:177–89. Epub 1995/04/21.
64. Sodek J, Chen J, Nagata T, Kasugai S, Todescan Jr R, Li IW, et al. Regulation of osteopontin expression in osteoblasts. Ann N Y Acad Sci. 1995;760:223–41. Epub 1995/04/21.
65. Cooper LF, Zhou Y, Takebe J, Guo J, Abron A, Holmen A, et al. Fluoride modification effects on osteoblast behavior and bone formation at TiO2 grit-blasted c.p. titanium endosseous implants. Biomaterials. 2006;27(6):926–36.
66. Guida L, Annunziata M, Rocci A, Contaldo M, Rullo R, Oliva A. Biological response of human bone marrow mesenchymal stem cells to fluoride-modified titanium surfaces. Clin Oral Implants Res. 2010;21(11):1234–41. Epub 2010/05/26.
67. Isa ZM, Schneider GB, Zaharias R, Seabold D, Stanford CM. Effects of fluoride-modified titanium surfaces on osteoblast proliferation and gene expression. Int J Oral Maxillofac Implants. 2006;21(2):203–11. Epub 2006/04/26.
68. Masaki C, Schneider GB, Zaharias R, Seabold D, Stanford C. Effects of implant surface microtopography on osteoblast gene expression. Clin Oral Implants Res. 2005;16(6):650–6. Epub 2005/11/26.
69. Valencia S, Gretzer C, Cooper LF. Surface nanofeature effects on titanium-adherent human mesenchymal stem cells. Int J Oral Maxillofac Implants. 2009;24(1):38–46. Epub 2009/04/07.
70. Goransson A, Arvidsson A, Currie F, Franke-Stenport V, Kjellin P, Mustafa K, et al. An in vitro comparison of possibly bioactive titanium implant surfaces. J Biomed Mater Res A. 2009;88(4):1037–47. Epub 2008/04/12.
71. Liu R, Lei T, Dusevich V, Yao X, Liu Y, Walker MP, et al. Surface characteristics and cell adhesion: a comparative study of four commercial dental implants. J Prosthodont. 2013;22:641–51. Epub 2013/06/04.
72. Ramis JM, Taxt-Lamolle SF, Lyngstadaas SP, Reseland JE, Ellingsen JE, Monjo M. Identification of early response genes to roughness and fluoride modification of titanium implants in human osteoblasts. Implant Dent. 2012;21(2):141–9. Epub 2012/03/03.
73. Santiago AS, Santos EA, Sader MS, Santiago MF, Soares Gde A. Response of osteoblastic cells to titanium submitted to three different surface treatments. Braz Oral Res. 2005;19(3):203–8. Epub 2005/11/26.
74. Guo J, Padilla RJ, Ambrose W, De Kok IJ, Cooper LF. The effect of hydrofluoric acid treatment of TiO2 grit blasted titanium implants on adherent osteoblast gene expression in vitro and in vivo. Biomaterials. 2007;28(36):5418–25. Epub 2007/09/18.
75. Monjo M, Petzold C, Ramis JM, Lyngstadaas SP, Ellingsen JE. In vitro osteogenic properties of two dental implant surfaces. Int J Biomater. 2012;2012:181024. Epub 2012/11/03.
76. Bhatavadekar NB, Hu J, Keys K, Ofek G, Athanasiou KA. Novel application of cytodetachment technology to the analysis of dental implant surfaces. Int J Oral Maxillofac Implants. 2011;26(5):985–90. Epub 2011/10/20.
77. Farley JR, Wergedal JE, Baylink DJ. Fluoride directly stimulates proliferation and alkaline phosphatase activity of bone-forming cells. Science. 1983;222(4621):330–2. Epub 1983/10/21.
78. Lau KH, Baylink DJ. Molecular mechanism of action of fluoride on bone cells. J Bone Miner Res. 1998;13(11):1660–7. Epub 1998/11/03.
79. Thor A, Rasmusson L, Wennerberg A, Thomsen P, Hirsch JM, Nilsson B, et al. The role of whole

blood in thrombin generation in contact with various titanium surfaces. Biomaterials. 2007;28(6):966–74. Epub 2006/11/11.
80. Kienapfel H, Sprey C, Wilke A, Griss P. Implant fixation by bone ingrowth. J Arthroplasty. 1999;14(3):355–68. Epub 1999/04/29.
81. Osborn JF, Newesely H. Dynamic aspects of the bone-implant interface. In: Heimke G, editor. Dental implants: materials and systems. Munich: Carl Hanser VErlag; 1980. p. 111–23.
82. Ellingsen JE, Johansson CB, Wennerberg A, Holmen A. Improved retention and bone-to-implant contact with fluoride-modified titanium implants. Int J Oral Maxillofac Implants. 2004;19(5):659–66. Epub 2004/10/29.
83. Berglundh T, Abrahamsson I, Albouy JP, Lindhe J. Bone healing at implants with a fluoride-modified surface: an experimental study in dogs. Clin Oral Implants Res. 2007;18(2):147–52. Epub 2007/02/03.
84. Abrahamsson I, Albouy JP, Berglundh T. Healing at fluoride-modified implants placed in wide marginal defects: an experimental study in dogs. Clin Oral Implants Res. 2008;19(2):153–9. Epub 2007/11/28.
85. Thor AL, Hong J, Kjeller G, Sennerby L, Rasmusson L. Correlation of platelet growth factor release in jawbone defect repair – a study in the dog mandible. Clin Implant Dent Relat Res. 2013;15(5):759–68. Epub 2012/01/13.
86. Monjo M, Lamolle SF, Lyngstadaas SP, Ronold HJ, Ellingsen JE. In vivo expression of osteogenic markers and bone mineral density at the surface of fluoride-modified titanium implants. Biomaterials. 2008;29(28):3771–80. Epub 2008/07/01.
87. Bressan E, Sivolella S, Urrutia ZA, Salata LA, Lang NP, Botticelli D. Short implants (6 mm) installed immediately into extraction sockets: an experimental study in dogs. Clin Oral Implants Res. 2012;23(5):536–41. Epub 2012/02/11.
88. Choi JY, Lee HJ, Jang JU, Yeo IS. Comparison between bioactive fluoride modified and bioinert anodically oxidized implant surfaces in early bone response using rabbit tibia model. Implant Dent. 2012;21(2):124–8. Epub 2012/03/03.
89. Coelho PG, Granato R, Marin C, Bonfante EA, Freire JN, Janal MN, et al. Biomechanical evaluation of endosseous implants at early implantation times: a study in dogs. J Oral Maxillofac Surg. 2010;68(7):1667–75. Epub 2010/06/22.
90. de Sanctis M, Vignoletti F, Discepoli N, Munoz F, Sanz M. Immediate implants at fresh extraction sockets: an experimental study in the beagle dog comparing four different implant systems. Soft tissue findings. J Clin Periodontol. 2010;37(8):769–76. Epub 2010/06/10.
91. de Sanctis M, Vignoletti F, Discepoli N, Zucchelli G, Sanz M. Immediate implants at fresh extraction sockets: bone healing in four different implant systems. J Clin Periodontol. 2009;36(8):705–11. Epub 2009/06/25.
92. Duyck J, Corpas L, Vermeiren S, Ogawa T, Quirynen M, Vandamme K, et al. Histological, histomorphometrical, and radiological evaluation of an experimental implant design with a high insertion torque. Clin Oral Implants Res. 2010;21(8):877–84. Epub 2010/06/10.
93. Johansson CB, Gretzer C, Jimbo R, Mattisson I, Ahlberg E. Enhanced implant integration with hierarchically structured implants: a pilot study in rabbits. Clin Oral Implants Res. 2012;23(8):943–53. Epub 2011/07/05.
94. Li Y, Zou S, Wang D, Feng G, Bao C, Hu J. The effect of hydrofluoric acid treatment on titanium implant osseointegration in ovariectomized rats. Biomaterials. 2010;31(12):3266–73. Epub 2010/02/06.
95. Vignoletti F, Discepoli N, Muller A, de Sanctis M, Munoz F, Sanz M. Bone modelling at fresh extraction sockets: immediate implant placement versus spontaneous healing: an experimental study in the beagle dog. J Clin Periodontol. 2012;39(1):91–7. Epub 2011/11/19.
96. Bilhan H, Geckili O, Mumcu E, Bozdag E, Sunbuloglu E, Kutay O. Influence of surgical technique, implant shape and diameter on the primary stability in cancellous bone. J Oral Rehabil. 2010;37(12):900–7. Epub 2010/06/10.
97. Kang IH, Kim CW, Lim YJ, Kim MJ. A comparative study on the initial stability of different implants placed above the bone level using resonance frequency analysis. J Adv Prosthodont. 2011;3(4):190–5. Epub 2012/01/20.
98. De Kok IJ, Chang KH, Lu TS, Cooper LF. Comparison of three-implant-supported fixed dentures and two-implant-retained overdentures in the edentulous mandible: a pilot study of treatment efficacy and patient satisfaction. Int J Oral Maxillofac Implants. 2011;26(2):415–26.
99. Stanford CM, Wagner W, Rodriguez YBR, Norton M, McGlumphy E, Schmidt J. Evaluation of the effectiveness of dental implant therapy in a practice-based network (FOCUS). Int J Oral Maxillofac Implants. 2010;25(2):367–73.
100. Geckili O, Bilhan H, Bilgin T. Impact of mandibular two-implant retained overdentures on life quality in a group of elderly Turkish edentulous patients. Arch Gerontol Geriatr. 2011;53(2):233–6.
101. Erkapers M, Ekstrand K, Baer RA, Toljanic JA, Thor A. Patient satisfaction following dental implant treatment with immediate loading in the edentulous atrophic maxilla. Int J Oral Maxillofac Implants. 2011;26(2):356–64.
102. Kleis WK, Kammerer PW, Hartmann S, Al-Nawas B, Wagner W. A comparison of three different attachment systems for mandibular two-implant overdentures: one-year report. Clin Implant Dent Relat Res. 2010;12(3):209–18.
103. Bressan E, Tomasi C, Stellini E, Sivolella S, Favero G, Berglundh T. Implant-supported mandibular overdentures: a cross-sectional study. Clin Oral Implants Res. 2012;23(7):814–9.
104. D'Haese J, De Bruyn H. Effect of smoking habits on accuracy of implant placement using mucosally

supported stereolithographic surgical guides. Clin Implant Dent Relat Res. 2013;15(3):402–11.
105. D'Haese J, Van De Velde T, Elaut L, De Bruyn H. A prospective study on the accuracy of mucosally supported stereolithographic surgical guides in fully edentulous maxillae. Clin Implant Dent Relat Res. 2012;14(2):293–303.
106. Goshima K, Lexner MO, Thomsen CE, Miura H, Gotfredsen K, Bakke M. Functional aspects of treatment with implant-supported single crowns: a quality control study in subjects with tooth agenesis. Clin Oral Implants Res. 2010;21(1):108–14.
107. Raes F, Cooper LF, Tarrida LG, Vandromme H, De Bruyn H. A case-control study assessing oral-health-related quality of life after immediately loaded single implants in healed alveolar ridges or extraction sockets. Clin Oral Implants Res. 2012;23(5):602–8.
108. Bressan E, Paniz G, Lops D, Corazza B, Romeo E, Favero G. Influence of abutment material on the gingival color of implant-supported all-ceramic restorations: a prospective multicenter study. Clin Oral Implants Res. 2011;22(6):631–7.
109. Raes F, Cosyn J, Crommelinck E, Coessens P, De Bruyn H. Immediate and conventional single implant treatment in the anterior maxilla: 1-year results of a case series on hard and soft tissue response and aesthetics. J Clin Periodontol. 2011;38(4):385–94.
110. Raes F, Cosyn J, De Bruyn H. Clinical, aesthetic, and patient-related outcome of immediately loaded single implants in the anterior maxilla: a prospective study in extraction sockets, healed ridges, and grafted sites. Clin Implant Dent Relat Res. 2013;15(6):819–35.
111. Tsuda H, Rungcharassaeng K, Kan JY, Roe P, Lozada JL, Zimmerman G. Peri-implant tissue response following connective tissue and bone grafting in conjunction with immediate single-tooth replacement in the esthetic zone: a case series. Int J Oral Maxillofac Implants. 2011;26(2):427–36.
112. van Brakel R, Noordmans HJ, Frenken J, de Roode R, de Wit GC, Cune MS. The effect of zirconia and titanium implant abutments on light reflection of the supporting soft tissues. Clin Oral Implants Res. 2011;22(10):1172–8.
113. Acocella A, Bertolai R, Sacco R. Modified insertion technique for immediate implant placement into fresh extraction socket in the first maxillary molar sites: a 3-year prospective study. Implant Dent. 2010;19(3):220–8.
114. Ferrus J, Cecchinato D, Pjetursson EB, Lang NP, Sanz M, Lindhe J. Factors influencing ridge alterations following immediate implant placement into extraction sockets. Clin Oral Implants Res. 2010;21(1):22–9.
115. Gokcen-Rohlig B, Meric U, Keskin H. Clinical and radiographic outcomes of implants immediately placed in fresh extraction sockets. Oral Surg Oral Med Oral Pathol Oral Radiol Endod. 2010;109(4):030.
116. Barbier L, Abeloos J, De Clercq C, Jacobs R. Peri-implant bone changes following tooth extraction, immediate placement and loading of implants in the edentulous maxilla. Clin Oral Investig. 2012;16(4):1061–70.
117. Collaert B, Wijnen L, De Bruyn H. A 2-year prospective study on immediate loading with fluoride-modified implants in the edentulous mandible. Clin Oral Implants Res. 2011;22(10):1111–6.
118. Donati M, La Scala V, Billi M, Di Dino B, Torrisi P, Berglundh T. Immediate functional loading of implants in single tooth replacement: a prospective clinical multicenter study. Clin Oral Implants Res. 2008;19(8):740–8.
119. Koutouzis T, Koutouzis G, Tomasi C, Lundgren T. Immediate loading of implants placed with the osteotome technique: one-year prospective case series. J Periodontol. 2011;82(11):1556–62.
120. Mertens C, Steveling HG. Early and immediate loading of titanium implants with fluoride-modified surfaces: results of 5-year prospective study. Clin Oral Implants Res. 2011;22(12):1354–60.
121. Schliephake H, Rodiger M, Phillips K, McGlumphy EA, Chacon GE, Larsen P. Early loading of surface modified implants in the posterior mandible – 5 year results of an open prospective non-controlled study. J Clin Periodontol. 2012;39(2):188–95.
122. Rismanchian M, Fazel A, Rakhshan V, Eblaghian G. One-year clinical and radiographic assessment of fluoride-enhanced implants on immediate non-functional loading in posterior maxilla and mandible: a pilot prospective clinical series study. Clin Oral Implants Res. 2011;22(12):1440–5.
123. Galindo-Moreno P, Nilsson P, King P, Becktor J, Speroni S, Schramm A, et al. Clinical and radiographic evaluation of early loaded narrow diameter implants – 1-year follow-up. Clin Oral Implants Res. 2012;23(5):609–16.
124. Cecchinato D, Bressan EA, Toia M, Araujo MG, Liljenberg B, Lindhe J. Osseointegration in periodontitis susceptible individuals. Clin Oral Implants Res. 2012;23(1):1–4.
125. Balleri P, Veltri M, Nuti N, Ferrari M. Implant placement in combination with sinus membrane elevation without biomaterials: a 1-year study on 15 patients. Clin Implant Dent Relat Res. 2012;14(5):682–9.
126. Galindo-Moreno P, Moreno-Riestra I, Avila G, Fernandez-Barbero JE, Mesa F, Aguilar M, et al. Histomorphometric comparison of maxillary pristine bone and composite bone graft biopsies obtained after sinus augmentation. Clin Oral Implants Res. 2010;21(1):122–8. Epub 2009/10/23.
127. Gulje F, Raghoebar GM, Ter Meulen JW, Vissink A, Meijer HJ. Mandibular overdentures supported by 6-mm dental implants: a 1-year prospective cohort study. Clin Implant Dent Relat Res. 2012;14(1):1708–8208.
128. Kahnberg KE, Wallstrom M, Rasmusson L. Local sinus lift for single-tooth implant. I: clinical and radiographic follow-up. Clin Implant Dent Relat Res. 2011;13(3):231–7.
129. Pieri F, Aldini NN, Fini M, Marchetti C, Corinaldesi G. Immediate fixed implant rehabilitation of the

atrophic edentulous maxilla after bilateral sinus floor augmentation: a 12-month pilot study. Clin Implant Dent Relat Res. 2012;14(1):1708–8208.
130. Støre G, Heyden A, Walaas L. Osseointegration surgery and implant stability in irradiated mandibles. Oral Surg. 2011;4(2):65–72.
131. Mertens C, Steveling HG, Seeberger R, Hoffmann J, Freier K. Reconstruction of severely atrophied alveolar ridges with calvarial onlay bone grafts and dental implants. Clin Implant Dent Relat Res. 2013;15(5):673–83. Epub 2011/10/20.
132. Vervaeke S, Collaert B, Vandeweghe S, Cosyn J, Deschepper E, De Bruyn H. The effect of smoking on survival and bone loss of implants with a fluoride-modified surface: a 2-year retrospective analysis of 1106 implants placed in daily practice. Clin Oral Implants Res. 2012;23(6):758–66. Epub 2011/05/07.
133. Fandridis J, Papadopoulos T. Surface characterization of three titanium dental implants. Implant Dent. 2008;17(1):91–9. Epub 2008/03/12.
134. Jarmar T, Palmquist A, Branemark R, Hermansson L, Engqvist H, Thomsen P. Characterization of the surface properties of commercially available dental implants using scanning electron microscopy, focused ion beam, and high-resolution transmission electron microscopy. Clin Implant Dent Relat Res. 2008;10(1):11–22. Epub 2008/02/08.
135. Svanborg LM, Andersson M, Wennerberg A. Surface characterization of commercial oral implants on the nanometer level. J Biomed Mater Res B Appl Biomater. 2010;92(2):462–9. Epub 2009/12/04.
136. Rupp F, Scheideler L, Eichler M, Geis-Gerstorfer J. Wetting behavior of dental implants. Int J Oral Maxillofac Implants. 2011;26(6):1256–66. Epub 2011/12/15.

Surface Modification of Titanium and Its Alloy by Anodic Oxidation for Dental Implant

7

Takashi Sawase and Ikuya Watanabe

Abstract

Anodic oxidation has been successfully used as a surface modification for orthopedic and dental implants in the past few decades. This chapter will overview the anodic oxidation of titanium and will discuss about processing parameters, microstructure, and composition. Finally, it will clarify the biological responses and the mechanism of enhanced osteoblast functions on the anodized titanium which is pertinent to dental implants.

Introduction

Titanium (Ti) spontaneously forms a surface oxide layer (TiO_2, 1.5–10 nm in thickness) when it is exposed to air and atmospheric water vapor [1, 2]. This surface oxide layer makes Ti passive with an excellent corrosion resistance. Since Ti is originally highly reactive metal, it can quickly and easily react with molecules with low atomic number such as oxygen. This thin passive oxide layer on Ti and its alloy surface provides their excellent biocompatibility characteristics because of good chemical stability, high corrosion resistance, and non-toxicity. Subsequently, Ti and its alloys are widely used as orthopedic and dental implant materials. Until now, machined commercially pure (c.p.) Ti implants with 5–10 nm of thin surface oxide layer have been documented as the most successful osseointegrated implants for a long time.

However, this thin natural oxide film may not be sufficiently protective in the aggressive biological environment since the titanium ion release from Ti implants has been reported after placement of the implants in muscles, long bones, and mandible. Furthermore, increased titanium-ion concentrations were found both in peri-implant tissues and in parenchymal organs (e.g., lung, liver, and spleen) [3–7]. Among several factors that may affect the titanium ion release, corrosion behavior and mechanical wear were discussed as the possible sources of tissue contamination by titanium [6, 8–10]. There are some evidences that early bone response to electropolished titanium with a thinner oxide layer showed less bone volume and bone-to-implant contact [11, 12].

T. Sawase, DDS, PhD (✉)
Department of Applied Prosthodontics, Graduate School of Biomedical Sciences, Nagasaki University, 1-7-1 Sakamoto, Nagasaki 852 8588, Japan
e-mail: sawase@nagasaki-u.ac.jp

I. Watanabe, PhD
Department of Biomaterials, Nagasaki University, Nagasaki, Japan

A. Wennerberg et al. (eds.), *Implant Surfaces and their Biological and Clinical Impact*,
DOI 10.1007/978-3-662-45379-7_7,

Hazan et al. [13] and Kitsugi et al. [14] demonstrated that the heat treatment of titanium alloy to make a relatively thick oxide layer could enhance the early bonding of alloy implant to bone. In addition, the natural TiO_2 layer is not bioactive enough to form a direct bonding with bone. According to the original Brånemark protocol, i.e., 3–6 months of healing period would be necessary to achieve osseointegration. There are two critical factors stated for successful implant treatment: (1) the certain primary stability that can maintain the implant stable until new bone formation and (2) good bone quality that can promise the enhanced bone formation around the implant. To consider the critical factors mentioned above, it is desirable that the surface oxide layer of the dental implant should be bioactive in order to promote bone formation around the implant.

In the last two decades, a great number of attempts were conducted to improve the surface properties such as topography, chemistry, and surface energy which influence the bone attachment to the implant. These surface modification techniques include mechanical methods (e.g., sand or hydroxyapatite (HA) blasting), chemical methods (e.g., acid etching), electrochemical methods (e.g., anodic oxidation), coatings (e.g., Ti or HA plasma spraying, ion beam–assisted deposition), etc. [12, 15–19]. It should be noted that each surface modification technique influences all of the surface properties such as topography, chemistry, and surface energy. For instance, the technique "sandblasting" will not only influence the surface topography but also can remove the surface chemical contaminations, resulting in high surface energy. However the chemical elements of the blasting particles remain. Anodic oxidation (anodization) which is the topic of this session also influences every surface property, namely, that can change the surface roughness, surface oxide composition and thickness, and wettability. Whatever surface modification technique is applied, it should be intensively considered that all surface properties will be varied with the type of modification.

In general, anodic oxidation is a well-established surface modification technique for valve metals in industry. Anodic oxidation allows the controlled formation of the protective oxide surface layer much thicker than that formed naturally. Controlling the thickness of the protective oxide layer on titanium (Ti) and its alloys could enhance the corrosion resistance and biocompatibility [20–26]. The coatings produced by anodic oxidation could make dense or porous surfaces with amorphous or crystalline structures depending on the treatment parameters, such as type of electrolyte, concentration of the electrolyte, and applied electrical potential applied [27]. The electrolytes most commonly used to anodize Ti and its alloys are sulfuric and phosphoric acids. Anodic oxidation has been successfully used as a surface modification for orthopedic and dental implants in the past few decades. This chapter will provide an overview on the anodic oxidation and will discuss processing parameters, microstructure, and composition. Beside it will clarify the biological responses and the mechanism of enhanced osteoblast functions on the anodized titanium which is pertinent to dental implants.

Anodic Oxidation of Titanium

Acid etching is usually performed before the anodic oxidation procedure in order to remove the natural titanium oxide and surface contaminants. The electrolyte anodic oxidation is carried out using three electrodes of titanium anode, platinum cathode, and Ag/AgCl reference electrode. When constant voltage or current is applied between the anode and cathode, reactions on Ti electrode surface lead to form an oxide layer on it. The final oxide layer thickness is proportional to the applied voltage. The properties of the oxide layer (such as roughness, morphology, chemical composition, etc.) after anodic oxidation was different depending on the applied voltage, current density, composition, pH, and temperature of electrolyte. The oxide layer formed on Ti anode grows up in accordance with the increasing voltage. After the applied voltage exceeds the dielectric breakdown limit of the oxide layer, the oxide layer cannot be sustained for further current flow;

so the sparking may occur at flaws and defects of the oxide layer. Finally, the dielectric barrier of the oxide layer will be broken down, resulting in porous surface morphology on the titanium surfaces produced for titanium implant. The typical morphology of the anodized oxide layer is a rough and porous texture. The size of the pores varies from a few hundred nanometers to a few micrometers depending on the used parameters. The pores are not uniformed on the same anodized surface. Moreover, these pores are interconnected and have a layered structure. The diameter of the porous layer was reported to increase with greater current density [28, 29], applied electrical potential [25], and concentration of the electrolyte [25]. The thickness of oxide film increases with oxidation time up to 10 μm.

Figure 7.1 shows the representative anodized dental implant surface (TiUnite®, Nobel Biocare). The typical porous surfaces (octopus-trap-like feature) indicate that the sparking has occurred to form oxide layer. According to the data sheets the TiUnite surface was modified by spark anodization in an electrolytic solution containing phosphoric acid. This manufacturing method efficiently produced thickened titanium oxide layer (up to 10 μm) and a moderately rough surface topography with nanopores and micropores (Ra1.2 μm). The TiUnite contains highly crystalline anatase and rutile which are the most important titanium oxides and is thereby highly crystalline biomaterial [30]. Since many studies have shown the presence of phosphorus in the oxide layer, the TiUnite may have both topography-related and chemistry-related effects on osseointegration. This newsletter explains how the TiUnite interacts with living tissue and accelerates the healing of wound tissue.

Figures 7.2 and 7.3 show the results of the chemical analyses of the anodized oxide layer of the TiUnite implant by means of cross-sectional transmission electron microscopy and energy-dispersed X-ray (EDX) spectroscopy. The surface has large undulations, and the thickness of the oxide layer is estimated to be approximately 3–10 μm. A large crack and a pore can be observed between the titanium base and the implant surface in Fig. 7.2. A protrusion and a depression are evident on the surface. Note that the depression located at the left top corner of implant surface (squared box). The dark-field transmission electron micrograph of the depression on the surface indicated that the left half of the micrograph shows an amorphous contrast, while the right half has crystalline structure. The diffraction patterns and EDX spectra taken from points b and c in Fig. 7.3a are shown in Fig. 7.3b, c. The diffraction pattern from the amorphous phase (point b) has halos. In contrast, the diffraction pattern taken from point c shows that the small crystals represent the TiO_2 phase of the anatase-type structure. The size of the anatase crystal is estimated to be around 10 nm. In the EDX spectra measured from the amorphous phase (Fig. 7.3b), a strong phosphorus peak was detected, which is considered to be derived from a phosphate anion (P) in a phosphoric solution during anodization process. The phosphate anion from the electrolyte is incorporated and concentrated into the amorphous phase of the oxide layer. Previous reports using XPS and AES [22, 32, 33] revealed similar results that P was incorporated into anodic oxide surfaces, whereas XRD study indicated that the titanium phosphates were identified in anodic oxide anodized in H_3PO_4 electrolyte (1 mol/l) at electrical potentials between 100 and 250 V [34]. Previous in vitro studies suggested that the phosphate

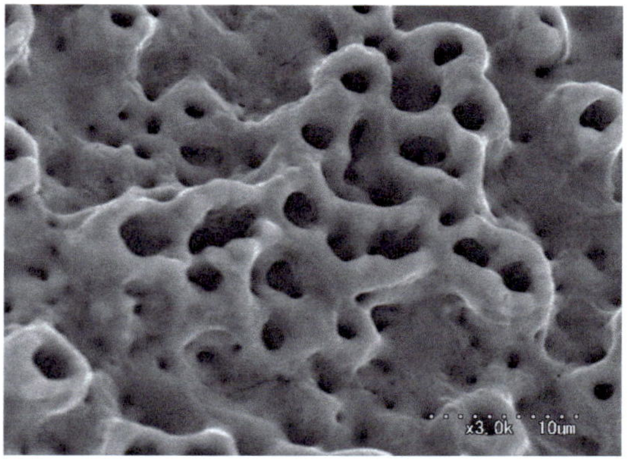

Fig. 7.1 Scanning electron micrograph of anodized TiUnite implant surface. The typical porous surfaces (octopus-trap-like feature) indicate that the sparking has occurred to form oxide layer

incorporation into anodic surface oxides on titanium and its alloys has beneficial effect that is capable of precipitation of bioactive Ca–P compounds during immersion in simulated body fluids (SBF) [35–38]. Sul et al. [39] demonstrated that the implant anodized in phosphoric acid showed strong bone reaction and provided direct chemical bonding sites for calcium ions and hydroxyapatite of the bone matrix during biologic mineralization.

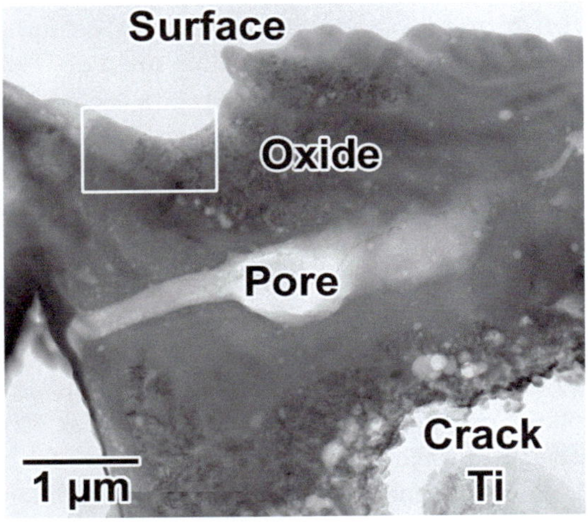

Fig. 7.2 Low-magnification transmission electron micrograph of the TiUnite surface. The *upper* portion of the photo shows the implant surface

The elemental ions contained in the electrolyte are usually present in the thick, porous ASD film oxide, and the ion concentration decreases from the outer layer inward the bulk substrate [40]. For example, phosphorous ion was found to be embedded in titanium oxide layer after anodization with a H_3PO_4 electrolyte [41], and its concentration decreased from outer surface inward the bulk substrate. Another approach to make the anodized titanium bioactive was reported to introduce apatite layers onto the surface. In SBF, the spark-discharged anodized titanium oxide could induce apatite formation on its surface [25]. One advantage of this method is that the composition and surface morphology of the resulting apatite layer is very similar to those of

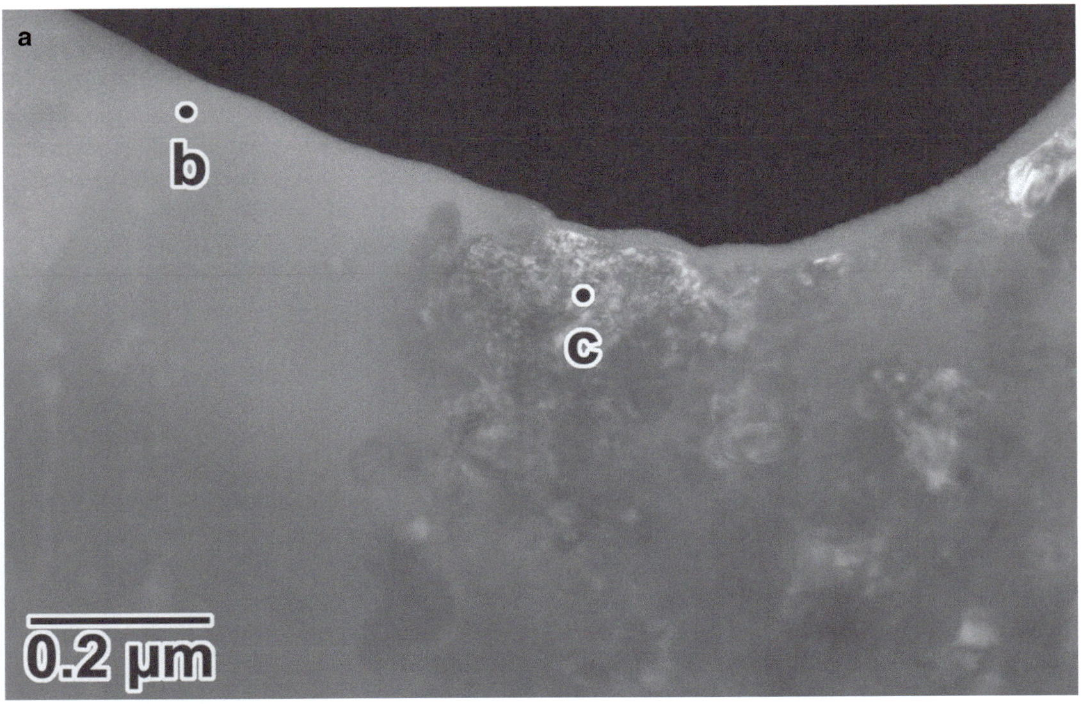

Fig. 7.3 (**a**) Dark-field transmission electron micrograph of the depression (*squared box*) on the surface shown in Fig. 7.2. Diffraction patterns and energy-dispersed X-ray spectra measured from points (**b**, **c**) in (a)

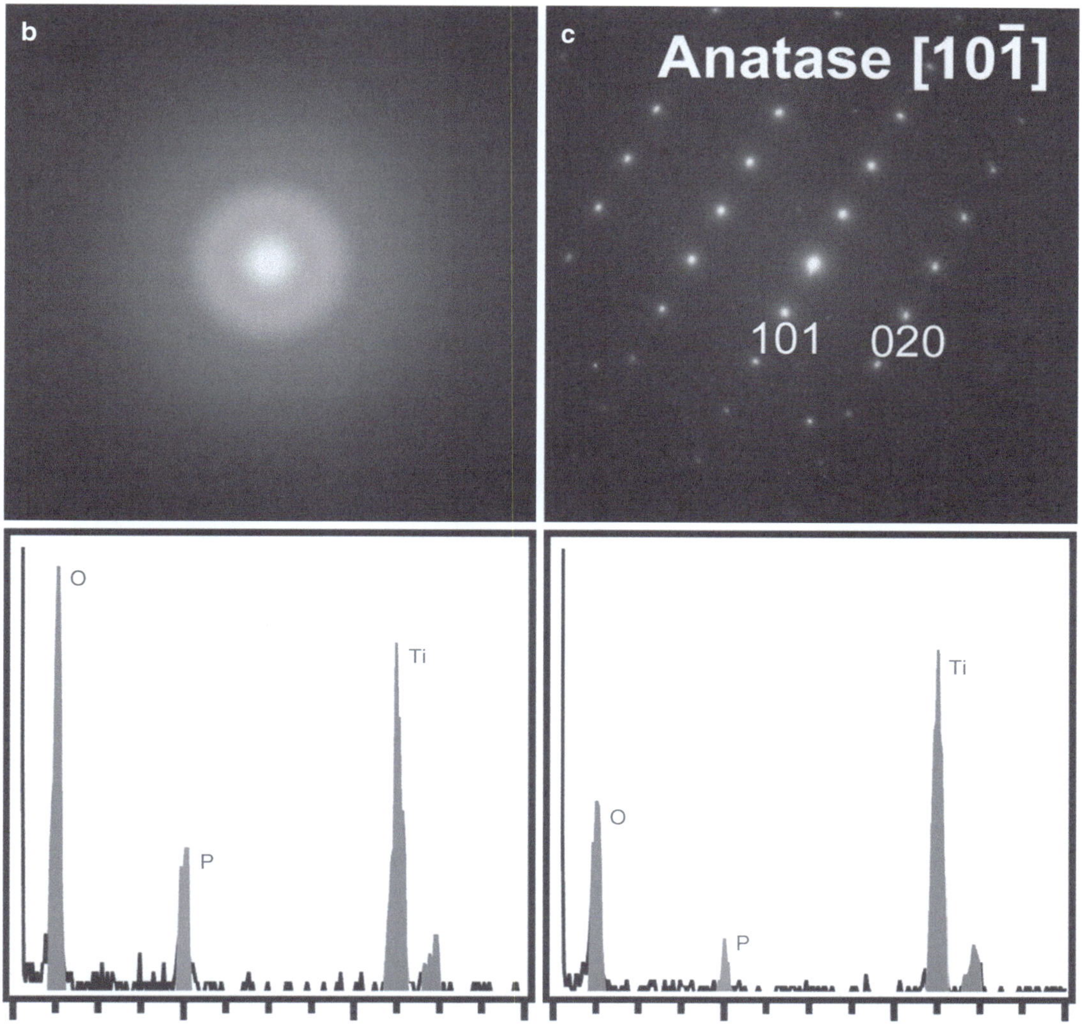

Fig. 7.3 (continued)

the apatite in natural bone. In the studies conducted by Ishizawa et al. [42, 43], c.p. titanium anodized in an electrolytic solution containing sodium beta-glycerophosphate (beta-GP) and calcium acetate (CA) formed a thin calcium phosphate layer having a Ca/P ratio equivalent to hydroxyapatite (HA) in natural bone. In these studies, the thin Ca–P layer formed on the anodized substrates subjected to the hydrothermal treatment at 300 °C to form HA crystals with fully coverage the surface.

Biological Properties of Anodized Titanium

In Vitro Studies

Numerous studies were carried out regarding the cell compatibilities on anodized titanium and its alloys surface. Especially, since these materials are supposed to be used for the bone-anchored apparatuses in the field of orthopedic and dental implant, bone cells such as osteoblast or bone marrow stromal cells were investigated for cell attachment, proliferation, and differentiation. In essence, there are two factors to influence the cell compatibilities for anodized titanium oxide. One is the special morphology with the micro- and nanopores, and another is the effect of surface chemistry of the anodic oxidized layer.

Rodriguez et al. [44] investigated in vitro osteoblast response to anodized titanium (A) and anodized titanium followed by hydrothermal treatment (AH). Due to the deposition of calcium and phosphorus ions on titanium oxide during anodization, the grown apatite-like crystals were observed after AH. Enhanced cellular function and mineralization, as indicated by total protein synthesis and osteocalcin production, respectively, were also observed after AH. Consequently, the phenotypic expression of osteoblast was enhanced by the presence of calcium phosphate or apatite-like crystals on anodized or hydrothermally treated Ti surfaces [45]. Zhu et al. [40, 46] investigated the effects of topography and composition of anodized titanium surfaces on cell behavior of osteoblast [40]. When the anodic oxidation was carried out in two kinds of electrolytes, H_3PO_4 or Ca–GP and CA, the P or Ca and P were incorporated into the anodized surfaces, respectively. Cell culture experiments demonstrated non-cytotoxicity and an increase of osteoblast adhesion and proliferation by the anodic oxides. Osteoblast cells on the surfaces with micropores showed an irregular and polygonal growth and had many lamellipodia, while osteoblasts on the smooth titanium surface or on anodic oxides formed at low voltages showed many thick stress fibers and intensive focal contacts. Therefore, porous structures with micrometer order supply positive guidance for anchorage-dependent cells to attach, leading to enhanced cell attachment. In contrast, the cells are attached to a smooth titanium surface by focal contacts as predominant adhesion structures.

The submicron-ordered structures are also important variables in determining osteoblast response to substrate topography [47]. Growth behavior of human osteoblast cell on control smooth and anodized titanium surfaces with a nonporous structure was studied using an osteoprecursor cell line [48]. Cell adhesions and differentiation on anodized surfaces were enhanced with vinculin protein and alkaline phosphatase production. The 3-(4,5-dimethylthiazol-2-yl)-2,5-diphenyl tetrazolium assays also showed an increase in living cell density and proliferation with anodized surfaces. It was obvious that nanosized rough surface morphology was one of the important factors to achieve good cell/materials interaction.

In addition to bone cell behaviors, the collagen fiber which is the major bone matrix was tightly immobilized and partially incorporated into the anodic oxide layer in SBF [30]. The geometry of type I collagen is a triple helix with 300 nm in length and 0.5 nm in width and has a periodicity of 67 nm. On the other hand, HA crystal is approximately 20–40 nm in length and deposits at the periodic gap of the collagen fiber [49]. This indicates the theoretical importance of nanosized topography of biomaterial surface.

Li et al. demonstrated the bioactivity and the biocompatibility of anodized nano-structure of the Ti by SBF soaking test and in vitro cell culture test, respectively [50]. The formation of nanostructures induced hydrophilicity, and bone-like apatite formation resulted in enhancement of cell adhesion and proliferation on the anodic oxidation. Surface energy and hydrophilicity were known to play an important role in subsequent cellular responses on biomaterials. Kim et al. [51] reported a test for Ti discs with two different surface topographies (machined and anodized), the surface energy, surface wettability, and osteoblast responses, including cell attachment capacity, cell proliferation rate, and cell differentiation level, significantly increased on anodized Ti surfaces immersed in modified SBF. The effects of biomimetic deposition with modified SBF on physiochemical surface characteristics and cell biological responses were greater on anodized surfaces than on machined surfaces.

Interestingly, Giordano et al. [52] demonstrated that the anodization treatment of pure titanium (applied voltage, 130 V) and Ti6Al4V alloy (applied voltage, 120 V) with higher voltage, compared to the untreated c.p. titanium and

Ti6Al4V and those anodized with low voltages, resulted in a greater decrease in bacterial attachment and biofilm formation in both in vitro and in vivo experiments. In contrast, the anodization with high voltages was found to promote osteoblast and fibroblast proliferation. These observations indicated that the anodization treatments with high voltages may contribute to preserve the tissue integration and to reduce bacteria colonization on titanium and titanium alloy for implant applications. Kang et al. [53] also indicated the antibacterial effect and cytocompatibility of anodized TiO_2 film that had nanostructures and contained Cl. They carried out two-step anodization, where a nanostructured titanium oxide film was formed by anodization in hydrofluoric acid and followed by NaCl solution. The Cl atoms were confirmed to incorporate into the coatings. The cell wall of the bacteria might be destroyed due to the antibacterial effect of Cl.

In Vivo Studies

The promising results from in vitro studies require conformations by in vivo studies to fully understand the relevance of anodization. From the survey of in vivo investigations, the clinical deployment was intended. Therefore, the screw-shaped implants with the size of clinical use were fabricated, and the efficacy of the surface modification was investigated by either histomorphometric analyses such as bone-to-implant contact and bone area around the vicinity of the implant or biomechanical tests such as pushout test and removal torque measurement. The surface modification of the titanium implant for in vivo studies was either spark anodization or spark anodization with hydrothermal treatment; hence, most studies provided similar porous surface morphology and their average roughness was 0.82–1.97 μm. These numbers are categorized as moderately roughened surface due to the high voltage of anodization. However, the surface chemical composition (mainly titanium oxide containing HA, P, S, and Ca) varied widely depending on the electrolyte used. Ishizawa and coworkers [42, 43] focused on anodized titanium enriched with Ca–P, and thin HA film (1–2 μm) was produced as described in in vitro study. The strong bone bonding was confirmed by pushout tests after 8 weeks of implantation into rabbits. Additionally, the histomorphometric analyses indicated much bone formation with anodized and hydrothermal-treated implant. Son et al. reported no significant difference in the percent bone contact for all samples but did find significantly increased removal torque strength for anodized implants after 6 weeks of implantation into a rabbit [54]. The chemical bonding between bone and deposited HA would be suggested. The electrolyte mixed with H_3PO_4/H_2SO_4 was introduced by several researchers [55–57]. Either special feature of tubular structure with interchanneled pores or incorporated P and S chemistry would provide significantly high pushout strength in the rabbit model.

A series of studies regarding anodized implant have been published by Sul and coworkers [56–59]. They systematically tried to prepare S-, P-, and Ca-incorporated implants by anodization with similar surface morphology and roughness. Prepared implants were inserted in the femora and tibiae of mature New Zealand white rabbits for 6 weeks [35]. Significantly higher removal torque value was shown in Ca-containing and S-containing anodized titanium implants compared to non-anodized titanium implants. The bone-to-implant contact was 186, 232, and 272 % higher in S, P, and Ca implants, respectively, when compared to the control groups. These results indicated that the ions incorporated into the titanium oxide layer during anodization had important roles in enhancing bone formation. Subsequently, magnesium (Mg)-incorporated anodic oxidized titanium implants were investigated in the same model. The result showed that the Mg-incorporated titanium implants significantly improved bone responses as compared with machine-turned control implants. When the differences and similarities of the surface oxide properties of controls and experimental implants were considered, the enhanced bone responses of Mg-incorporated implants could be explained by the Mg surface chemistry of the experimental implants [58].

Intriguingly, we found that anodized porous TiO_2 implants acquire photoinduced hydrophilicity when irradiated with ultraviolet (UV) light [31]. The water contact angle for the ordinary anodized porous TiO_2 implants (TiUnite) was 44°, whereas it dramatically decreased to 11° after 24 h of UV irradiation, which indicates that the anodized porous TiO_2 implants have inherent photoinduced hydrophilicity. However, no significant enhancement of bone regeneration around the anodized porous TiO_2 implants irradiated with UV could be seen after 4 weeks of healing in the rabbit tibiae. Subsequently, further improvement of the photoinduced hydrophilicity of the anodized porous TiO_2 implant was attempted by fluoride modification [59]. The result showed that the anodized porous TiO_2 implants modified with fluoride demonstrated significantly greater degrees of bone-to-metal contact than control implants after 2 and 6 weeks of healing. These results proved that the enhanced photoinduced hydrophilicity of the anodized implants modified with NH_4HF_2 promoted bone apposition during early stages of osseointegration.

It is noteworthy that plaque accumulation and subsequent periimplantitis are suspected to be due to the rough surfaces with pore structure of anodized surface. Albouy [60] alerted to take precautions against more plaque accumulation and periimplantitis progress of anodized TiUnite implant than machine-turned implant in the ligature-induced periimplantitis dog model. Clinical verification would be necessary to clarify the risk of acquiring periimplantitis on anodized implant.

Anodized Implant: Clinical Trials

The most well-known anodized commercial dental implant is TiUnite which is spark anodized in H_3PO_4-containing electrolyte. The surface properties of the oxide layer were characterized as several micrometer thickness and porous topography with 4–5 μm-sized pores; chemical elements containing Ti (15 %), O (55 %), C (20 %), P (5 %), S (1 %), and Si (1 %); the presence of anatase and rutile crystal of TiO_2, and an average roughness (Ra) of approximately1.2 μm [61]. The TiUnite was launched on the market in 2001, and the surface design was combined with various implant designs in Nobel Biocare implant systems. As there are a lot of clinical studies regarding the TiUnite implant, either randomized clinical trial (RCT) or long-term prospective clinical studies more than 10 years were selected to clarify the clinical relevance of TiUnite implant. Five RCTs and two long-term prospective studies were found from the electrical search [62–66]. However, three out of five RCTs were reported from same group and research subjects; hence the results were rounded up as follows. Quirynen and coworkers [62–64] carried out prospective randomized controlled trial and compared the clinical, microbiological, and biochemical outcome of machine-turned and anodic oxidized implant (TiUnite) in a split-mouth design. After 3 years' follow-up of 14 subjects, no statistically significant differences were found in survival rate, marginal bone resorption, and subgingival biofilm formation. Moreover microbiota were observed between above two implants surfaces. They stated that minimally and moderately rough implant surfaces perform clinically and microbiologically in similar manner. The results suggested that risk of periimplantitis on anodized implant could be avoided by proper oral hygiene protocol.

The advantages of anodized TiUnite implant comparing to machine-turned implant was provided by Rocci et al. [66]. The anodized TiUnite implant and machine-turned implant were compared for 9 years' survival rate in immediate-loading protocol by RCT. Three out of 66 TiUnite and 8 out of 55 machine-turned implants failed within 7 weeks of loading, resulting in a cumulative survival rate of 95.5 and 85.5 %, respectively, after 9 years of load. The TiUnite implants obtained a 10 % higher success rate compared with machine-turned implant, indicating that the validity of the anodized implant was suggested in terms of immediate loading. Similarly, Jokstad and Alkumru [65] reported the feasibility of reducing healing period using TiUnite implant. Patients with fully healed edentulous mandible were recruited to partake in a blinded two-arm parallel RCT. The changes of crestal bone level over 5 years were identical in the immediate- and conventional-loading groups, that is, 1.2 mm (SD=0.7). There were no differences between the two study arms with regard to incidence of biological and technical adverse events. The results suggested that anodized TiUnite implant could contribute to reduce healing period of the implant.

POI implant (Kyocera, Kyoto, Japan) is another anodized implant on the market and made of Ti6Al4V alloy spark anodized in H3PO4-containing electrolyte. Nevertheless two in vitro studies [67, 68] regarding surface analyses were found, and no in vivo and clinical studies are available.

Future Directions

Both surface chemical and topographical properties are the lifeblood of the biomaterials. Among several surface modification techniques for the bone-anchored biomaterials, anodic oxidation can modify both surface chemistry and topography. According to the review focusing on oral implant surfaces [69], anchorage mechanisms of oral implants were classified as (i) biomechanical bonding, (ii) biochemical bonding, and (iii) doped surfaces having the potential of enhancing bone genesis.

(i) Biomechanical Bonding
Anodization provides not only micrometer topography but also nanosized features depending on the electrical conditions and electrolyte. Webster and Ejiofor [70] reported that increased viable osteoblast density was observed at a surface modified with submicron particles compared with a surface modified with micrometer particles. The importance and validity of nano-feature surface were suggested by three-dimensional nanotopography of the bone tissue. Both collagen type I and apatite crystal dimensions are in nanometer size, and apatite crystal precipitates at the gap zone in between the collagen molecules. Currently, several researches are focusing on biologically inspired nanometer surface structures of biomaterials. It was reported that nanoporous structures can be created by titanium anodization in chromic acid at 10–40 V [71]. Interestingly, self-ordered nanotubular structures could be obtained by titanium anodization [72, 73]. For these studies, fluorine electrolyte solutions were used and the applied voltage was much lower than the dielectric breakdown. The technology of fluoride-modified TiO_2-blasted implant, the so-called OsseoSpeed™ implant (Astra Tech), is based on fluoride ions to form nanoporous structures on a titanium surface. Nanostructures after the fluoride modification correlate rapid bone formation around the OsseoSpeed™ implant.

(ii) Biochemical Bonding
Anodization has a strong potential to incorporate Ca and P into Ti coatings. Moreover, the HA deposition onto the anodized titanium can be achieved from anodization followed by hydrothermal treatment. Biochemical bonding can be therefore accomplished by coating with these calcium phosphates. One problem that still needs to be fully investigated is the bonding strength between apatite crystals and anodic oxides.

(iii) Doped Surfaces
Finally, porous ASD surfaces can be used as substrate for drug storage and release; the pore structures could fulfill a role as reservoirs of cytokine, such as bone morphogenetic protein-2 (BMP-2) and osteogenic protein-1(OP-1) [74]. However, they are still under developmental stage. Further investigations are necessary to apply for the patient.

References

1. Sul YT, Johanson CB, Jeong Y, Albrektsson T. The electrochemical oxide growth behaviour on titanium in acid and alkaline electrolytes. Med Eng Phys. 2001;23:329–46.
2. Diamanti MV, Pedeferri MP. Effect of anodic oxidation parameters on the titanium oxide formation. Corros Sci. 2007;49:939–48.
3. Woodman JL, Jacobs JJ, Galante JO, Urban RM. Metal ion release from titanium-based prosthetic segmental replacements of long bones in baboons: a long-term study. J Orthop Res. 1984;1:421–30.

4. Osborn JF, Willich P, Meenen N. The release of titanium into human bone from a titanium implant coated with plasma-sprayed titanium. In: Heimke G, Soltesz U, Lee AJC, editors. Clinical implant materials, Advances in Biomaterials, vol. 9. Amsterdam: Elsevier; 1990. p. 75–80.
5. Lodding AR, Fischer PM, Odelius HA, et al. Secondary ion mass spectrometry in the study of biomineralizations and biomaterials. Anal Chim Acta. 1990;241:299–314.
6. Solar RJ, Pollack SR, Korostoff E. In vitro corrosion testing of titanium surgical implant alloys: an approach to understanding titanium release from implants. J Biomed Mater Res. 1979;13:217–50.
7. Ektessabi AM, Otsuka T, Tsuboi Y, Yokoyama K, Albrektsson T, Sennerby L, Johansson C. Application of micro beam PIXE to detection of titanium ion release from dental and orthopaedic implants. Int J PIXE. 1994;4:81–91.
8. Ducheyne P, Willems G, Martens M, Helsen J. In vivo metal-ion release from porous titanium-fiber material. J Biomed Mater Res. 1984;18:293–308.
9. Healy KE, Ducheyne P. The mechanisms of passive dissolution of titanium in a model physiological environment. J Biomed Mater Res. 1992;26:319–38.
10. Schliephake H, Reiss G, Urban R, Neukam FW, Guckel S. Metal release from titanium fixtures during placement in the mandible: an experimental study. Int J Oral Maxillofac Implants. 1993;8:502–11.
11. Larsson C, Thomsen P, Lausmaa J, Rodahl M, Kasemo B, Ericson LE. Bone response to surface modified titanium implants: studies on electropolished implants with different oxide thicknesses and morphology. Biomaterials. 1994;15:1062–74.
12. Larsson C, Thomsen P, Aronsson BO, Rodahl M, Lausmaa J, Kasemo B, Ericson LE. Bone response to surface-modified titanium implants: studies on the early tissue response to machined and electropolished implants with different oxide thicknesses. Biomaterials. 1996;17:605–16.
13. Hazan R, Brener R, Oron U. Bone growth to metal implants is regulated by their surface chemical properties. Biomaterials. 1993;14:570–4.
14. Kitsugi T, Nakamura T, Oka M, Yan WQ, Goto T, Shibuya T, Kokubo T, Miyaji S. Bone bonding behavior of titanium and its alloys when coated with titanium oxide (TiO_2) and titanium silicate (Ti5Si3). J Biomed Mater Res. 1996;32:149–56.
15. Brunette DM, Tengvall P, Textor M, Thomsen P. Mechanical, thermal, chemical and electrochemical surface treatment of titanium. In: Thomsen P, editor. Titanium in medicine. New York: Springer; 2001. p. 232.
16. Kim HM, Miyaji F, Kokubo T, Nakamura T. Effect of heat treatment on apatite-forming ability of Ti metal induced by alkali treatment. J Mater Sci Mater Med. 1997;8:341–7.
17. Kokubo T, Kim HM, Kawashita M, Nakamura T. Bioactive metal: preparation and properties. J Mater Sci Mater Med. 2004;15:99–107.
18. Sittig C, Textor M, Spencer ND, Wieland M, Vallotton PH. Surface characterization of implant materials c.p. Ti, Ti-6Al-7Nb and Ti-6Al-4 V with different pretreatments. J Mater Sci Mater Med. 1999;10:35–46.
19. Bordji K, Jouzeau JY, Mainard D, Payan E, Netter P, Rie KT, Stucky T, Hage-Ali M. Cytocompatibility of Ti-6Al-4 V and Ti-5Al-2.5Fe alloys according to three surface treatments, using human fibroblasts and osteoblasts. Biomaterials. 1996;17:929–40.
20. Oh HJ, Lee JH, Jeong Y, Kim YJ, Chi CS. Microstructural characterization of biomedical titanium oxide film fabricated by electrochemical method. Surf Coat Technol. 2004;198:247–52.
21. Kim HM, Miyaji F, Kokubo T, Kitsugi T, Nakamura T. Preparation of bioactive titanium and alloys via simple chemical surface treatment. J Biomed Mater Res. 1996;32:409–17.
22. Marino CEB, Nascente PAP, Biaggio SR, Rocha-Filho RC, Bocchi N. XPS characterization of anodic titanium oxide films grown in phosphate buffer solution. Thin Solid Films. 2004;468:109–12.
23. Kokubo T, Kim HM, Kawashita M. Novel bioactive materials with different mechanical properties. Biomaterials. 2003;24:2161–75.
24. Jon.šov L, Müller FA, Helebrant A, Strnad J, Greil P. Hydroxyapatite formation on alkali-treated titanium with different content of Na+ in the surface layer. Biomaterials. 2002;23:3095–101.
25. Yang B, Uchida M, Kim HM, Zhang X, Kukobo T. Preparation of bioactive titanium metal via anodic oxidation treatment. Biomaterials. 2004;25:1003–10.
26. Brunette DM, Tengvall P, Textor M, Thomsen P. Mechanical, thermal, chemical and electrochemical surface treatment of titanium. In: Thomsen P, editor. Titanium in medicine. New York: Springer; 2001. p. 171.
27. Jaeggi C, Kern P, Michler J, Zehnder T, Siegenthaler H. Anodic thin films on titanium used as masks for surface micropatterning of biomedical devices. Surf Coat Technol. 2005;200:1913–9.
28. Chiesa R, Sandrini E, Santin M, Rondelli G, Cigada A. Osteointegration of titanium and its alloys by anodic spark deposition and other electrochemical techniques: a review. J Appl Biomater Biomech. 2003;1:91.
29. Delplancke JL, Winand R. Galvanostatic anodization of titanium – I. Structures and composition of the anodic films. Electrochim Acta. 1973;33:1539–47.
30. Schüpbach P, Glauser R, Rocci A, Martignoni M, Sennerby L, Lundgren A, Gottlow J. The human bone-oxidized titanium implant interface: a light microscopic, scanning electron microscopic, backscatter scanning electron microscopic, and energy-dispersive x-ray study of clinically retrieved dental implants. Clin Implant Dent Relat Res. 2005;7 Suppl 1:S36–43.
31. Sawase T, Jimbo R, Wennerberg A, Suketa N, Tanaka Y, Atsuta M. A novel characteristic of porous titanium oxide implants. Clin Oral Implants Res. 2007;18:680–5.

32. Lausmaa J, Kasemo B, Mattson H. Surface spectroscopic characterization of titanium implant materials. Appl Surf Sci. 1990;44:133–46.
33. Lausmaa J, Kasemo B, Mattson H, Odelius H. Multitechnique surface characterization of oxide films on electropolished and anodically oxidized titanium. Appl Surf Sci. 1990;45:189–200.
34. Park YL, Shin KH, Song HJ. Effects of anodizing conditions on bond strength of anodically oxidized film to titanium substrate. Appl Surf Sci. 2007;253:6013–8.
35. Sul YT. The significance of the surface properties of oxidized titanium to the bone response: special emphasis on potential biochemical bonding of oxidized titanium implant. Biomaterials. 2003;24:3893–907.
36. Hanawa T, Kaga M, Itoh Y, Echizenya T, Oguchi H, Ota M. Cytotoxicities of oxides, phosphates and sulphides of metals. Biomaterials. 1992;13:20–4.
37. Lee JH, Kim SE, Kim YJ, Chi CS, Oh HJ. Effects of microstructure of anodic titania on the formation of bioactive compounds. Mater Chem Phys. 2006;98:39–43.
38. de Sena LA, Rocha NCC, Andrade MC, Soares GA. Bioactivity assessment of titanium sheets electrochemically coated with thick oxide film. Surf Coat Technol. 2003;166:254–8.
39. Sul YT, Johansson CB, Kang Y, Jeon DG, Albrektsson T. Bone reactions to oxidized titanium implants with electrochemical anion sulphuric acid and phosphoric acid incorporation. Clin Implant Dent Relat Res. 2002;4:78–87.
40. Zhu X, Chen J, Scheideler C, Reichl R, Geis-Gerstorfer J. Effects of topography and composition of titanium surface oxides on osteoblast responses. Biomaterials. 2004;25:4087–103.
41. Kurze P, Krysmann W, Schneider HG. Application fields of ANOF layer and composites. Cryst Res Technol. 1986;21:1603–9.
42. Ishizawa H, Ogino M. Mechanical and histological investigation of hydrothermally treated and untreated anodic titanium oxide films containing Ca and P. J Biomed Mater Res. 1995;29:1071.
43. Ishizawa H, Ogino M. Formation and characterization of anodic titanium oxide films containing Ca and P. J Biomed Mater Res. 1995;29:65.
44. Rodriguez R, Kim K, Ong JL. In vitro osteoblast response to anodized titanium and anodized titanium followed by hydrothermal treatment. J Biomed Mater Res A. 2003;65:352–8.
45. Suh JY, Jang BC, Zhu X, Ong JL, Kim K. Effect of hydrothermally treated anodic oxide films on osteoblast attachment and proliferation. Biomaterials. 2003;24:347.
46. Zhu X, Chen J, Scheideler L, Altebaeumer T, Geis-Gerstorfer J, Kern D. Cellular reactions of osteoblasts to micron- and submicron-scale porous structures of titanium surfaces. Cells Tissues Organs. 2004;178:13–22.
47. Zhao G, Zinger O, Schwartz Z, Wieland M, Landolt D, Boyan BD. Osteoblast-like cells are sensitive to submicron-scale surface structure. Clin Oral Implants Res. 2006;17:258–64.
48. Das K, Bose S, Bandyopadhyay A. Surface modifications and cell-materials interactions with anodized Ti. Acta Biomater. 2007;3:573–85.
49. Bronzino JD. Biomedical engineering handbook. New York: CRC Press; 1995. p. 274.
50. Li B, Li Y, Li J, Fu X, Li H, Wang H, Xin S, Zhou L, Liang C, Li C. Influence of nanostructures on the biological properties of Ti implants after anodic oxidation. J Mater Sci Mater Med. 2014;25:199–205.
51. Kim MH, Lee SY, Kim MJ, Kim SK, Heo SJ, Koak JY. Effect of biomimetic deposition on anodized titanium surfaces. J Dent Res. 2011;90:711–6.
52. Giordano C, Saino E, Rimondini L, Pedeferri MP, Visai L, Cigada A, Chiesa R. Electrochemically induced anatase inhibits bacterial colonization on titanium grade 2 and Ti6Al4V alloy for dental and orthopedic devices. Colloids Surf B Biointerfaces. 2011;88:648–55.
53. Kang MK, Moon SK, Kim KM, Kim KN. Antibacterial effect and cytocompatibility of nanostructured TiO(2) film containing Cl. Dent Mater J. 2011;30:790–8.
54. Son WW, Zhu X, Shin HI, Ong JL, Kim KH. In vivo histological response to anodized and anodized/hydrothermally treated titanium implants. J Biomed Mater Res B Appl Biomater. 2003;66B:520–5.
55. Henry P, Tan AE, Allan BP. Removal torque comparison of Tiunite and turned implants in the Greyhound dog mandible. Appl Osseointegration Res. 2000;1:15–7.
56. Sul YT, Johansson CB, Jeong Y, Wennerberg A, Albrektsson T. Resonance frequency and removal torque analysis of implants with turned and anodized surface oxide. Clin Oral Implants Res. 2002;13:252–9.
57. Sul YT, Johansson CB, Roser K, Albrektsson T. Qualitative and quantitative observations of bone tissue reactions to anodized implants. Biomaterials. 2002;23:1809–17.
58. Sul YT, Johansson P, Chang BS, Byon ES, Jeong Y. Bone tissue responses to Mg-incorporated oxidized implants and machine-turned implants in the rabbit femur. J Appl Biomater Biomech. 2005;3:18–28.
59. Jimbo R, Ono D, Hirakawa Y, Odatsu T, Tanaka T, Sawase T. Accelerated photo-induced hydrophilicity promotes osseointegration: an animal study. Clin Implant Dent Relat Res. 2011;13:79–85.
60. Albouy JP, Abrahamsson I, Berglundh T. Spontaneous progression of experimental peri-implantitis at implants with different surface characteristics: an experimental study in dogs. J Clin Periodontol. 2012;39:182–7.
61. Hall J, Lausmaa J. Properties of a new porous oxide surface on titanium implants. Appl Osseointegration Res. 2001;1:5–8.
62. Quirynen M, Van Assche N. RCT comparing minimally with moderately rough implants. Part 2: microbial observations. Clin Oral Implants Res. 2012;23:625–34.
63. Van Assche N, Coucke W, Teughels W, Naert I, Cardoso MV, Quirynen M. RCT comparing minimally with moderately rough implants. Part 1: clinical observations. Clin Oral Implants Res. 2012;23:617–24.

64. Nicu EA, Van Assche N, Coucke W, Teughels W, Quirynen M. RCT comparing implants with turned and anodically oxidized surfaces: a pilot study, a 3-year follow-up. J Clin Periodontol. 2012;39: 1183–90.
65. Jokstad A, Alkumru H. Immediate function on the day of surgery compared with a delayed implant loading process in the mandible: a randomized clinical trial over 5 years. Clin Oral Implants Res. 2013. doi:10.1111/clr.12279 [Epub ahead of print].
66. Jokstad A, Alkumru H. Immediate function on the day of surgery compared with a delayed implant loading process in the mandible: a randomized clinical trial over 5 years. Clin Oral Implants Res. 2013;28:891–5.
67. Sawase T, Wennerberg A, Hallgren C, Miyamoto I, Albrektsson T. Atomic force microscopic study of commercially available implant abutments. Clin Implant Dent Relat Res. 1999;1:92–7.
68. Sawase T, Wennerberg A, Hallgren C, Albrektsson T, Baba K. Chemical and topographical surface analysis of five different implant abutments. Clin Oral Implants Res. 2000;11:44–50.
69. Albrektsson T, Wennerberg A. Oral implant surfaces: part 1–review focusing on topographic and chemical properties of different surfaces and in vivo responses to them. Int J Prosthodont. 2004;17:536–43.
70. Webster TJ, Ejiofor JU. Increased osteoblast adhesion on nanophase metals: Ti, Ti6Al4V, and CoCrMo. Biomaterials. 2004;25:4731–9.
71. Baun WL. Formation of porous films on titanium alloys by anodization. Surf Technol. 1980;11:421–30.
72. Gong D, Grimes CA, Varghese OK, Hu W, Singh RS, Chen Z, Dickey EC. Titanium oxide nanotube arrays prepared by anodic oxidation. J Mater Res. 2001;16:3331–4.
73. Raja KS, Misra M, Paramguru K. Formation of self-ordered nanotubular structure of anodic oxide layer on titanium. Electrochim Acta. 2005;51:154–65.
74. Varkey M, Gittens SA, Uludag H. Growth factor delivery for bone tissue repair: an update. Expert Opin Drug Deliv. 2004;1:19–36.

Novel Surfaces for Clinical Usage: The Use of Dual Acid Etching, a Historical Review, and Current Applications

8

Pär-Olov Östman and Hugo De Bruyn

Abstract

The introduction of dual acid-etched surface led to a change in treatment protocol, predominantly with respect to shortening treatment time. Clinically, implant displayed more predictable outcomes compared to turned surfaces from the same company. Over time, clinicians and industry collaborated to optimize and simplify treatment protocols in order to improve the prognosis in terms of implant survival and peri-implant health. Implant and protocol modifications aimed for shortening the treatment time and widening of the indications for implant treatment in conjunction with improvement of functional as well as aesthetical outcomes. These protocol modifications had the ultimate aim of increasing patient satisfaction. This chapter describes the outcome of dual acid-etched surface alteration in a historical perspective and present finding in terms of implant success and peri-implant outcome. Moreover, modification of the dual acid-etched implant with nanomodified surfaces is described.

Early Implant: Surface Modification

Dental implants were introduced in the 1950s. They consisted of subperiosteal frames, blade implants, or transmandibular devices. At that time, there was no clinical or scientific evidence available to support these treatment protocols. The results were rather poor, although individual successful cases were reported. In the 1960s, Brånemark conducted experimental studies that led to the introduction of the concept of osseointegration [1]. The term was first defined by Albrektsson and coworkers as direct contact between a living bone and an implant at the light microscope level [2]. Later, a more biomechanical definition was suggested, and osseointegration was coined as "a process whereby clinically asymptomatic rigid fixation of alloplastic materials, typically titanium, is achieved and maintained, in bone during functional loading" [3]. During the first era of modern oral implantology, turned (machined) surfaces predominated. This was not a result of extensive surface topography research, but rather an empirical choice based on the

P.-O. Östman, DDS, PhD (✉)
H. De Bruyn, DDS, MSc, PhD
Department Periodontology and Oral Implantology, University of Ghent, University Hospital Dental School, Ghent, Belgium
e-mail: po@holmgatan.se

A. Wennerberg et al. (eds.), *Implant Surfaces and their Biological and Clinical Impact*, DOI 10.1007/978-3-662-45379-7_8, © Springer-Verlag Berlin Heidelberg 2015

extensive animal research followed by the clinical introduction showing that turned titanium implants had the ability to osseointegrate and remain functional with a good prognosis. Brånemark implemented his research findings in clinical dentistry for the treatment of edentulous patients with commercially pure, turned, turned titanium, and screw-shaped implants [4]. The first patient was treated with their approach in Sweden in 1965 and died by the beginning of our new millennium with all original implants still in function. In those days implants were predominantly used for mandibular full-arch rehabilitations, with prolonged submerged healing times. The classic treatment protocol consisted of a two-stage delayed approach, where implants were kept unloaded for several months, allowing a stress-free healing period [4–7]. It was believed that premature loading, compromising direct bone healing, would result in non-integration of the implants. Hence, a second-stage surgery was necessary to uncover the implants prior to assure a transmucosal connection and allow functional loading. In the 1970s, a one-stage delayed treatment protocol was introduced by Schroeder [8]. In this treatment concept, a transmucosal healing abutment is placed immediately after implant installation to secure the connection between the implant and the oral cavity, avoiding a second surgery. Despite this one-stage approach, the Swiss treatment protocol still advocated delayed loading.

The initial success of osseointegrated implants may have been due to treatment being mainly administered at universities with strict protocols [9]. Furthermore, clinicians received extensive preclinical training and courses prior to implant surgery or prosthodontics. Following this strict approach, Brånemark demonstrated 90 % survival rate for implants used to restore edentulous jaws and followed for 5–9 years [10]. Recent studies yield an above 20 years clinical survival rate of 91.5 % when using the turned implants in single-tooth restorations and less than 5 % of the implants showing progressive bone loss over time [11].

Over time, clinicians and industry collaborated to optimize and simplify treatment protocols in order to improve the prognosis in terms of implant survival and peri-implant health. Implant and protocol modifications aimed for shortening the treatment time and to widen the indication for implant treatment in conjunction with improvement of functional as well as aesthetical outcomes. All this was done with the ultimate goal of increasing patient satisfaction.

In this context, it became clear that implants with turned surfaces had lower survival rates when placed in soft bone [12]. It must be noted that in those days no compensatory surgical protocol was used in sites with soft bone. Most likely, an adaptive surgical protocol, employed to achieve an increased primary stability in sites with poor bone quality, would have resulted in fewer implant failures. Others used the approach of undersizing the implant bed and as such enhancing lateral bone compression and increasing initial implant stability. Even when using turned implants, they only reported 3.3 % of implant failure after 3 years of function for immediate loading of edentulous mandibles [13].

One of the earliest strategies to enhance osseointegration was to roughen the implant surface. When compared to the relatively smooth, anisotropic turned titanium surface, a roughened surface was found to increase bone-to-implant contact and to improve the strength of the bone-to-implant interface [14]. From the 1980s on, implant manufacturers developed various techniques for roughening implant surfaces. These included titanium plasma spraying (TPS) [15], grit blasting with titanium dioxide particles [16], and coating with hydroxyapatite (HA) [17]. Histological research showed de novo bone formation on surface-modified implants. In contrast, osseointegration of turned-surface implants mainly was achieved by distance osteogenesis.

While these early surface alterations were effective at improving aspects of osseointegration in terms of bone-to-implant contact and healing response, they often caused unforeseen problems. Mucosal and other peri-implant complications such as delamination of HA coatings were reported for this first generation of roughened dental implants. This led to efforts to better understand the effect of surface roughness on bone biology and on risk assessment for biological complications. Research demonstrated that it was possible to influence the anchorage of implants by altering the surface structure morphology [18]. In this context, Wennerberg and coworkers described and classified surface roughness in a series of animal studies using among others histomorphometry and mechanical testing. These experiments provided clear evidence that the bone response to moderately roughened surfaces was significantly stronger than bone responses to smoother or more rougher ones [19–21].

Modification of Surfaces

Early attempts on additive surface treatments such as TPS or hydroxyapatite coatings were identified as biologically problematic because unexpected bone loss with peri-implant complications occurred due to the surface texture or delamination of the coating [22, 23]. Methods to alter the texture of an implant surface based on surface reduction were explored. One reductive approach to surface roughening is the use of acid etching which yields a complex surface that is isotropic and pitted. The pits are created by removal of grains. Because certain phases and impurities in the titanium surface are more sensitive to the etching process, a selective removal of material occurs. The resulting roughness is dependent on the bulk material, the surface microstructure, the type of acid, and the contact time. Hence changing one or more parameters in this process allows for creating a wide variability of roughness. The commercially available acid-etched surfaces are by and large minimally rough with typical average surface area (Sa) values ranging from 0.3 to 1.0 μm [24].

Dual Acid Etching

The OSSEOTITE® surface, introduced by BIOMET 3i (Palm Beach Gardens, FL, USA) in 1996, is created with a dual-etching process that consecutively involves application of three acids: hydrofluoric acid (HF), hydrochloric acid (HCl), and sulfuric acid (H_2SO_4). The implant is first treated with the hydrofluoric acid, which removes the oxide layer and creates the large-scale (macro) roughness. The hydrochloric and sulfuric acid are then applied, creating the submicron complexity. The OSSEOTITE® surface on a grade IV titanium has an average surface roughness with an Sa value around 0.7 μm and a surface area ratio (Sdr) of 28 % [25] (Fig. 8.1).

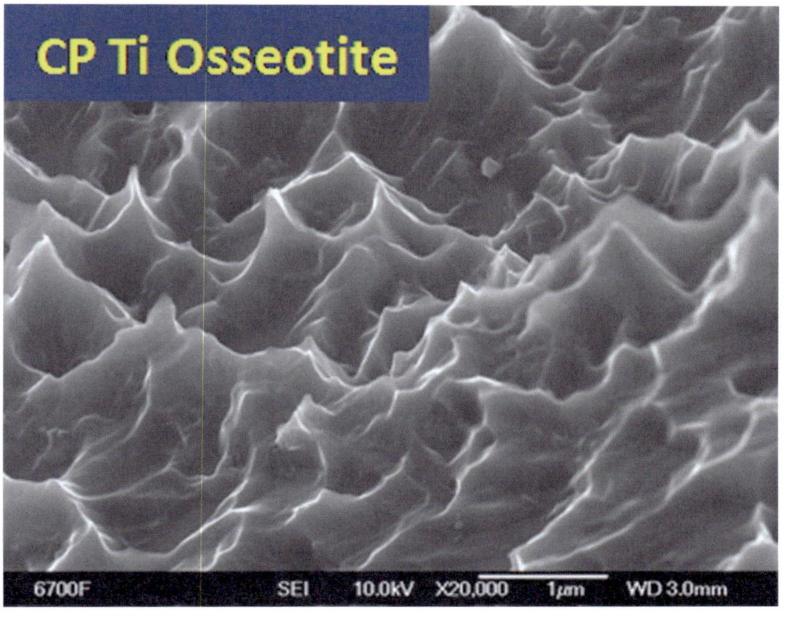

Fig. 8.1 CP grade IV titanium OSSEOTITE® in 20,000× magnification

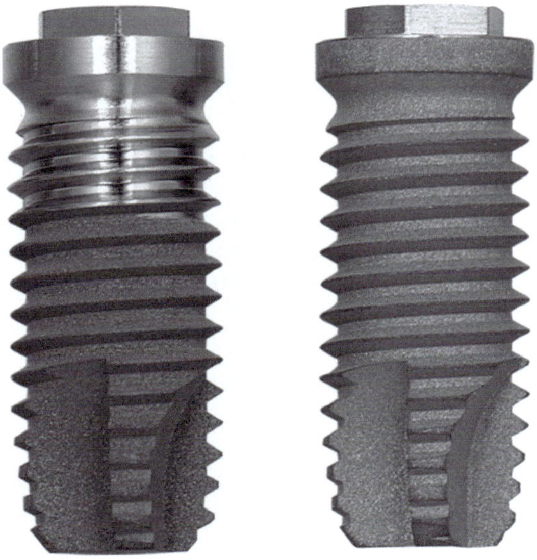

Fig. 8.2 The hybrid and fully OSSEOTITE® implant with dual acid-etched surface

The OSSEOTITE® surface was first commercialized as a hybrid designed implant, with DAE from the implant apex up to approximately the third coronal thread, and had from thereon a turned surface up to the restorative platform (Fig. 8.2). This different surface texture approach was chosen because it was believed it would prevent or decrease the risk for peri-implantitis. Indeed, contemporaneous observations of catastrophic failures of implants with first-generation HA- and TPS-coated surfaces had led to the hypothesis that a rough surface in close contact with the mucosal lining of the peri-implant attachment as found near to the seating platform would contribute to mucosal complications and adverse events. First-generation plasma-sprayed implants were clearly rougher than modern surfaces [26–29].

This hypothesis was strongly influenced by clinical model studies indicating that submucosal or supramucosal initial plaque accumulation and composition was different on smooth versus rough healing abutments [30, 31]. Most of these early studies involved low patient numbers and short follow-up time. As such they did not evaluate the possible occurrence of peri-implantitis but only evaluated plaque accumulation and localized mucosal inflammation. Peri-implantitis defined as peri-implant bone loss and pocket formation with inflammation related to bleeding and/or pus evacuation is known to occur first after some time in situ, and hence it was simply not tested in these short-term studies. Later studies revealed that commercially pure titanium, titanium plasma-sprayed, hydroxyapatite-coated, and acid-etched surface textured implants were equally prone to artificially provoked ligature-induced peri-implantitis with comparable microbial composition and no difference in peri-implant bone loss [32].

The DAE implant was compared to the standard BIOMET 3i turned implant regarding peri-implant soft and hard tissue healing in a dog study. Histomorphometry revealed that the peri-implant soft tissues and the marginal level of bone-to-implant contact were similar for both implants but bone-to-implant contact was significantly larger at the DAE surface [33]. In preclinical studies it was concluded that the mean torque value after 8 weeks of healing was four times greater for DAE-surfaced implants than the mean for turned BIOMET 3i implants [34]. Khang and colleagues presented clinical outcomes from a study evaluating both turned and hybrid DAE implants placed in the same patient, with an outcome of 86.7 % for turned BIOMET 3i surfaced implants and 95 % for DAE implants [35]. In soft bone, the survival rate leapt 10 %, going from 88 to 98 % for a turned versus DAE surface [36]. The introduction of DAE OSSEOTITE® surface led to a change in treatment protocol, predominantly with respect to shortening treatment time. The historically recommended 3–6 months between implant placement and functional loading of implants in respectively mandible and maxilla using a two-stage surgical approach was revised based on human histologic and experimental studies, showing increased bone-to-implant contact with the DAE surface compared to the turned ones. A human histologic study [37] evaluated bone-to-implant contact (BIC) for DAE versus BIOMET 3i turned implant surfaces. Miniscrews with a split-surface design were installed in the posterior maxilla of 11 patients allowing bone-implant biopsies. One side of the implant received the BIOMET 3i DAE surface modification and the opposite side maintained a turned surface. Histologic analysis indicated that the mean BIC value for the OSSEOTITE® (DAE) surfaces (72.96 % ± 25.13 %) was statistically significantly higher ($P<0.05$) than the mean BIC value for the turned surfaces (33.98 % ± 31.04 %). The results of this study indicated that in the poorer quality bone typically found in the posterior maxilla, the DAE surface increased bone contact compared to opposing machined surfaces on the same implant.

A further step in treatment involved the introduction of early loading. A 1-year multicenter clinical trial by Lazzara and coworkers showed that the DAE implant could be safely loaded after 2 months of placement. This early loading study involved 429 OSSEOTITE® implants placed in 155 patients using a one-stage approach and early loading. The cumulative implant survival rate was 98.5 % at 1 year [38]. In a 4-year multicenter study, the cumulative implant survival rate for DAE implants placed with a two-stage protocol was 98.7 %, with a 99.4 % survival rate in the posterior mandible and 98.4 % survival rate in the posterior maxilla. All implant failures occurred prior to loading and were categorized as early implant failures. When the clinical success of implants 10 mm or shorter was compared to that of implants greater than 10 mm in length, the shorter implants performed similarly to longer implants [39]. Later reports of DAE implants loaded within 2 months after surgery in posterior areas of both mandible and maxilla showed cumulative 3-year implant survival rates of 97.5 and 98.4 %, respectively. This again suggested that microtextured OSSEOTITE® implants in the posterior jaws could safely bear functional load applied 2 months after insertion. When the DAE implants were immediately loaded in mandibles, a cumulative survival rate of 98.9 % was achieved for up to 48 months of follow-up, while the prosthetic cumulative survival rate for the same period was 100 %. Marginal bone loss at the immediately loaded implants was within the generally accepted conventional limits for standard delayed loading protocols [40]. Additional human biopsies revealed that under immediate loading the DAE may yield above 78 % of BIC after 4 months [41]. Browaeys and coworkers evaluated immediately loaded implants in fully edentulous maxillae and mandibles. Information was retrospectively retrieved from 83 patients' records with 749 OSSEOTITE® implants supporting immediately loaded semipermanent full-arch restorations. Five hundred sixty-eight (75.8 %) implants were placed in healed bone and 181 (24.2 %) in augmented bone. The latter included sinus lifting and/or onlay/inlay grafts with/without biomaterials and membranes. Implant survival and success based on radiological peri-implant bone loss were registered. The implant survival was 96.8 % in the maxilla and 98.8 % in the mandible which is in line with the current evidence that immediate loading has become a predictable treatment procedure provided implant stability is sufficient and cross-arch stabilization of the implants is realized by means of a rigidly connected and screw-retained rehabilitation. Figure 8.3 gives an overview of all the radiographic bone level measurements in relation to function time [42], and Fig. 8.4 shows bone level changes of 100 immediately loaded DAE implants up to 5 years indicative of crestal bone stability after 2 years.

Hybrid Dual Acid-Etched to Fully Etched Design

The recognition of the DAE surface's benefits with respect to clinical outcome compared to the turned BIOMET 3i surface, improved implant survival in compromised bone, and faster and increased osseointegration lead to a challenging interest to further extend the DAE surface further coronally up to the seating platform. The potential benefits of having the DAE surface complexity on the entire implant surface in contact with bone were weighed against the possibility of increasing the incidence of peri-implantitis. A series of animal investigations were initiated in beagle dogs to further elucidate the safety of the roughened surface when in contact with the peri-implant soft tissue lining. Abrahamsson and

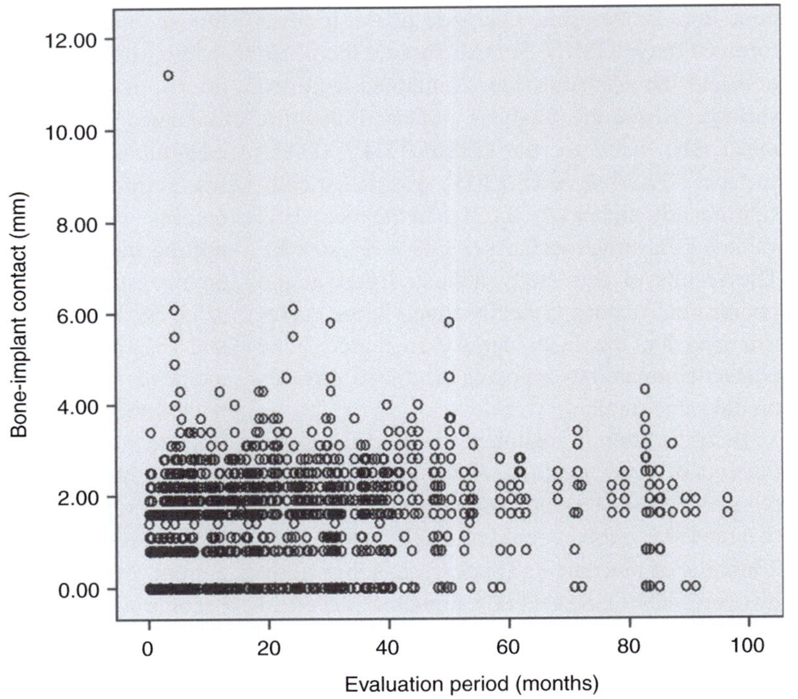

Fig. 8.3 Overview of bone level measurements of 749 immediately loaded DAE implants in relation to function time (From Browaeys et al. [42] © 2011 Wiley Periodicals, Inc. Reprinted with permission)

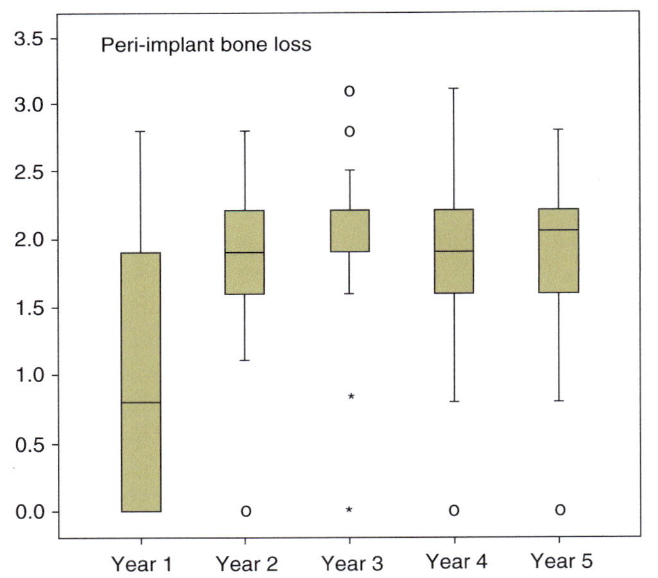

Fig. 8.4 The bone level changes over time for 100 immediately loaded DAE implants, whereby from all time point's radiographs were available for crestal bone level evaluation (From De Bruyn et al. [73]. © 2013 John Wiley & Sons A/S. Reprinted with permission)

coworkers [43] performed an experiment to study the composition of the soft tissue barrier that formed to turn or DAE surface healing abutments. At the end of a 6-month period during which proper plaque control had been maintained, biopsies including the implant and the surrounding soft and hard tissues were obtained. The attachment between the peri-implant mucosa and abutment was similar from both a quantitative and a qualitative aspect. The attachment comprised a barrier epithelium and a zone of connective tissue attachment of similar dimension, and hence it was concluded that soft tissue attachment that formed was not influenced by the roughness of the titanium surface. A similar experiment, but with 6 months plaque accumulation, resulted in the establishment of an inflammatory lesion in the connective tissue of the peri-implant mucosa that did not differ between DAE or turned abutments within respect to location, size, and cell composition. Hence it was concluded that the different surface characteristics failed to influence plaque formation and inflammatory response in the peri-implant mucosa [44].

To assess the risk for peri-implantitis, a long-term randomized-controlled multicenter study of hybrid versus full OSSEOTITE® implants was designed. In that study, the control implants had the hybrid design, while the entire surface of the test implants received the DAE treatment. All implants were placed in a one-stage surgical approach, and prosthetic rehabilitation was in function 6 weeks after surgery with insertion of a provisional restoration. Final prostheses were delivered within 6 months and followed for up to 5 years. A declaration of peri-implantitis included scoring all of the following criteria: severe mucositis with positive findings of bleeding and/or suppuration upon probing, a probing depth increase measuring greater than 5 mm, and crestal bone loss that was progressive, i.e., greater than 5 mm and confirmed by radiography. The outcome of the study after 5 years with 139 control and 165 test implants showed one implant being declared as having peri-implantitis (0.7 %) with none of the fully etched implants showing an increased risk. For both groups, there were no increases in probing depths, besides the infected control implant, greater than or equal to 3 mm. Zetterqvist and coworkers demonstrated that the fully etched surface reduced crestal bone loss compared to the hybrid design (0.6 mm versus 1.0 mm, $P < 0.0001$) [45]. This result was consistent with the 2009 1-year results of Baldi et al. [46], who found a statistically significant reduction in bone loss for fully etched versus hybrid implants (0.6 mm versus 1.5 mm, $P < 0.02$). The DAE surface performs well in more challenging treatment protocols. Prospective multicenter studies on immediate loading showed results ranging from 98.5 to 99.4 % survival rate [38, 40, 47–50]. Galli and coworkers reported a randomized-controlled, prospective, multicenter study on a group of 52 OSSEOTITE® implants loaded at 2 months (early) and a group of 52 implants loaded within 48 h [49]. Periapical radiographs were taken at implant placement and 2, 8, and 14 months afterward to determine marginal bone level changes. Soft tissue stability (height of the clinical crown) was measured on plaster casts poured from alginate impressions taken at 8 and 14 months. After 14 months, crestal bone loss for both groups averaged 1.1 mm, and there were no statistically significant changes in soft tissue parameters from the baseline.

Dual Acid-Etched Surface with Discrete Crystalline Deposition (DCD)

With the different surface modifications, the traditional Brånemark protocol slowly evolved. The change from a two-stage to a one-stage surgical approach, accelerated loading protocols, and later immediate loading dramatically reduced the discomfort and inconvenience experienced by patients undergoing implant treatment.

To further enhance early osseointegration, the application of nanometer-scale crystals of calcium phosphate (CaP) onto the DAE surface was investigated in early 2000. Such crystals were deposited with coverage of approximately 50 % of the OSSEOTITE® surface's peaks and valleys (Fig. 8.5).

In contrast to plasma-sprayed surfaces that can show as many as 20,000 μg of CaP, the newer discrete crystalline deposition (DCD) process deposits less than 20 μg of CaP on the DAE surface. This process increases the surface area by approximately 200 %, providing greater complexity, which may play a role in early bone formation. A series of animal studies evaluating the contribution of the CaP nanocrystals to enhancing

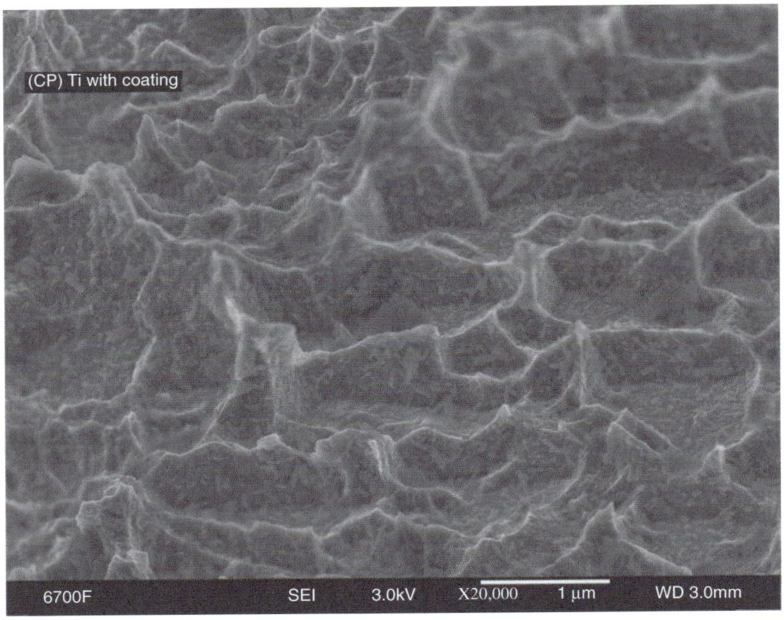

Fig. 8.5 CP grade IV titanium NanoTite™ in 20,000× magnification

the DAE surface has shown entirely positive outcomes for the combination of DAE and DCD. After 2 weeks of healing, the DAE surface exhibited 25 % linear contact, whereas the DAE/DCD surface showed more than 50 % linear bone-to-implant contact. Biomechanical studies indicate that the DAE/DCD surface's effect takes place early in the bone-healing process. This could positively affect implant-treatment outcomes, as a reduction in time before new bone is formed on the surface might reduce the decrease in stability typically observed shortly after implant placement. Two weeks after placement in rabbit tibias, bullet-shaped DAE/DCD implants required forces 189 % greater than those required to detach DAE control implants [51]. This suggests that the effects are occurring early in the osseointegration process when de novo bone formation is most susceptible to micromotion. Nishimura and colleagues [52] demonstrated the early fixation properties of the same nanosurface in a rat push-in model, with the ability to resist mechanical loads increasing by 76 % after 2 weeks. Further fixation studies corroborate these findings, demonstrating forces required to disrupt nanosurfaced implants at 9 days in a rat model to be more than 450 % greater than that for non-coated control implants. These high percentages of detachment force actually represent the force needed to break the bone, as the implant/bone interface was still intact. Histological and histomorphometric outcomes of nanotopographic implants placed in humans in comparison to those with dual-etched surfaces also demonstrated significant effects [53]. Using a previously described model, Orsini and colleagues placed custom 2 × 10 mm site-evaluation implants (SEIs) in posterior maxillae of 15 patients and measured bone-to-implant contact (BIC) after 2 months of healing [54]. The results showed a 70 % increase in BIC of the nanosurface in comparison with the control surface and were statistically significant. Further human histomorphometric investigations using a similar protocol measured a 194 % increase in BIC on SEIs at 4 weeks and a 148 % increase at 8 weeks for the nanosurface in comparison to control surfaces [53]. The results of these preclinical and human histomorphometric studies indicate that the nanosurface-mediated effects occur early.

Good clinical outcomes have been reported for NanoTite™ PREVAIL implants (BIOMET 3i). In Glibert et al.'s follow-up evaluation (mean 6.2 years; range 5.4–9.8 years) of 122 NanoTite™

PREVAIL implants, one implant had failed early, presenting an overall cumulative survival rate of 99.2 %. Average mean bone loss for the 121 surviving implants was 0.31 mm (SD 0.54). This study also found few mucosal complications, a low incidence of peri-implant infections, and stable bone levels [55]. Martens and coworkers evaluated 33 periodontally compromised patients in a prospective 5-year follow-up clinical study whereby immediate loading was performed in edentulous maxillae or mandibles. In total 163 implants (130 in the maxilla and 33 in the mandible) were placed whereof 132 were NanoTite™ and 31 were OSSEOTITE®. The survival rate was 96.3 % and the mean crestal bone loss was 1.6 mm for the whole group. The mean overall and interproximal probing depths were 3.4 and 3.6 mm, respectively. Only 4.6 % of the implants had a mean interproximal probing depth of more than 5 mm. Only 6 % of the implants were detected with peri-implantitis based on total bone loss from the day of surgery of more than 2 mm and probing depths above 4 mm. The bone loss around full DAE implants without or with discrete deposition of Cap was respectively 1.56 and 1.40 mm when pairwise compared within 11 patients who had both implants in equal number. This difference was not statistically significant ($P = 0.68$). The authors concluded that NanoTite™ and OSSEOTITE® implants without a gradient in surface roughness did not appear to be prone to peri-implant disease [56].

During the last decade, implant treatment has progressed from the traditional two-stage surgical protocol with long healing times to accelerated loading protocols. This change coincided with the shift from minimally to moderately rough surface textured implants to implants designed with macro-, micro-, and nanosurface modification. Besides a better biologic understanding of the concept of osseointegration and more clinical expertise in daily clinical practice, implant components have been improved to perform in a predictable way under challenging clinical situations. The tapered implant design has grown in popularity and is used today mainly because of a standardized drill protocol with ability to gain good primary stability. Good primary stability is one of the most important factors when applying immediate loading and is based on torque resistance during implant placement. An insertion torque of 30–40 Ncm before the implant is fully seated seems to be a good indicator that the implant has reached sufficient stability for immediate loading. Implant surface topography may be another important factor for proper integration in challenging situations, such as immediate loading. The minimally rough surface NanoTite™ (BIOMET 3i, Palm Beach Gardens, FL, USA) featuring nanotopography with calcium phosphate nanoparticles added to the dual acid-etched titanium surface was presented in 2007. Only limited information is available on short- and long-term outcome of immediately loaded tapered implants, and to the knowledge of the authors, no information specifically on NanoTite™ Tapered implants is currently available [57]. With regard to surface topography, several studies have reported an improved survival rate for moderately rough implants, especially in demanding conditions such as poor quality bone compared with turned [58, 59]. Furthermore, the introduction of nanotechnology to implant surfaces may enhance the osteoconductivity of the implant which is the assumed reason why many implant producers have presented nanotopographically altered surfaces [60]. Theoretically, the bioactive topographical feature, which enhances the initial osseointegration cascade, may enhance implant success [60–62]. Additionally, the difference in peri-implant bone loss between implants with a different surface topography and design has been evaluated. The clinical outcome of the immediately loaded normal-diameter implants with a provisional bridge has not been published yet but is discussed below.

OSSEOTITE® and NanoTite™ implants were placed in a split jaw study to allow comparison of both surfaces within the same patient. From the boxplot one can see that a few implants lost more bone than accepted. There was no significant difference in bone loss between implants with an OSSEOTITE® or NanoTite™ topography. This is in agreement with earlier studies of Hinze et al. and Tealdo

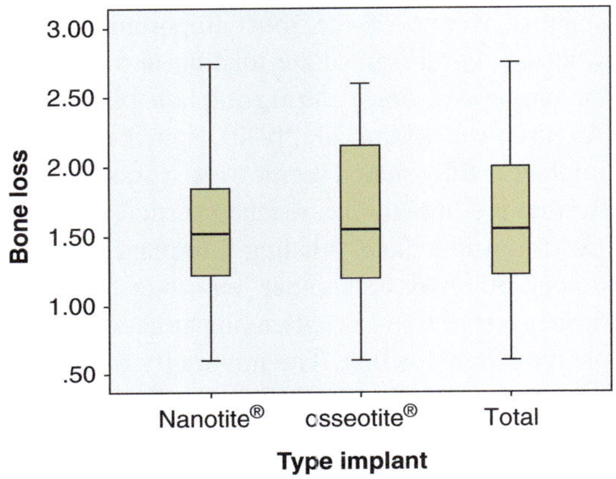

Fig. 8.6 Boxplot showing bone loss expressed in mm and divided in 25 % percentile range at the final examination. The total group ($n=44$) split up in both OSSEOTITE® ($n=22$) and NanoTite™ ($n=22$) surfaces is given. In the total material, 75 % of all implants have bone loss below 2 mm

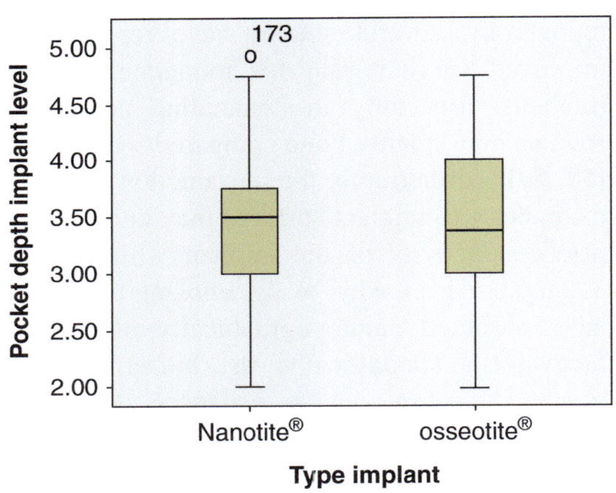

Fig. 8.7 The probing depth (mm) around each implant

et al. [63, 64]. The mean bone loss on 22 OSSEOTITE® (1.56 mm) and 22 NanoTite™ (1.40 mm) implants was pairwise compared in 11 patients who had both implants in equal number and was not statistically significantly different ($P=0.68$) (Fig. 8.6).

The mean overall and interproximal probing depths were 3.5 mm (range 2–5; SD 0.72) and 3.7 mm (range 3.0–6 5.5; SD 0.73), respectively (Fig. 8.7). Seventy-five percent of all implants had a mean probing depth below 4 mm and only 2.3 % had a probing depth above 5 mm. Despite the stable bone condition and low probing depths, sulcus bleeding was present around 66 % of the implants on one or more sites but only one implant presented with pus. 45.5 % of the implants showed plaque accumulation in contact with the mucosal tissues explaining the high mucositis prevalence, the consequence of an imperfect oral hygiene level. There was no difference in peri-implant health between the two surfaces. If one takes 5 mm as a threshold level for acceptable marginal bone loss, as recently suggested by the International Team for Implantology consensus conference [65], only 2.3 % of the implants were diagnosed with peri-implantitis.

Grit-Blasted and DAE/DCD Implant Surfaces

The majority of dental implants in use today are moderately rough at the micro level, with a Sa value in the range of 1–2 μm. One way of increasing the roughness but retaining the documented effect of DAE is to first grit blast the surface and then etch it to obtain a dual surface roughness and remove any embedded blasting particles. The etching also reduces the highest peaks while creating smaller pits, leading to a more complex surface texture. Clinical comparative studies have shown a tendency toward better clinical results with moderately roughened surfaces than minimally rough ones, e.g., less than 1 μm Sa. However, this difference is seldom significant, except in compromised bone sites [60]. Östman and coworkers showed excellent short-term results for immediately loaded NanoTite™ PREVAIL and Tapered implants with a Sa value of under 0.4 μm [57, 66]. Cordioli et al. reported no benefits by increasing coarse surface roughness at 5 weeks in a rabbit reverse-torque (RTQ) model, specifically demonstrating that a dual acid-etched surface (minimally rough) had significantly higher RTQ values than grit blasted (moderately rough) and plasma sprayed (rough) [67]. These findings are consistent with those of Klokkevold et al., who measured reverse torque (RTQ) for dual acid-etched and moderately rough-surfaced implants 1 month after placement in rabbit tibias [68]. The latter study included additional time points for testing reverse torque and showed that the rougher-surfaced implants had significantly higher RTQ results at 2 and 3 months after placement. The authors attributed the higher RTQ to the moderately rough surfaces' increased depth of topography and subsequent void volume, which permitted additional bone ingrowth for mechanical interlocking.

In recent years, studies on submicron, micron, and coarse roughness properties have been presented. It seems that all three layers play an important role in overall osseointegration, with each layer addressing bone formation at different time points. In vitro studies have evaluated the surface topography effects on bone formation through osteoconduction, including the steps of protein absorption, fibrin clot retention, and platelet interaction [69–72]. For example, Davies reported that enhanced surface topographies, due to blasting or acid etching, displayed significantly greater fibrin-retention forces than machined surfaces [71]. Kikuchi et al. have documented that microtopographic surfaces, defined as those exhibiting features in the scale range of platelets (≤3 μm), displayed greater platelet activation than smoother surfaces [69].

The new T3 implant (BIOMET 3i) (Fig. 8.8) has a surface (Fig. 8.9) addressing different aspects of osseointegration and peri-implant health. The coronal aspect of the implant has a microtopography similar to the fully etched OSSEOTITE® implant, consisting of submicron features superimposed on 1–3 μm pitting, overlaid on a minimally rough surface topography (Sa <1.0 μm). From the base of the collar to the apical tip, the T3 implant has greater roughness. The resulting trilevel surface consists of submicron features of CaP nanoparticles superimposed on 1–3 μm pitting, overlaid on a moderately rough surface topography (Sa ~1.4 μm).

The apical surface is designed to enhance osseointegration. As such, the included surface features have been researched to assess their potential impacts on de novo bone formation and the strength of the resulting bone-to-implant interface at different time points: nanoroughness to initiate osseointegration, DAE for the next osseointegrative time point, and course micron features for long-term bone locking. Preliminary clinical results are promising in different bone qualities and locations. However, further follow-up is needed before definitive conclusions can be drawn about this implant surface.

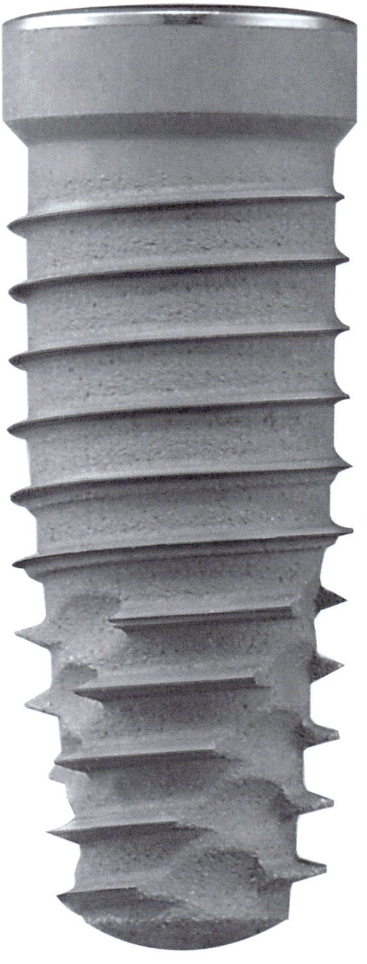

Fig. 8.8 The novel 3i T3 implant from BIOMET 3i with a hybrid design: grit blasted/DAE in the apical portion and DAE in the coronal portion. ©BIOMET 3i

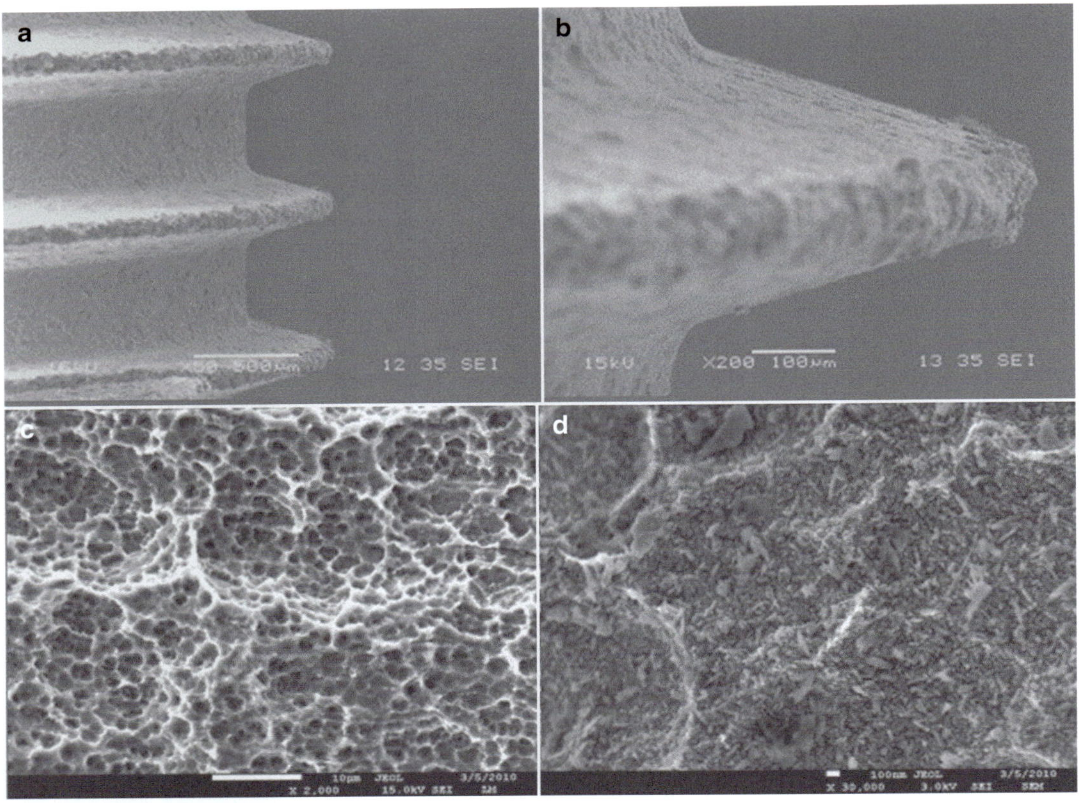

Fig. 8.9 The 3i T3 implant surface in different magnification (**a**) 50×, (**b**)100×, (**c**) 2,000×, (**d**) 30,000×. ©BIOMET 3i

References

1. Brånemark PI, Adell R, Breine U, Hansson BO, Lindstrom J, Ohlsson A. Intra-osseous anchorage of dental prostheses. I. Experimental studies. Scand J Plast Reconstr Surg. 1969;3:81–100.
2. Albrektsson T, Brånemark PI, Hansson HA, Lindström J. Osseointegrated titanium implants. Requirements for ensuring a long-lasting, direct bone anchorage in man. Acta Orthop Scand. 1981;52:155–70.
3. Zarb G, Albrektsson T. Osseointegration – a requiem for the periodontal ligament? – An editorial. Int J Periodont Restor Dent. 1991;11:88–91.
4. Brånemark PI, Hansson BO, Adell R, Breine U, Lindstrom J, Hallen O, et al. Osseointegrated implants in the treatment of the edentulous jaw. Experience from a 10 year period. Scand J Plast Reconstr Surg Suppl. 1977;16:1–132.
5. Adell R, Lekholm U, Rockler B, Branemark PI. A 15 year study of osseointegrated implants in the treatment of the edentulous jaw. Int J Oral Surg. 1981;10: 387–416.
6. Schnitman PA, Wohrle PS, Rubenstein JE, Da Silva JD, Wang NH. Ten-year results for Branemark implants loaded with fixed prostheses at implant placement. Int J Oral Maxillofac Implants. 1997;12:495–503.
7. Ericsson I, Johansson CB, Bystedt H, Norton MR. A histomorphometric evaluation of bone-to-implant contact on machine-prepared and roughened titanium dental implants. A pilot study in the dog. Clin Oral Implants Res. 1994;5(4):202–6.
8. Schroeder A. The Herskovits implant. Preliminary report on a new implantation method. SSO Schweiz Monatsschr Zahnheilkd. 1974;84:742–7.
9. Albrektsson T, Zarb G. The Brånemark osseointegrated implant. Chicago: Quintessence Publishing Co; 1989. ISBN 0-86715-208-7.
10. Brånemark PI. Osseointegration and its experimental background. J Prosthet Dent. 1983;50(3):399–410.
11. Dierens M, Vandeweghe S, Kisch J, Nilner K, De Bruyn H. Long-term follow-up of turned single implants placed in periodontally healthy patients after 16–22 years: radiographic and peri-implant outcome. Clin Oral Implants Res. 2012;23(2):197–204.
12. Jaffin RA, Berman CL. The excessive loss of Brånemark fixtures in type IV bone: a 5-year analysis. J Periodontol. 1991;62(1):2–4.
13. Van de Velde T, Collaert B, De Bruyn H. Immediate loading in the completely edentulous mandible: tech-

nical procedure and clinical results up to 3 years of functional loading. Clin Oral Implants Res. 2007;18: 295–303.
14. Wennerberg A, Albrektsson T. Effects of titanium surface topography on bone integration: a systematic review. Clin Oral Implants Res. 2009;20 Suppl 4:172–8.
15. Buser D, Weber HP, Lang NP. Tissue integration of non-submerged implants. 1-year results of a prospective study with 100 ITI hollow-cylinder and hollow-screw implants. Clin Oral Implants Res. 1990;1(1): 33–40.
16. Ericsson I, Randow K, Glantz PO, Lindhe J, Nilner K. Clinical and radiographical features of submerged and nonsubmerged titanium implants. Clin Oral Implants Res. 1994;5:185–9.
17. Block MS, Kent JN, Kay JF. Evaluation of hydroxylapatite-coated titanium dental implants in dogs. J Oral Maxillofac Surg. 1987;45(7):601–7.
18. Gotfredsen K, Wennerberg A, Johansson C, Skovgaard LT, Hjørting-Hansen E. Anchorage of TiO2-blasted, HA-coated, and machined implants: an experimental study with rabbits. J Biomed Mater Res. 1995;29(10):1223–31.
19. Wennerberg A, Albrektsson T, Andersson B. An animal study of c.p. titanium screws with different surface topographies. J Mater Sci Mater Med. 1995;6: 302–9.
20. Wennerberg A, Albrektsson T, Andersson B, Krol J. A histomorphometric and removal torque study of screw-shaped titanium implants with three different surface topographies. Clin Oral Implant Res. 1996;6: 24–30.
21. Wennerberg A, Ektessabi A, Albrektsson T, Johansson C, Andersson B. A 1-year follow-up of implants of differing surface roughness placed in rabbit bone. J Oral Maxillofac Implants. 1997;12:486–94.
22. Biesbrock AR, Edgerton M. Evaluation of the clinical predictability of hydroxyapatite-coated endosseous dental implants: a review of the literature. Int J Oral Maxillofac Implants. 1995;10:712–20.
23. Liao H, Fartash B, Li J. Stability of hydroxyapatite-coatings on titanium oral implants (IMZ). 2 retrieved cases. Clin Oral Implants Res. 1997;8:68–72.
24. Ballo A, Omar O, Xia W, Palmquist A. Dental implant surfaces – physicochemical properties, biological performance, and trends, implant dentistry – a rapidly evolving practice. In: Turkyilmaz I, editor. ISBN: 978-953-307-658-4, InTech 2011.
25. Sul YT, Byon E, Wennerberg A. Surface characteristics of electrochemically oxidized implants and acid-etched implants: surface chemistry, morphology, pore configurations, oxide thickness, crystal structure, and roughness. Int J Oral Maxillofac Implants. 2008;23(4):631–40.
26. Block MS, Gardiner D, Kent JN, Misiek DJ, Finger IM, Guerra L. Hydroxyapatite-coated cylindrical implants in the posterior mandible: 10-year observations. Int J Oral Maxillofac Implants. 1996;11(5):626–33.
27. Hanisch O, Cortella CA, Boskovic MM, James RA, Slots J, Wikesjö UM. Experimental peri-implant tissue breakdown around hydroxyapatite-coated implants. J Periodontol. 1997;68(1):59–66.
28. Piattelli A, Cosci F, Scarano A, Trisi P. Localized chronic suppurative bone infection as a sequel of peri-implantitis in a hydroxyapatite-coated dental implant. Biomaterials. 1995;16(12):917.
29. Becker W, Becker B, Ricci A. A prospective multicenter trial comparing one- and two stage titanium screw shaped fixtures with one-staged plasma sprayed solid-screw fixtures. Clin Implant Dent Relat Res. 2000;2:159–65.
30. Quirynen M, Bollen CM. The influence of surface roughness and surface-free energy on supra- and subgingival plaque formation in man. A review of the literature. J Clin Periodontol. 1995;22(1):1–14.
31. Quirynen M, van der Mei HC, Bollen CM, Schotte A, Marechal M, Doornbusch GI, Naert I, Busscher HJ, van Steenberghe D. An in vivo study of the influence of the surface roughness of implants on the microbiology of supra- and subgingival plaque. J Dent Res. 1993;72(9):1304–9.
32. Shibli JA, Martins MC, Lotufo RF, Marcantonio Jr E. Microbiologic and radiographic analysis of ligature-induced peri-implantitis with different dental implant surfaces. Int J Oral Maxillofac Implants. 2003;18(3):383–90.
33. Abrahamsson I, Zitzmann NU, Berglundh T, Wennerberg A, Lindhe J. Bone and soft tissue integration to titanium implants with different surface topography: an experimental study in the dog. Int J Oral Maxillofac Implants. 2001;16(3):323–32.
34. Klokkevold PR, Nishimura RD, Adashi M, Caputo AM. Osseointegration enhanced by chemical etching of the titanium surface. A torque removal study in the rabbit. Clin Oral Implants Res. 1997;8:442–7.
35. Khang W, Feldman S, Hawley CE, Gunsolley J. A multi-center study comparing dual acid-etched and machined-surfaced implants in various bone qualities. J Periodontol. 2001;72(10):1384–90.
36. Stach RM, Kohles SS. A meta-analysis examining the clinical survivability of machined-surfaced and Osseotite® implants in poor-quality bone. Implant Dent. 2003;12(1):87–96.
37. Lazzara RJ, Testori T, Trisi P, Porter SS, Weinstein RL. A human histologic analysis of Osseotite® and machined surfaces using implants with 2 opposing surfaces. Int J Periodontics Restorative Dent. 1999;19(2):117–29.
38. Lazzara RJ, Porter SS, Testori T, Galante J, Zetterqvist L. A prospective multicenter study evaluating loading of Osseotite® implants two months after placement: one-year results. J Esthet Dent. 1998;10(6):280–9.
39. Testori T, Wiseman L, Woolfe S, Porter SS. A prospective multicenter clinical study of the Osseotite® implant: four-year interim report. Int J Oral Maxillofac Implants. 2001;16(2):193–200.
40. Testori T, Del Fabbro M, Szmukler-Moncler S, Francetti L, Weinstein RL. Immediate occlusal loading of Osseotite® implants in the completely edentulous mandible. Int J Oral Maxillofac Implants. 2003;18:544–51.

41. Testori T, Szmukler-Moncler S, Francetti L, Del Fabbro M, Scarano A, Piattelli A, Weinstein RL. Immediate loading of Osseotite® implants: a case report and histologic analysis after 4 months of occlusal loading. Int J Periodontics Restorative Dent. 2001;21(5):451–9.
42. Browaeys H, Defrancq J, Dierens MC, Miremadi R, Vandeweghe S, Van de Velde T, De Bruyn H. A retrospective analysis of early and immediately loaded Osseotite® implants in cross-arch rehabilitations in edentulous maxillas and mandibles up to 7 years. Clin Implant Dent Relat Res. 2013;15(3):380–9. Epub 2011 Jul 11.
43. Abrahamsson I, Zitzmann NU, Berglundh T, Linder E, Wennerberg A, Lindhe J. The mucosal attachment to titanium implants with different surface characteristics: an experimental study in dogs. J Clin Periodontol. 2002;29(5):448–55.
44. Zitzmann NU, Abrahamsson I, Berglundh T, Lindhe J. Soft tissue reactions to plaque formation at implant abutments with different surface topography. An experimental study in dogs. J Clin Periodontol. 2002;29(5):456–61.
45. Zetterqvist L, Feldman S, Rotter B, Vincenzi G, Wennström JL, Chierico A, Stach RM, Kenealy JN. A prospective, multicenter, randomized-controlled 5-year study of hybrid and fully etched implants for the incidence of peri-implantitis. J Periodontol. 2010;81(4):493–501.
46. Baldi D, et al. Plaque accumulation on exposed titanium surfaces and peri-implant tissue behavior: a preliminary one-year clinical study. Int J Prosthodont. 2009;22(4):447–55.
47. Ibanez JC, Tahhan MJ, Zamar JA, Menendez AB, Juaneda AM, Zamar NJ, Monqaut JL. Immediate occlusal loading of double acid-etched surface titanium implants in 41 consecutive full-arch cases in the mandible and maxilla: 6- to 74-month results. J Periodontol. 2005;76:1972–81.
48. Sullivan D, Vincenzi G, Feldman S. Early loading of Osseotite® implants after placement in the maxilla and mandible: a five-year report. Int J Oral Maxillofac Implants. 2005;20:905–12.
49. Galli F, Capelli M, Zuffetti F, Testori T, Esposito M. Immediate non-occlusal versus early loading of dental implants in partially edentulous patients: a multicentre randomized clinical trial. Periimplant bone and soft-tissue levels. Clin Oral Implants Res. 2008;19:546–52.
50. Testori T, Meltzer A, Del Fabbro M, Zuffetti F, Troiano M, Weinstein RL. Immediate occlusal loading of Osseotite® implants in the lower edentulous jaw. A multicenter prospective study. Clin Oral Implants Res. 2004;15:278–84.
51. Kenealy JN, Stach RM, Berckmans B. Nanometer-scale CaP enhances early implant-bone fixation in an animal model. Clin Oral Implants Res. 2006;17:cxxi.
52. Nishimura I, Huang Y, Butz F, Ogawa T, Lin A, Wang CJ. Discrete deposition of hydroxyapatite nanoparticles on a titanium implant with predisposing substrate microtopography accelerated osseointegration. Nanotechnology. 2007;18(24).
53. Goené RJ, Testori T, Trisi P. Influence of a nanometer-scale surface enhancement on de novo bone formation on titanium implants: a histomorphometric study in human maxillae. Int J Periodontics Restor Dent. 2007;3:210–9.
54. Orsini G, Piattelli M, Scarano A, et al. Randomized, controlled histologic and histomorphometric evaluation of implants with nanometer-scale calcium phosphate added to the dual acid-etched surface in the human posterior maxilla. J Periodontol. 2007;78:209–18.
55. Glibert M, Östman PO, De Bruyn H. Immediate-loading of NanoTite™ PREVAIL implants: six-year evaluation of radiographic, clinical and mucosal outcomes. Int J Oral Maxillofac Implants. Accepted for publication 2014.
56. Martens F, Vandeweghe S, Browaeys H, De Bruyn H. Peri-implant outcome of immediately loaded OSSEOTITE® and NanoTite™ implants with a fully arched implant fixed denture: a 5-year prospective case series. Int J Periodontics Restorative Dent. 2014;34:189–97.
57. Ostman PO, Wennerberg A, Ekestubbe A, Albrektsson T. Immediate occlusal loading of NanoTite™ ™ tapered implants: a prospective 1-year clinical and radiographic study. Clin Implant Dent Relat Res. 2013;15(6):809–18.
58. Buser D, Weber HP, Bragger U, Balsiger C. Tissue integration of one-stage ITI implants: 3-year results of a longitudinal study with Hollow-Cylinder and Hollow-Screw implants. Int J Oral Maxillofac Implants. 1991;6:405–12.
59. Weng D, Jacobson Z, Tarnow D, Hurzeler MB, Faehn O, Sanavi F, Barkvoll P, Stach RM. A prospective multicenter clinical trial of 3i machined-surface implants: results after 6 years of follow-up. Int J Oral Maxillofac Implants. 2003;18:417–23.
60. Wennerberg A, Albrektsson T. On implant surfaces: a review of current knowledge and opinions. Int J Oral Maxillofac Implants. 2010;25:63–74.
61. Mertens C, Steveling HG. Early and immediate loading of titanium implants with fluoride-modified surfaces: results of 5-year prospective study. Clin Oral Implants Res. 2011;22:1354–60.
62. Ostman PO, Hupalo M, del Castillo R, Emery RW, Cocchetto R, Vincenzi G, Wagenberg B, Vanassche B, Valentin A, Clausen G, Hogan P, Goene R, Evans C, Testori T. Immediate provisionalization of NanoTite™ implants in support of single-tooth and unilateral restorations: one-year interim report of a prospective, multicenter study. Clin Implant Dent Relat Res. 2010;12 Suppl 1:e47–55.
63. Hinze M, Thalmair T, Bolz W, Wachtel H. Immediate loading of fixed provisional prostheses using four implants for the rehabilitation of the edentulous arch: a prospective clinical study. Int J Oral Maxillofac Implants. 2010;25:1011–8.
64. Tealdo T, Bevilacqua M, Pera F, Menini M, Ravera G, Drago C, Pera P. Immediate function with fixed

implant-supported maxillary dentures: a 12-month pilot study. J Prosthet Dent. 2008;99:351–60.
65. Heitz-Mayfield LJ, Needleman I, Salvi GE, Pjetursson BE. Consensus statements and clinical recommendations for prevention and management of biologic and technical implant complications. Int J Oral Maxillofac Implants. 2014;29 Suppl:346-50. doi: 10.11607/jomi.2013.g5.
66. Ostman PO, Wennerberg A, Albrektsson T. Immediate occlusal loading of NanoTite™ PREVAIL implants: a prospective 1-year clinical and radiographic study. Clin Implant Dent Relat Res. 2010;12(1):39–47.
67. Cordioli G, Majzoub Z, Piattelli A, Scarano A. Removal torque and histomorphometric investigation of 4 different titanium surfaces: an experimental study in the rabbit tibia. Int J Oral Maxillofac Implants. 2000;15(5):668–74.
68. Klokkevold PR, Johnson P, Dadgostari S, Caputo A, Davies JE, Nishimura RD. Early endosseous integration enhanced by dual acid etching of titanium: a torque removal study in the rabbit. Clin Oral Implants Res. 2001;12(4):350–7.
69. Kikuchi L, Park JY, Victor C, Davies JE. Platelet interactions with calcium phosphate-coated surfaces. Biomaterials. 2005;26(26):5285–95.
70. Park JY, Gemmell CH, Davies JE. Platelet interactions with titanium: modulation of platelet activity by surface topography. Biomaterials. 2001;22(19): 2671–82.
71. Davies JE. Understanding peri-implant endosseous healing. J Dent Educ. 2003;67(8):932–49.
72. Kuzyk PR, Schemitsch EH. The basic science of peri-implant bone healing. Indian J Orthop. 2011;45(2): 108–15.
73. Bruyn D, et al. Radiographic evaluation of modern oral implants with emphasis on crestal bone level and relevance to peri-implant health. Periodontology. 2000;2013:256–70.

Sandblasted and Acid-Etched Implant Surfaces With or Without High Surface Free Energy: Experimental and Clinical Background

9

Stefan K. Roehling, Bo Meng, and David L. Cochran

Abstract

The scientifically most investigated technique for creating a micro-rough surface topography on dental implants is the sandblasting and acid-etching procedure, creating the well-known, moderately rough SLA surface topography. The sandblasting procedure induces a macro-rough surface topography and is followed by an acid-etching procedure that superimposes the micro-rough topography. This SLA surface can be produced on commercially pure titanium as well as on titanium-zirconium alloys or on zirconium dioxide ceramics. In recent years, this hydrophobic SLA surface has been further developed, by a completely new and elaborated production process, creating a similar SLA topography but with increased chemical activity resulting in surface hydrophilicity and surface energy (modSLA surface). In vitro studies have shown that osteoblasts grown on the SLA surface exhibit properties of highly differentiated bone cells, which suggest that this surface is more osteoconductive compared to smoother surfaces. Compared to SLA, modSLA titanium surfaces further decreased cell proliferation and osteoclast activity and additionally enhanced osteoblastic cell differentiation and production of angiogenic factors. In vivo studies have demonstrated that, in comparison to implants

S.K. Roehling, DDS
Department of Periodontics, The University of Texas Health Science Center at San Antonio, Dental School, 7703 Floyd Curl Drive, MSC 7894, San Antonio, TX 78229-3900, USA

Department of Oral and Cranio-Maxillofacial Surgery, Hightech Research Center, University Hospital Basel, University of Basel, Basel, Switzerland

B. Meng, DDS, PhD
Department of Periodontics, The University of Texas Health Science Center at San Antonio, 7703 Floyd Curl Drive, San Antonio, TX 78229, USA

Oral Implantology Center, Guangdong Provincial Stomatological Hospital, Southern Medical University, 366 South Jiangnan Avenue, Guangzhou, Guangdong 510280, People's Republic of China

D.L. Cochran, DDS, MS, PhD, MMSci, Drhc (✉)
Department of Periodontics, The University of Texas Health Science Center at San Antonio, Dental School, 7703 Floyd Curl Drive, MSC 7894, San Antonio, TX 78229-3900, USA
e-mail: COCHRAN@uthscsa.edu

A. Wennerberg et al. (eds.), *Implant Surfaces and their Biological and Clinical Impact*, DOI 10.1007/978-3-662-45379-7_9, © Springer-Verlag Berlin Heidelberg 2015

with turned/machined surfaces, the increased roughness topography enhances bone tissue responses, such as greater bone–implant contact (BIC) and increased removal torque-out values (RTQ). These implants with increased surface hydrophilicity revealed accelerated bone (significantly increased BIC, RTQ) and soft tissue healing within the first 4 weeks after placement compared to implants with an SLA surface. Clinically, it has been shown that implants with an SLA surface topography can be successfully loaded 6–8 weeks after implant placement, thus, significantly reducing the healing period compared to implants with a turned or machined surface topography. With regard to the modSLA surface, it has been demonstrated that implants can successfully be loaded immediately or 3–6 weeks after placement, thus, further reducing the healing time. The SLA as well as the modSLA implant surface revealed comparable survival and success rates of more than 95 % up to and after 3 years of investigation; however, for SLA, also similar survival and success rates up to and after 10 years are available. Thus, both types of implant surfaces (SLA and modSLA) show highly successful comparable clinical outcomes; however, the modSLA surfaces allow for earlier bone and soft tissue healing and implant loading without compromising the overall survival and success rates.

Introduction

The use of dental implants to replace missing teeth has become a routine procedure in dentistry and relies on a biological stabilization of the implant in bone tissue called osseointegration. Furthermore, it has been found out that, besides implant material, implant design, bone status, surgical technique, and loading protocol, the implant surface itself is one of the most critical factors for the achievement of a successful and long-lasting osseointegration [1]. Immediately after the placement of the implant, proteins, ions, sugars, and lipids that are present in the blood and tissue fluids of the peri-implant soft and bone tissue condition the implant's surface. In this context, it has been stated that the most important implant surface properties affecting this process during initial osseointegration are surface topography, surface chemistry, surface charge, and surface hydrophilicity [2].

During the initial phase of dental implantology in the 1970s and 1980s, implants with a machined, rather smooth surface (mechanical polished) and implants with a rather rough, microporous titanium plasma-sprayed (TPS) surface dominated the market. At the beginning of the 1990s, preclinical studies started to investigate the influence of the surface topography of titanium implants on the osseointegration process in detail. In general, it has been demonstrated that roughening of the implant surface up to a certain degree led to an accelerated and increased osseous integration within healing periods up to 12 weeks [3, 4]. Additionally, it has been found out that titanium implants with a moderately rough sandblasted with large grits and acid-etched surface topography (SLA), which showed distinctively increased surface roughness values compared to machined surfaces but slightly decreased roughness values compared to TPS surfaces, demonstrated the best osseointegrative capacity compared to implants with a machined or TPS surface topography; however, the TPS implants were similar to the SLA implants [3, 4]. Clinical studies confirmed these results and showed survival and success rates of 97 % and more for investigation periods of 10 years for commercially pure titanium (c.p. Ti) implants with a hydrophobic sandblasted and ad acid-etched surface [5].

Due to these excellent clinical results of the c.p. Ti implants with a hydrophobic SLA surface, since the beginning of the 2000s, the demands of clinicians and patients for successful and fast treatment procedures have further increased. Thus, within the past 10 years, experimental studies have started to focus not only on surface topography but also on surface chemistry resulting in surface hydrophilicity and surface free energy on the titanium implant to improve and accelerate the osseointegration process even more and to provide treatment protocols that allow an even earlier functional loading of the implants.

In the literature, several procedures have been described to affect the surface chemistry and to induce an increased surface hydrophilicity and surface free energy of titanium implant surfaces, for example, surface treatment with alkali or hydrogen peroxide in combination with heat [6], implant surface treatment with ultraviolet light for 15 min just prior to implant placement ("photofunctionalization" [7, 8]), implant surface conditioning with a highly diluted sodium hydroxide solution just prior to implant placement [9, 10], or, after sandblasting and acid-etching, rinsing the implant under N_2 protection and continuously storing of implant in isotonic sodium chloride (NaCl) solution [2, 11, 12]. The latter procedure describes the further developed manufacturing process (SLActive®, Institut Straumann AG, Basel, Switzerland) of the well-known and highly successful SLA® implant surface. A lot of experimental in vitro and in vivo as well as many clinical studies have been performed to investigate this chemically active and hydrophilic SLA implant surface (SLActive®, described as modSLA in the following chapter), which is produced on titanium implants of exactly the same geometrical design compared to implants with an SLA® surface (compare below). Thus, differences with regard to osseointegrative capacity or clinical performance can directly be attributed to the differences in surface chemistry, surface hydrophilicity, and surface free energy and are not influenced by a different geometrical implant design. For that reasons, the following chapter describes the most current experimental and clinical studies on the SLA® and SLActive® implant surfaces and examines the application of both types of surfaces in the clinical daily routine.

Most recently, the process of sandblasting and acid-etching has not only been applied to c.p. Ti; it has also been applied to some specific titanium alloys, such as one specific combination of titanium-zirconium alloy (TiZr [13]), or to oxide ceramics, such as zirconium dioxide (zirconia, ZrO_2; see Fig. 9.2). Thus, the production of sandblasted and acid-etched implant surfaces, with or without enhanced surface chemistry resulting in surface hydrophilicity and surface free energy, not only is a unique manufacturing process for c.p. titanium but can also be applied to other materials to stimulate an enhanced osseointegration process for dental implants. On this account, the following chapter presents current scientific results from studies investigating the SLA and modSLA surface on c.p. Ti and the similar SLA-like surface topography on implants made of a specific TiZr alloy and on a dental implant made of zirconium dioxide.

SLA Implant Surfaces

Physical and Chemical Properties

The sandblasted and acid-etched (SLA) surface is characterized by a primary roughness produced by the sandblasting procedure that creates "valleys," whereas the acid-etching procedure attacks the titanium surface, producing micropits superimposed on the rough-blasted surface (Fig. 9.1) [14]. The sandblasting procedure may be performed using either medium-grit or large-grit aluminum oxide particles. Literature reports have shown that the acid-etching process can employ either a hydrochloric acid or sulfuric acid mixture (HCl/H_2SO_4) or pickling in 2 % hydrofluoric acid/10 % nitric acid (HF/HNO_3) [3, 14–16]. Grit-blasted and acid-etched surfaces have a complex morphology consisting of craters ranging from 20 to 100 μm in diameter and overlaid with micropits approximately 0.5–2 μm in diameter [17]. In addition to increasing surface roughness, surface blasting and acid-etching can

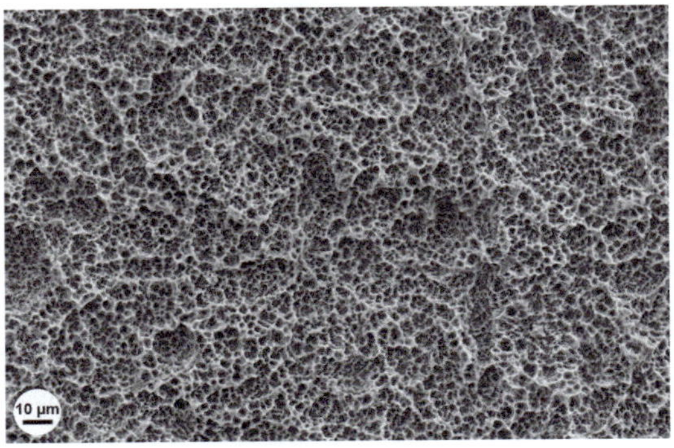

Fig. 9.1 Electron micrograph of titanium sandblasted and acid-etched surface (SLA)

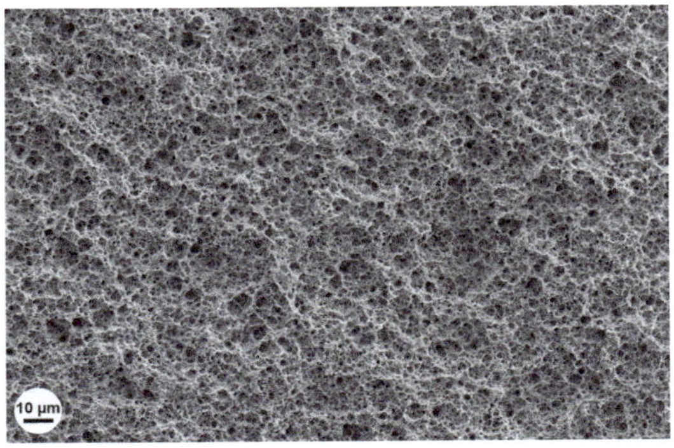

Fig. 9.2 Electron micrograph of zirconia sandblasted and acid-etched surface (ZLA). Similar surface topography compared to zirconia implants that were produced by low-pressure injection molding followed by acid etching [28–31]

remove surface contaminants and increase the surface reactivity of the metal.

Many researchers studied the SLA surface commercially produced by Institut Straumann AG, Basel, Switzerland, and found that the Sa value (the arithmetic mean of deviations in the roughness profile from mean line in 3 dimensions) is 1.79 ± 0.2 µm (evaluated at the top of the thread) [18] and the Ra value (the mean height of the roughness based on only 2 dimensions) is 2.93 ± 0.46 µm [19]. Additionally, the difference between the Sa and Ra value with regard to these 2 studies can be related to the fact that the Sa value was measured by optical profilometry [18] while the Ra value was determined by evaluating scanning electron micrographs from implants using image analysis software [19]. Such a titanium oxide surface exhibits low surface energy because of adsorbed hydrocarbons and carbonates from ambient air [2]. Taborelli et al. confirmed the water contact angle of the SLA surface about 117° ± 2.7 [20], while Buser et al. measured the dynamic contact angle (DCA) of the SLA surface and the results indicated that the SLA surface was hydrophobic (DCA = 138.3° ± 4.2) [11]. During acid-etching, the titanium oxide layer is dissolved, and small native hydrogen ions diffuse into the unprotected implant surface, which enrich the implant surface with hydrogen and precipitate into titanium hydride (TiH) [21]. X-ray diffraction (XRD) analysis of SLA-treated titanium samples showed the presence of 20–40 % of titanium hydride (d-TiH2-x) in addition to titanium [22, 23].

It has been reported that the etching process modifies the titanium surface composition of SLA-treated implants. Observation has shown that the dull SLA surface is soft [24], particularly when compared with a titanium plasma–sprayed (TPS) surface. The SLA surface consists mainly of TiO_2 with some carbon containing contamination (like hydrocarbons) due to the exposure to air. X-ray photoelectron spectroscopy (XPS) analysis indicated that the SLA surface had a 44.2 ± 1.9 at% (atomic concentration) oxygen (O) concentration, an 18.4 ± 1.6 at% titanium (Ti) concentrations [11], and a 37.3 ± 3.4 at% carbon (C) concentration, which is comparable to the result of Kang et al. with 47.1 at% O, 20.1 at% Ti, and 32.0 % C [25].

Besides pure titanium, SLA surfaces can also be produced on other materials, such as titanium-zirconium alloys [13] and zirconium dioxide ceramics (Fig. 9.2). Due to the similar crystal structure of titanium and zirconium, the TiZr alloy can be sandblasted and acid-etched, exactly like commercially pure titanium (compare 3.1 in this chapter), to create a micro-rough SLA surface (Fig. 9.3). In contrast to that, with regard to zirconia ceramics, it has been shown that surface treatment procedures that create micro-rough surface topographies, like conventional sandblasting or uncontrolled machining processes, might reduce the fracture strength of zirconia

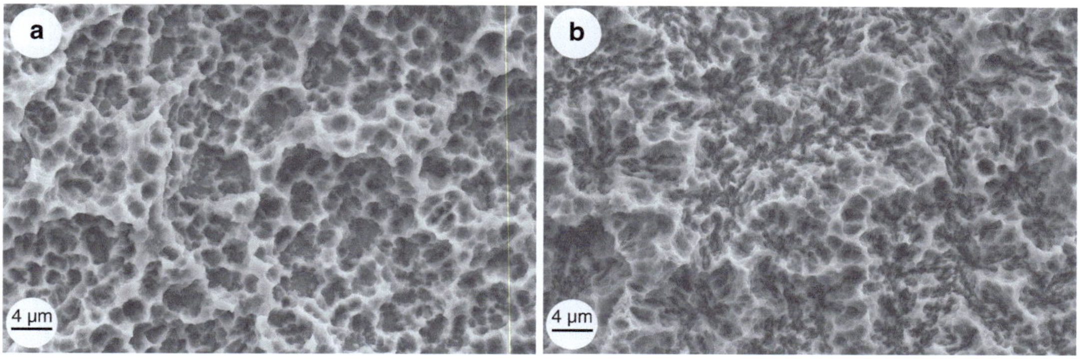

Fig. 9.3 SEM image of SLA/modSLA surface on c.p. titanium (**a**) and on TiZr alloy (**b**)

dental implants and lead to implant fractures [26, 27]. Thus, the manufacturing processes of creating micro-rough surfaces on commercially pure titanium or titanium alloy implants cannot simply be transferred to zirconia but must accurately be attuned to the material properties of the zirconia ceramics. The first manufacturing process that created a micro-rough surface topography on zirconia implants that was similar to the SLA surface on titanium implants, without compromising the zirconia implant fracture strength, was a low-pressure injection molding technique, using a mold showing an SLA-like surface topography, followed by an etching procedure with hot hydrofluoric acid [28–31]. Later on, for zirconia dental implants, the manufacturing and surface treatment procedures have been further developed so that currently a micro-rough surface topography can be produced on zirconia implants by using a specially designed, mild sandblasting procedure followed by an etching procedure with hydrofluoric acid (zirconia large-grit sandblasted and acid-etched, ZLA™ surface, Straumann® PURE Ceramic Implant, Institut Straumann AG, Basel, Switzerland, Fig. 9.2), again without compromising the resistance to fracture of the ZLA-treated zirconia implants. The sandblasted and acid-etched surface on zirconia implants has a similar surface topography compared to the SLA surface on titanium implants (Figs. 9.1 and 9.2); however, with regard to quantitative surface analysis, the micro-rough zirconia implant surface shows a reduced arithmetic mean value (Sa = 0.70 µm). Calculations were performed with the use of a Gaussian filter with a cutoff wavelength of 30 µm (information provided by Institut Straumann AG, Basel, Switzerland) and compared to implants with an SLA surface (Sa = 1.15 µm, Table 9.1).

Table 9.1 Roughness parameters of SLA and modSLA surfaces [11]

Roughness parameter	SLA	modSLA
S_a [µm]	1.15 ± 0.05	1.16 ± 0.04
S_q [µm]	1.45 ± 0.06	1.45 ± 0.04
S_t [µm]	7.83 ± 0.47	7.65 ± 0.31
S_k [µm]	4.44 ± 2.33	4.51 ± 2.26

S_a arithmetic mean deviation of the surface, S_q root-mean-square deviation of the surface, S_t maximum peak-to-valley height of the surface, S_k amplitude distribution skew. Calculations were performed with the use of a Gaussian filter with a cutoff wavelength of 31 µm. Results presented as mean ± SD; $n = 10$ for each surface. Analysis of variance (ANOVA) was performed; for all parameters, no significant differences were seen between implant types ($p > 0.05$)

Preclinical In Vitro Studies

SLA: Osteoblast Activity

Bone formation on implant surfaces requires recruitment of osteoblast precursor cells, their differentiation into secretory osteoblasts, production of unmineralized extracellular matrix (osteoid), and calcification of the extracellular matrix [32], which finally lead to osseointegration. Initial interactions between implant surfaces and cells in the early stages of healing are believed to predetermine later events in the process of osseointegration of dental implants [32, 33]. Baschong et al. [34] investigated the influence of SLA surfaces on the differentiation of human mesenchymal progenitor cells (HMPC), i.e., the type of cells immigrating to colonize the implant surface upon implant insertion [35, 36], from adult bone marrow and demonstrated that SLA surfaces promotes osteogenic differentiation of HMPC, which could explain in vivo observations of enhanced bone–implant integration.

It is widely recognized that SLA surfaces increase osteoblast attachment, differentiation, and biomineralization, in comparison with smoother topographies, which promote adhesion formation, spreading, and proliferation [37]. Zinger et al.'s study showed that for hemispherical cavities, the minimal width for bone cell response is around 30 μm, and interestingly, cells cultured on the SLA surfaces preferentially occupied the shallow hollows existing in the SLA rough topography, which measured around 20–30 μm [38]. Osteoblasts also appear to be sensitive to surface roughness and exhibit greater initial attachment to rough titanium surfaces [39]. Sammons et al. demonstrated that rat calvarial osteoblasts attached and spread on the SLA surfaces more rapidly than on smoothed, anodized, or acid-etched surfaces [19]. It has also been shown that osteoblasts exhibit a more differentiated phenotype when grown on titanium substrates with micron-scale roughness than when grown on smooth titanium substrates or on tissue culture polystyrene [40]. Schwartz et al. found that osteoblasts exhibited a decrease in cell number and increase in osteocalcin when grown on SLA surfaces. A number of in vitro laboratory studies have shown that SLA surfaces could increase the response of osteoblast-like cells to systemic hormones [41] and promote osteoblast and chondrocyte differentiation [15]. Interactions with the SLA surface may facilitate mechanical interlocking of cells with the surface, allowing the ingress of vascular tissue and favoring osseointegration.

The osteophilic properties of the SLA surface were confirmed in a series of in vitro studies examining various titanium surfaces in tissue culture with osteoblast-like cells [15, 41–43]. In vitro studies have shown that SLA surfaces also influence a number of events in the process of osteoblast differentiation including spreading and proliferation; the production of alkaline phosphatase, collagen, proteoglycans, and osteocalcin; and synthesis of cytokines and growth factors (TGF-β1 and PGE_2). Osteoblasts grown on SLA surfaces enhance osteointegration by producing local factors that regulate bone formation as well as bone remodeling, including the RANK ligand decoy receptor osteoprotegerin (OPG). In addition to producing a collagen-rich extracellular matrix [44], increased alkaline phosphatase activity, and elevated levels of osteocalcin [42], osteoblasts produce increased levels of local factors on these surfaces, including prostaglandins E_1 and E_2 (PGE_2) [41] and transforming growth factor beta-1 (TGF-β1) [45]. Levels of latent and active TGF-β1 were increased in the conditioned media of cultures grown on the SLA surfaces, which then increase the levels of OPG [2]. The SLA surface induced an accelerated gene expression of the bone matrix molecules osteopontin and osteonectin, along with an upregulation of bone sialoprotein, collagen type III, and integrins in the initial healing stages up to 1 week [46]. These studies demonstrated that, in vitro, the SLA surface could accelerate the bone formation that occurs at the cell-implant surface.

SLA: Osteoclast Activity

Osteoclasts are also important in the process of osseointegration. Osteoclasts and osteoblasts show a close interplay, called coupling, regulated through multiple signaling pathways. Lossdorfer et al. showed that the SLA surface can enhance the phenotypic maturation of MG63 osteoblast-like cells towards a more differentiated osteoblast cell type expressing local factors that inhibit osteoclastogenesis [17]. In addition, Brinkmann et al. found that osteoclast differentiation on SLA surfaces seems to be comparable with differentiation on native bone, which will attract osteoblasts and then mineralize the bone around the implant [47].

Preclinical In Vivo Studies

SLA: Characteristics

The key events that lead to osseointegration of an implant occur largely at the bone-implant surface. Various publications have demonstrated that bone contact differs when different titanium implant surfaces are used. In several in vivo studies, SLA surfaces were found to produce better bone fixation than smooth surfaces [3, 48–50], and the SLA surfaced implants also showed a more than 5 % higher interfacial stiffness than machine surfaced implants [51]. A histometric study by Buser et al. [3] evaluated 5 different titanium surfaces in miniature pigs and found that the SLA surfaced implant revealed the best bone apposition to the implant surface among the titanium surfaces, with 52 % and 58 % of bone-to-implant contact (BIC) after 3 and 6 weeks of healing, respectively. This surface also was evaluated in a separate animal system in the oral cavity under loaded and non-loaded conditions and compared to implants with a titanium plasma-sprayed surface. The SLA implant surface produced favorable results in this study as well, with the BIC level of about 72.33 % after 12 weeks of healing [50]. Perrin et al. acquired 82.12±6.1 % BIC by using SLA surfaced implants in Landrace pigs in a submerged way after 10 weeks [23]. Data from these in vivo animal studies suggest that implants with SLA surfaces produce a more rapid bone response and/or more bone-to-implant contact than ones with smooth or turned surfaces.

Besides animal studies, a human study was performed by Lang et al. [52], during which SLA surfaced implants were placed in the volunteers' mandibular retromolar area and retrieved with the surrounding tissues after healing periods of 7, 14, 28, and 42 days. The histological analysis showed that osseointegration took place with an increasing BIC from 7 to 42 days at which time it reached 62 % of the implant surface exposed to the parent bone. The authors pointed out that osseointegration appeared to be slower in humans when compared with animals, which is consistent with bone formation rates. Nevertheless, with a BIC of 62 % after 4 weeks of healing, the osseointegration may have developed to a sufficient degree to fully carry functional load [53]. The results of these tests show that the SLA surface has a high potential to form bone-to-implant contact in humans.

A significantly higher removal torque value has been demonstrated for SLA implants compared to smooth implant surfaces [14]. A removal torque study by Buser et al. in the maxillae of miniature pigs compared SLA surfaces with the machined and the TPS surface and confirmed that the machined surface had 8 to 10 times lower removal torque values when compared with the SLA surface and that the SLA surface showed slightly higher removal torque values than the TPS surfaces [14]. A biomechanical study by Wilke et al. tested removal torque values (RTVs) of unloaded titanium implants with various surface characteristics in the tibia of sheep. This study demonstrated that the RTVs for the SLA surface clearly exceed the mean RTVs of polished or fine-textured implant surfaces during the course of the study period. Further studies [4, 14, 54] using functional assays demonstrated that this same SLA surface resulted in significantly higher removal torque values than did smoother surfaces (e.g., machined surface). Thus, it appears that implants with an SLA surface might be able to be restored after shorter healing times than those associated with implants with a machined surface.

Less loss of bone height at the preload evaluation, as well as after a loading period, has been demonstrated for SLA implants. Cochran and coworkers [16, 50] found significantly less coronal bone loss in arches in which SLA surfaced implants had been placed, and this may be the result of the higher osteoconductive properties of the SLA surface. In a study conducted by Cochran et al. [16], an SLA implant was compared radiographically to a TPS implant under unloaded and loaded conditions in the canine mandible for up to 15 months. Radiographic assessment of the bone response to the implants was carried out by measuring the distance between the implant shoulder and the most coronal bone-to-implant contact (DIB) and by evaluation of bone density changes using computer-assisted densitometric image analysis (CADIA). DIB measurements revealed that SLA implants had significantly less bone height loss (0.52 mm) than TPS implants (0.69 mm) at the preload evaluation ($p=0.0142$) as well as at 3 months of loading (0.73 mm/1.06 mm; $p=0.0337$). The same trend was also evident for CADIA measurements with SLA implants showing higher crestal bone density values when comparing preload to baseline data ($p=0.0890$) and 3 months to baseline data ($p=0.0912$). Arlin also found that the frequency of crestal bone loss was lower for SLA implants than for TPS implants [55]. Moreover, they also found that cumulative survival rates were equally good for SLA and TPS implants; additionally, the failure rate for SLA implants was lower than that for TPS implants. In an additional study, Perrin et al. found that surface composition did not play a significant role in the bone response to the SLA surface, and they concluded that the osteophilic properties of the SLA surface are due to its surface topography and not to its specific surface composition [23].

SLA: Bone Growth

It has been demonstrated that SLA surfaces allowed for "contact osteogenesis" to take place [56]. Cochran et al. demonstrated that remodeling processes were "fully occurring" already after 3 months of healing of a 200-mm-wide gap that occurred between the bone wall and the screw threads of an implant with an SLA surface [50]. Botticelli et al. [57–60] have published the results from 4 experimental studies in the dog. In these studies, they created defects lateral to the implants to simulate implants placed in extraction sockets. The histological analysis indicated that defects lateral to implants with an SLA surface heal with adequate osseointegration and demonstrated that the healing of a wide marginal defect around an SLA implant is characterized by appositional bone growth from the lateral and apical bone walls of the defect. In another one of Botticelli's publications [61], a model was described which allowed the study of bone formation adjacent to endosseous implants. In this model, prior to implant placement, a large defect was prepared in the marginal bone compartment of the recipient site. In biopsies obtained after 4 months of healing, it was observed that the defects adjacent to the implants had been filled with newly formed bone. In addition, the degree of bone-to-implant contact that had been established between the newly formed bone tissue and the SLA surfaced implant was high and not different from those characterizing similar implants placed in a recipient site without defects of the alveolar bone crest. The SLA surface appeared to have the ability to close the marrow spaces with new bone when inserted in rather spongious bone, leading to a quasi-continuous layer of bone running along the implant surface. This property could explain the higher BIC level recorded at SLA surfaces when compared to TPS surfaces [3]. This SLA surface appeared to express its osteophilic properties more readily in spongious bone rather than in cortical bone.

SLA: Bone Graft Materials

Guided bone regeneration (GBR) has been successfully applied to treat bone defects associated with implants, and bone grafting materials have often been placed around dental implant surfaces to simultaneously reduce treatment time. Freilich et al. [62] tested the vertical bone-forming capacity of demineralized bone matrix (DBM) around SLA surfaced implants in membranous bone in a rabbit model and demonstrated that the DBM, in combination with the implant and scaffold retention screw which kept the scaffold in a stable, non-compressed position during healing, was successful at inducing new bone formation around the SLA roughened surface. The mean supracrestal bone height determined via histomorphometric analysis was 2.4 ± 0.6 mm and that by micro-CT was 2.1 ± 0.9 mm. They also pointed out that the high bone contact value obtained (58.1 ± 14 %) within the new supracrestal bone indicates successful implant placement into alveolar bone by clinical standards, and these data illustrate the potential for vertical bone-guiding capacity of sandblasted and acid-etched implants. Carmagnola et al. [63] demonstrated that the SLA implants placed in rabbit tibiae previously grafted with 3 different biomaterials, i.e., Bio-Oss®, Ostims-Pastes®, and PerioGlas®, obtained a larger extent of osseointegration, although not statistically significant, than implants placed in non-grafted bone. De Vicene et al. [64] evaluated the efficacy of collagen membranes (Bio-Gide®, Geistlich Pharma), either alone or combined with a human demineralized freeze-dried bone allograft (DFDBA) or natural bovine bone graft, in bone defects around dental implants with an SLA surface, and it was observed that the mean bone-to-implant contact was 35.3 %, and was even higher, 75.6 %, when the defects were filled with inorganic bovine bone. They pointed out that although no statistically significant differences were found in this study between the membrane and non-membrane groups, bone defects augmented with anorganic bovine bone and membranes showed the most promising results from a histological and histomorphometric perspective. Retzepi et al. [65] demonstrated that de novo alveolar bone formation can be achieved around SLA surfaced implants via application of the GBR principle in experimentally induced diabetic rats; however, there was higher outcome variability and an increased rate of infectious complications in these diabetic animals. These studies demonstrate the value of this surface to help promote vertical bone growth by providing an osteoconductive surface to support osteoblast cell adhesion and growth [66]. Therefore, the SLA surface has osteoconductive characteristics, which have the capacity to guide bone growth when placed in conjunction with bone grafting materials.

SLA-like Surface on Zirconia

As described above, recently a micro-rough surface topography has been produced on zirconia implants by using a specially designed sandblasting and acid-etching procedure (Fig. 9.2). However, the first generation of these micro-rough zirconia implants was produced by a low-pressure injection molding technique, using a mold showing an SLA-like surface topography, followed by an acid-etching procedure [28–31], creating a similar surface topography compared to the current sandblasting and acid-etching procedure (Fig. 9.2). At present, only experimental data from the first generation of these micro-roughened zirconia implants are available [28–31]. Histological and biomechanical animal studies in miniature pigs investigated the bone tissue response to these first-generation micro-roughened zirconia implants and compared it to titanium implants with an SLA surface [28–31]. The authors demonstrated comparable bone-to-implant contact ratio and bone density values for zirconia implants (BIC range between 67.7 ± 21.1 % and 70 ± 14.5 %; bone density range between 60.4 ± 9.9 % and 63.3 ± 21.5 %) and titanium SLA implants (BIC range between 64.7 ± 9.4 % and 83.7 ± 10.3 %, bone density range between 61.1 ± 6.2 % and 68.2 ± 5.8 %) after 4, 8, and 12 weeks of unloaded healing. No statistically significant differences could be detected at any investigated time point [30]. With regard to biomechanical testing, mean torque-out values ranged between 97.4 ± 29.3 and 139.6 ± 56.63 Ncm for zirconia and between 131.6 ± 35.6 and 177.6 ± 51.6 Ncm for titanium SLA at corresponding time intervals. After 4 and 12 weeks of healing, no significant differences could be evaluated between both materials [31]. Thus, it can be suggested that the micro-roughened zirconia implants with an SLA-like surface topography have a comparable osseointegrative capacity as titanium implants with an SLA surface topography.

Clinical Studies

SLA: Bone Formation

The concept of enhanced bone formation around the SLA implant surface in humans was demonstrated by a clinical human study [67], during which the SLA surfaced implants were placed in extraction sockets. This occurred both in the maxilla and the mandible and all implants were not loaded. Four months later, surgical re-entry procedures were performed, and it could be observed that the majority of the extraction sockets were almost completely filled by bone. Based on these results, the authors concluded that marginal gaps following placement of the SLA surfaced implants into extraction sockets may predictably heal with bone formation and defect resolution. Barewal et al. measured the resonance frequency of SLA implant stability in vivo and found that there was no significant difference in the pattern of stability changes among different bone types (type I–IV) after 5 weeks of healing; however, the dip in stability which occurs around 2–3 weeks in patients is lower in more cancellous bone types [68]. The results of another evaluation show that the SLA surfaced implants have a significantly higher survival rate than machine-surfaced implants in autogenous grafted maxillary bone [69]. Stricker et al. [70] demonstrated that placement of SLA surfaced implants, in combination with autografts for sinus floor elevation, is a safe and predictable procedure for the reconstruction of the severely resorbed posterior aspect of the maxilla.

SLA: Reducing Time to Loading

A formal prospective, multicenter clinical trial [71] was initiated to determine whether the advantages of increased bone formation and osseointegration demonstrated for SLA surfaced implants seen in experimental in vitro and animal studies could be translated into benefits for patients. It was reasoned that if greater bone contact and a stronger bond to the bone occurred at earlier times around implants with an SLA surface, then patients should be able to have their implants restored after shorter healing periods than those considered conventional (3–6 months) which were established in studies with smooth machined surfaced implants. In this clinical study, SLA implants were loaded after 6 weeks when placed in class I, II, or III bone or after 12 weeks if in class IV bone. The results demonstrated that, under these defined conditions, the SLA surfaced implants can be restored after approximately 6 weeks of healing with a high predictability of success, defined by abutment placement at 35 Ncm without counter torque [71]. This represented a significant advancement in the restoration of missing teeth with implants by directly providing the patient benefit of reduced treatment time. However, one possible shortcoming of this trial was that the patients were selected carefully and monitored closely. As such, their treatment represented ideal conditions in which to evaluate the reduced healing time. However, the successful abutment placement that has been demonstrated in this clinical trial, and the subsequent implant success, provides further evidence that the SLA surface has significant clinical advantages such as shorter restoration times than those used in earlier studies on implant restoration [71]. At both 1- and 2-year follow-up, 99 % of the implants were successful. An identical success rate (i.e., 99 %) was also reported at 3 years [72], which indicated that no so-called "late failures" occurred in the 3-year time frame.

The possibility of reduced healing times was also examined in another larger multicenter, prospective human clinical study, in which the patients were not as carefully selected and monitored. The success of early abutment placement was again assessed without counter torque, based on the documented advantages of the SLA titanium surface, which has both high percentages of bone-to-implant contact in descriptive histomorphometric studies [50] and high removal torque values in functional studies based on the strength of the bone-to-implant contact [4, 73]. The implants in this less-controlled environment could be placed and restored successfully with reduced healing times (approximately half the conventional healing time) without a consequent increase in failure or complication. The results of this multicenter clinical trial clearly established the capacity of implants characterized by the SLA surface to withstand abutment torquing and consequent loading within the experimental time frame. Therefore, SLA surfaced implants have a benefit for patient care which is a shorter healing time than that historically recommended. By reducing the time required for osseointegration and loading, patient acceptance and rehabilitation options were improved.

As shown above, early loading of SLA implants have demonstrated clinical outcomes equivalent to conventional loading [71, 74]. A healing time of 6 weeks for implants placed in good-quality bone has been recommended for SLA surfaced implants [71, 75]. Bornstein et al. used an early loading protocol with 6 weeks of healing to demonstrate that titanium implants with the SLA surface can achieve and maintain successful tissue integration with high predictability for at least 5 years of follow-up in selected patients and sites [76]. Salvi et al. pointed out that loading of titanium implants with an SLA surface as early as 2 weeks did not appear to jeopardize the osseointegration healing process in the posterior mandible [77]. Quinlan used 48 SLA surfaced implants in a canine model and indicated that no statistically significant differences existed between conventionally loaded, early loaded, and immediately loaded SLA implants by clinical, radiographic, and histologic data [78]. Immediate or early loading of SLA implants in single-tooth replacement [79], splinted crowns and fixed prostheses [80–82], full-arch prostheses [83], and overdentures [84] have demonstrated success and survival rates comparable with those obtained using older standard conventional loading protocols (6–9 months).

Due to the 2 levels of micro-roughness of the SLA surface, osseointegration of SLA implants has been improved, and time to loading has been reduced to at least 50 % of conventional healing times. The biologic reasons for the early loading capacity of the SLA implants are based on the osteoconductive nature of the surface and the physical characteristics of the titanium surface resulting from the subtractive techniques of producing the SLA implant surface. Electron micrographs show bone cells with their cell bodies located over the 20- to 40 μm pits created by the sandblasting procedure, whereas the cell extensions reach out to the 1- to 2 μm roughness of the acid-etching procedure. Apparently, osteoid is laid down under the cell bodies, calcifies, and acts as retentive areas for the implant to resist forces applied to the implant [54, 85]. These mechanisms may explain why the implants can resist 35 Ncm of force without counter torque at 6–8 weeks and allow for restoration of the implant at reduced healing times. This suggests that the early bone-to-implant contact that is formed is sufficiently strong to resist occlusal forces on the restorations.

SLA: High Survival and Success Rate

A meta-analysis of longitudinal descriptive implant experiences in patients has suggested that, in certain indications, the advantages of rough titanium surfaces can also be reflected in better success rates for patients [86]. A prospective, multicenter, human clinical observational study was conducted by Cochran et al. [87] which was performed in a prospective fashion involving 92 practitioners in 16 countries. Most implants were placed in posterior locations and were placed in intermediate-quality (type II and III) bone. The implants were to be placed and restored in predominantly private practice settings around the world. Ninety-two practitioners in 16 countries agreed to participate, and 86 followed the study design. Very high survival and success rates were documented in this field trial. The cumulative survival rate was 99.56 % at 3 years and 99.26 % at 5 years. The overall success rate was 99.12 % at 3 years and 97.38 % after 5 years. Typical of many studies, the majority of lost implants occurred as early failures, with only 1 implant lost as a late failure. Additionally, the implant complications were typical and included inflammation, infection, and discomfort of a few implants on yearly recall. Thus, although many variables were uncontrolled, the predictability of the procedure with the SLA surfaced implant was not affected compared to rates in a carefully controlled, prospective, multicenter human clinical trial [71] using the same implant.

A retrospective study conducted by Buser et al. [5] assessed the 10-year outcomes of 511 titanium implants with the SLA surface in 303 partially edentulous patients. Over the 10-year period, no implant fracture was noted, whereas 6 implants (1.2 %) were lost. Two implants (0.4 %) showed signs of suppuration at the 10-year examination, whereas 7 implants had a history of peri-implantitis (1.4 %) during the 10-year period but presented healthy peri-implant soft tissues at the final examination. This retrospective analysis resulted in a 10-year implant survival rate of 98.8 % and a success rate of 97.0 %. In addition, the prevalence of peri-implantitis in this large cohort of orally healthy patients was low with 1.8 % during the 10-year period.

As periodontitis is one of the main reasons for tooth loss, Roccuzzo et al. [88] compared the long-term outcomes of SLA implants in patients previously treated for periodontitis and in periodontally healthy patients (PHP). After clinical measurement of the pocket depths at 4 sites per tooth, patients with an initial diagnosis of periodontitis were classified according to a special score, which was calculated according to a defined formula: S = number of pockets (5–7 mm) +2× (number of pockets (≥8 mm)). Patients with a score >25 were considered as severe periodontally compromised patients (PCP). The results showed that at the 10-year follow-up, the implant survival rate was 100 % for PHP and 97.1 % even for severe PCP. They pointed out that SLA implants, placed under a strict periodontal control, offer predictable long-term results and patients should be informed, from the beginning, of the value of the supportive periodontal therapy (SPT) in enhancing long-term outcomes of implant therapy, particularly those affected by periodontitis.

Besides partially edentulous patients, Fischer et al. [89] also evaluated the totally edentulous maxilla of 24 patients with SLA surfaced implants and found that after a 10-year follow-up, the implant survival rate was 95.1 %, with a 1.07 mm mean value of bone loss. This confirmed the prospective study above that evaluated implants that had been restored in half the conventional healing time over a period of 5 years, and the life table analyses demonstrated a 99.1 % survival rate and a 98.8 % success rate for the SLA surfaced implants in a formal, carefully and externally monitored, multicenter, multinational clinical study [90]. A further clinical study conducted by Dam [91] evaluated the crestal bone loss (CBL) around dental implants by measuring radiographs after 5–6 years and found that SLA surfaced implants had less CBL than TPS implants. Lethaus et al. [92] conducted a prospective study to examine the long-term outcome of early loading of SLA implants in the edentulous mandible and reported a 5-year cumulative success rate of 96.7 %, with a 0.77 mm mean loss of crestal bone height. In a clinical follow-up report, Luongo et al. [81] presented favorable 3-year results of a prospective multicenter study with healing times between 0 and 11 days. In particular, Baker and coworkers [93] suggested that the early integration strength of SLA implants could be particularly advantageous in single-stage surgical protocols.

SLA: Summary of Clinical Studies

Taken together, these studies demonstrated that SLA surfaced titanium implants have a high survival and success rate and a very small number of implant failures occur during follow-up. Implant failures can be divided into early failures and late failures. Early failures are those occurring prior to and at the time of restoration, while late failures are those occurring after restoration [55]. Many studies have shown that the majority of implant failures occur as early failures during the healing period, and very few implant losses are observed after the onset of loading or during the follow-up period [71, 87, 92, 94]. Implant failure is to be expected in patients exhibiting risk factors such as systemic diseases causing wound-healing problems, heavy smoking, increased periodontal susceptibility, and anatomic factors such as poor bone density or extreme atrophy [95]. In spite of these many variables during the healing time and loading phase time, the predictability of the SLA surfaced implants in the listed studies was not affected. This suggests that the preclinical findings of large amounts of bone-to-implant contact and high interfacial strength with SLA implants have long-term advantages in patients.

In conclusion, these clinical studies of early loaded SLA implants reinforce that, under well-controlled clinical conditions and in less well-controlled private practice conditions, using a variety of indications, SLA implants can achieve very high success rates when abutments are torqued to 35 Ncm without counter torque at a healing time of 6 weeks. Furthermore, the osseointegration also allows the SLA surfaced implants to be highly successful in the longer term, with 10-year follow-up in some studies with very few late-term failures and very few implants with peri-implantitis.

ModSLA Implant Surfaces

Physical and Chemical Properties

As detailed above, titanium implants, intended for placement in osseous host tissue, can have different physical surface properties that are defined by the manufacturing process of the implants. Thus, titanium implants with different surface topographies, like relatively smooth surfaces created by the machining process or turning of the metal rod or a moderately rough surface topography [96] after sandblasting and acid-etching, can be produced [3]. The type of surface topography directly influences bone apposition, since it has been demonstrated that roughening of the implant's surface up to a certain degree induced significantly increased osseous integration [3, 4]. Besides different physical properties, titanium surfaces can also show different chemical properties, defined by the atoms and molecules that are attached to the implant surface (chemical composition). Thus, the chemical properties of the titanium implant-bone complex are not defined only by the material itself but also by the dioxide layer that is automatically and immediately formed on the titanium implant surface when exposed to air if the surface atmosphere is not controlled and/or protected [97]. It has been stated that "It is thus a combination of the microarchitecture and the chemical composition of the surface that is expected to determine the overall, mutual interaction between implant and biological system" [98]. In this context, it is important to know that the chemical properties of the implant surface directly influence surface wettability and surface free energy [99] and that an increased surface free energy can further promote the interaction between the implant surface and the aqueous peri-implant biologic environment [100, 101]. Moreover, it has been shown that an increased surface free energy was correlated with increased surface hydrophilicity [12]. Pure titanium dioxide surfaces show a high initial hydrophilicity, since the oxide layer that is formed on the surface (as noted above) is intrinsically hydrophilic and immediately hydroxylated under room temperature and when aqueous solutions or its vapors have contact to the surface. Those binding OH groups are amphoteric in character as they can react as an acid or a base [102]. Unfortunately, when exposed to air, this clean and initial hydrophilic TiO_2 surface is contaminated with hydrocarbons and carbons from the atmosphere and air, leading to a hydrophobic character and a reduced surface wettability and surface free energy [20].

Many experimental studies have demonstrated that the sandblasted, large-grit, and acid-etched titanium (commercially pure titanium (c.p. Ti)) implant surface (SLA®, Institut Straumann AG, Basel, Switzerland) is highly osteoconductive [16, 50], but as a possibly restrictive feature, it has a hydrophobic character [12]. As described above, native titanium dioxide surfaces are initially hydrophilic and chemically reactive. One goal for further development of the c.p. Ti-SLA surface was to fabricate a surface that has a hydrophilic character like in its native, uncontaminated state. In this context, a modified SLA surface with a high hydrophilicity and surface free energy has been developed and established on the market (SLActive®, Institut Straumann AG, Basel, Switzerland). The modified SLA surface is similarly produced like SLA, but after the same sandblasting and acid-etching procedure, the titanium implants (or experimental disks) are rinsed under N_2 protection and directly stored in isotonic NaCl solution at pH 4–6, again protected by N_2 filling [2, 11, 12]. Qualitative examinations using scanning electron microscopy (SEM) and quantitative evaluations by confocal white-light microscopy to calculate three-dimensional roughness parameters [2, 11] showed no differences between both types of surfaces concerning surface topography and surface roughness parameters (Fig. 9.3a, Table 9.1). However, more detailed SEM investigations of both surfaces clearly identified nanostructures only on the modSLA surface, leading to a significantly increased surface development on modSLA compared to SLA surfaces [103].

When investigating surface wettability and surface free energy, significant differences have been found between modSLA and SLA surfaces. Rupp et al. investigated the surface hydrophilicity and the surface wettability from both surfaces by dynamic contact angle analysis (DCA) and determined the surface free energy [12]. The main outcome of these evaluations was that modSLA showed significantly increased initial hydrophilicity and a complete wettability documented by water contact angles of 0°, compared to SLA that was rather hydrophobic with initial contact angles of 139.9° (Fig. 9.4). Furthermore,

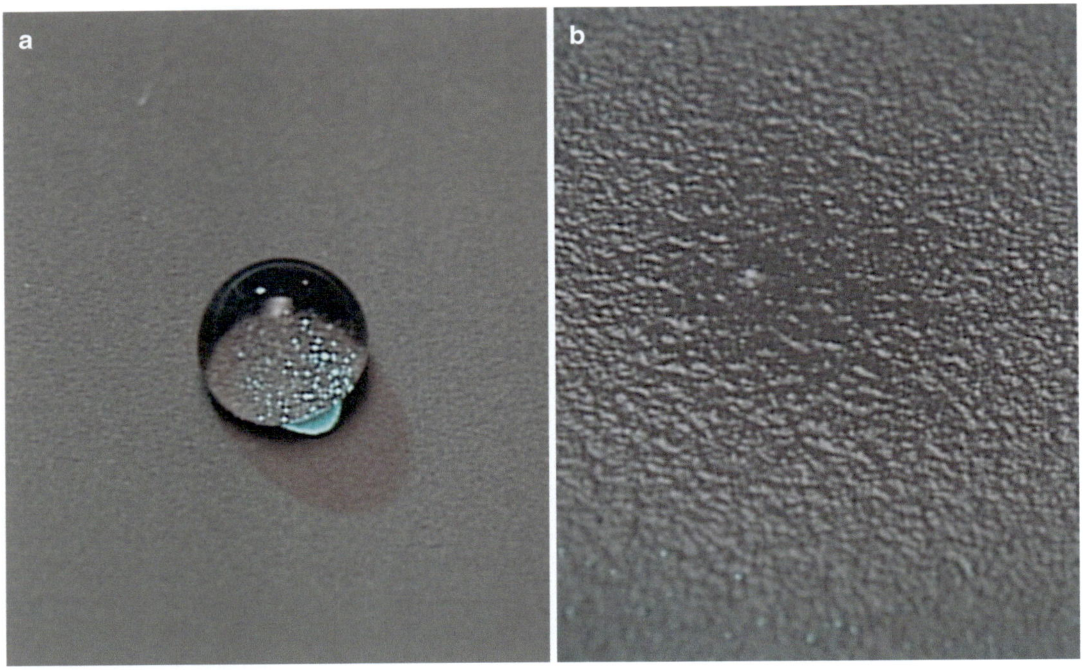

Fig. 9.4 Drop of water on hydrophobic SLA surface (**a**) and on hydrophilic modSLA surface (**b**). Increased hydrophilicity on modSLA surface indicated by complete dispersion of waterdrop (**b**, no measurable contact angle between water drop and surface); however, no dispersion of waterdrop on hydrophobic SLA surface (**a**, obvious measurable contact angle between waterdrop and surface)

the authors demonstrated that an "increased initial hydrophilicity of modSLA could be clearly correlated with increased surface free energy" [12]. Analogous results could also be demonstrated from different authors using similar methods [2, 11, 103].

The increased surface hydrophilicity can also induce an accelerated covering of the implant surface with blood from the peri-implant soft and bone tissue during placement of the implant (Fig. 9.5), compared to hydrophobic SLA surfaces, thus accelerating the initial implant healing period.

Additionally, by using x-ray photoelectron spectroscopy (XPS) to investigate the chemical composition of both surfaces, it could be evaluated that modSLA showed increased oxygen and titanium concentrations and reduced carbon concentrations compared to SLA (Table 9.2). Before analysis, the modSLA surfaces were taken from the containment ampule, rinsed with ultrapure water, and dried with N_2 to remove electrostatically bound ions from the surface. The results indicated an increased concentration of hydroxylated groups bound to the modSLA surface in comparison to SLA and a decreased adsorption of potential contaminants (carbons, hydrocarbons) from the atmosphere [11, 12, 103].

Another study evaluated the chemical composition of the modSLA surface as received from the manufacturer without rinsing the implant surface with ultrapure water prior to XPS analysis. The results showed similar values for C (16.8 %) and N (1.1 %) but slightly different values for Ti (11.6 %) and O (28.6 %). Furthermore and expectedly, they could detect Na (25.2 %) and Cl (16.1 %) ions indicating a surface coating with NaCl crystals due to the storage of the implant in NaCl solution [104]. After drying up of the solution, the water evaporated but the NaCl that was in the solution remained on the implant surface.

Besides commercially pure titanium, also titanium alloys were used for the production of dental implants with a sandblasted and acid-etched

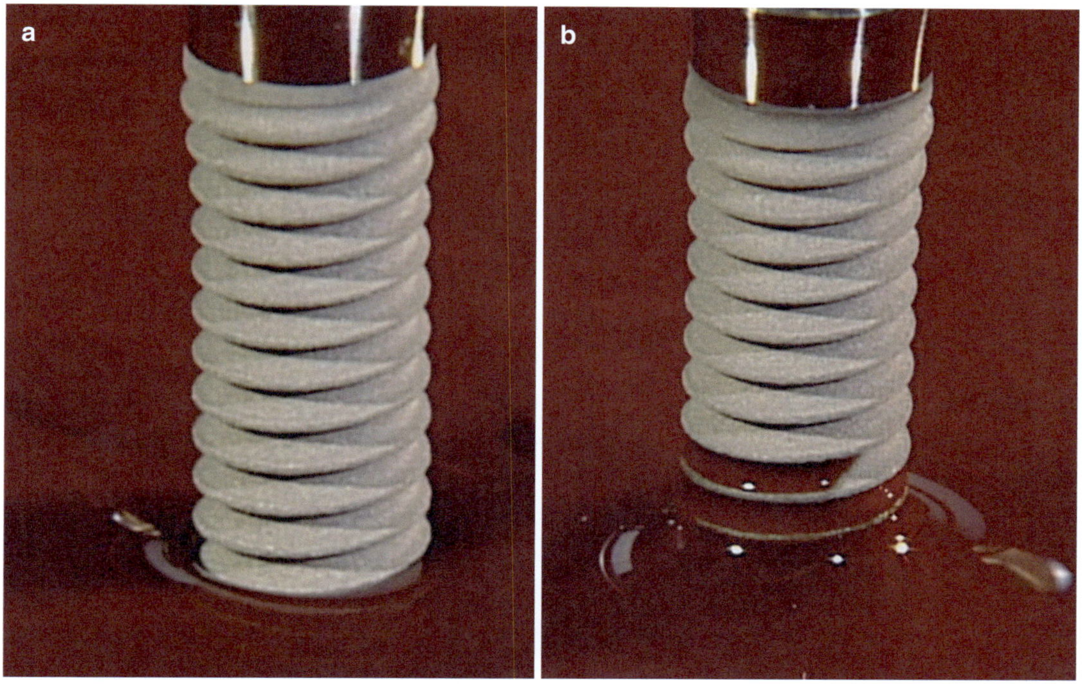

Fig. 9.5 Accelerated covering of the implant surface with blood on implant with hydrophilic modSLA surface (**b**) compared to implant with hydrophobic SLA surface (**a**)

Table 9.2 Chemical surface composition [12]

	Chemical composition [%]	
Element	SLA	modSLA
O	49.2 ± 2.1	61.1 ± 0.9
Ti	14.3 ± 1.3	22.5 ± 0.9
N	1.3 ± 0.4	0.7 ± 0.3
C	35.2 ± 2.2	14.2 ± 1.2

Results presented as mean ± SD, $n = 5$ for each surface

surface with or without high surface free energy. However, due to the chemical composition of the implants, not every alloy can be sandblasted and acid-etched like c.p. Ti. For example, it has been shown that acid-etching of the alloys Ti-6Al-4V and Ti-6Al-7Nb resulted in different surface microstructures than acid-etching of c.p. titanium [105]. These differences were related to the different crystal structures of c.p. titanium and these 2 alloys. At room temperature and pressure, c.p. titanium shows a hexagonal closed-packed (α) crystal structure, while at high temperatures, it adopts a body-centered cubic (β) structure [106]. The addition of Al stabilizes the α structure, while addition of Nb or V stabilizes the β structure [105]. In the case of these 2 alloys, the etching induced a selective dissolution of the α-phase and an enrichment of the β-phase, resulting in different surface microstructures compared to c.p. titanium [105]. Recently, a new titanium-zirconium (TiZr) alloy with a modSLA surface has been established on the market (Roxolid® SLActive®, Institut Straumann AG, Basel, Switzerland) that consists of titanium and 13–17 % zirconium [13, 107]. In comparison to c.p. titanium, it has been found that titanium-zirconium alloys show superior biomechanical properties, identified by increased hardness and tensile strength [108]. Since titanium, zirconium, as well as the TiZr alloy show the α-phase crystal structure at room temperature and pressure [106], the manufacturing procedure (sandblasting and acid-etching, rinsing under N_2 protection, storage in isotonic NaCl solution) for creating the modSLA surface on c.p titanium can be transferred to this particular TiZr alloy [107]. Thus,

Table 9.3 Roughness parameters for modSLA surfaces [109]

Roughness parameter	c.p. titanium	TiZi
S_a [μm]	1.00±0.02	1.30±0.09
S_t [μm]	6.73±0.18	8.90±0.36
S_{Sk} [μm]	0.14±0.03	0.21±0.06
S_{dr} [%]	29.6±1.2	39.0±3.3

S_a arithmetic mean deviation of the surface, S_t maximum peak-to-valley height of the surface, S_{Sk} skewness of the surface, S_{dr} developed surface area. Results presented as mean ± SD; $n=9$ for each surface. Calculations were performed with the use of a moving average Gaussian filter with a cutoff wavelength of 30 μm. A two-tailed student *t*-test (unequal variance) was performed to compare the surfaces. Significant differences were evaluated for all parameters ($p<0.01$) [109]

Table 9.4 Chemical surface composition of modSLA surfaces [107]

	Chemical composition [%]	
Element	c.p. titanium	TiZr
O	52.20±1.7	50.87±2.7
Ti	21.11±1.2	17.94±1.4
N	1.21±0.4	0.80±0.1
C	24.79±3.1	24.63±4.5
F	0.83±0.6	0.61±0.2
Al	–	2.56±0.0
Zr	–	2.79±0.2

Results presented as mean ± SD, $n=3$ for each surface

one specific advantage of this TiZr alloy is its increased biomechanical strength compared to c.p. titanium combined with the ability to create a modSLA surface topography.

SEM investigations on both materials show a similar micro-rough surface topography (Fig. 9.3). When investigating surface roughness parameters by performing quantitative surface analysis using confocal white-light microscopy (Table 9.3, [109]) and blue light laser and interferometer [107], significant differences have been observed for the number of samples measured. However, the c.p. Ti and the TiZr-modSLA surface both have similar characteristic roughness parameters between 1 and 2 μm (e.g., both surfaces are moderately rough [96]).

When investigating the chemical composition of the modSLA surfaces of both materials, no significant differences were observed. On the modSLA surface of TiZr, additional amounts of aluminum and zirconium were detected, and besides TiO_2 molecules, also ZrO_2 molecules were found (Table 9.4) [107]. The presence of Al can be explained by Al_2O_3 residuals due to the sandblasting process [103].

These results suggest that manufacturing a sandblasted and acid-etched surface with high surface free energy is not specific for one certain material, as the manufacturing process can be applied on commercially pure titanium as well as on this particular titanium-zirconium alloy, creating a similar moderately rough surface topography with an analogue chemical surface composition and similar surface roughness parameters.

ModSLA: Summary of Physical and Chemical Properties

In summary, due to the same sandblasting and acid-etching procedure, there were no differences in surface topography or surface roughness parameters between SLA and modSLA surfaces; however, nanostructures could only be found on the modSLA surface. Due to the different rinsing and storage procedures, differences were found in the chemical surface composition of the surfaces. In comparison to SLA, after rinsing with ultrapure water, the modSLA surfaces showed decreased adsorption of contaminants from the atmosphere and an increased concentration of hydroxylated groups on the surface, thus resulting in an increased surface hydrophilicity, surface wettability, and surface free energy. This is a result of the shared chemical bonding of the oxygen molecules from the native dioxide surface. Furthermore, the modSLA surface can be created on c.p. Ti as well as on a specific TiZr alloy, resulting in similar moderately rough microsurface topographies, with an analogue chemical surface composition and similar surface roughness parameters.

In Vitro Studies

In vitro investigations on cell-implant interactions provide valuable and detailed information about single cells and factors that affect the initial osseointegration process at the implant-bone interface. Therefore, it has been concluded that an "in vitro approach provides a powerful tool to elucidate the detailed biological events that take place at such an interface and has permitted the compositional and structural characteristics of the interface to be defined" [110]. Previous in vitro investigations have demonstrated that an increased surface roughness decreased cell proliferation (identified by a decreased number of cells on the surface) and increased cell attachment and differentiation of osteoblast-like cells that were cultured on titanium disks [15, 39, 41]. Due to the increased amount of hydroxylated groups bound to the dioxide layer (see above), the modified SLA surface is chemically more reactive than the SLA surface. Thus, it could be hypothesized that not only surface roughness but also surface free energy can directly influence cellular behavior and growth factor or cytokine production of cells, which are involved in the osseointegration process. One part of the goal of this review was to present current in vitro studies that investigated single cells and factors, which are involved in the implant healing process. Most findings on the modSLA surface were directly compared to findings on the SLA surface so that only differences due to the change in surface chemistry could be evaluated.

ModSLA: Bone Tissue Healing and Remodeling

The first part of implant healing consists of the recruitment and the migration of osteogenetic cells to the implant surface through the fibrin network of the peri-implant blood clot. This process is mainly initiated by platelet activation (release of cytokines, growth factors) within the first 3 days of healing [32, 35]. In this context, it was demonstrated that whole blood collected from human patients in direct contact with modSLA surfaces revealed significantly increased degrees of platelet binding, platelet activation, and intrinsic coagulation system activation, when compared to SLA surfaces [111]. The activated platelets not only stimulate factors that enhance osteogenetic cells but also release factors that activate leukocytes and macrophages (between 24 and 48 h after implant placement), which are involved in the demolition of the peri-implant blood clot [35], thus probably delaying the healing process. An attenuated pro-inflammatory response of the activated macrophages that might indicate a faster and improved wound healing was identified on modSLA compared to SLA. Whereas there were no significant differences in cellular macrophage attachment or proliferation on both surfaces, differences were found concerning the regulation of pro-inflammatory genes for cytokines and chemokines. Surface roughness induced activation of pro-inflammatory genes on both surfaces, but in contrast to SLA, on modSLA the expression of many genes was also significantly downregulated after 24 h and 3 days of investigation [112, 113].

Following recruitment and migration, osteogenetic cells attach to an implant surface and begin to proliferate [32, 35]. When investigating the attachment of MG63 osteoblast-like cells by seeding a defined number of cells on modSLA and SLA surfaces and evaluating the number of attached cells after 4 h of incubation, no differences in cell attachment levels could be evaluated between both surfaces [114]. The same results were found after cell attachment analysis of human mesenchymal stem cells and human mesenchymal stromal cells after 3 h of incubation [115, 116] and for human periodontal ligament cells after 5 h of incubation [117]. In contrast to that, when evaluating the number of attached human osteoblast cells, the modSLA surface demonstrated significantly increased cell attachment rates after 1 and 3 h of seeding in comparison to SLA [118]. Furthermore, integrin β_1 and α_V gene expression analysis of human osteoblast indicated a higher initial cell adhesion rate, and a strongly enhanced gene expression after 24 and 48 h was demonstrated on modSLA surfaces in comparison to SLA surfaces [119]. Thus, the increased attachment effect on modSLA implant surfaces appears to be cell specific for human osteoblasts.

With regard to cell proliferation, previous studies have shown that an increased surface roughness decreased the proliferation of MG63 osteoblast-like cells [15, 41]. When investigating these bone-producing cells, a higher surface free energy and wettability induced a further significant decrease of cell proliferation on modSLA in comparison to SLA [2, 114, 120–123]. Moreover, it was shown that the addition of 10^{-9} M calcitriol ($1\alpha,25(OH)_2D_3$) further significantly decreased the cell number on SLA, whereas no effects were noticed on modSLA [2]. Cell proliferation was also investigated using human osteoblast cells. The results again demonstrated a significantly reduced cell proliferation on modSLA compared to SLA surfaces [123, 124]. In general, cell number is decreased when cells begin to differentiate, indicating a change from a mainly proliferative to a more differentiated cell state [125, 126]. Thus, with regard to new bone formation, cell differentiation can be considered as a more decisive factor than initial cell proliferation.

Initial cell morphology has additionally been investigated on modSLA and SLA surfaces. It was shown that there were no significant differences between single MG63 osteoblast-like cells grown on modSLA or SLA surfaces. The shape of the cells was described as polygonal, elongated with many thin filopodia, attached to the surface [2, 118, 120]. By using time-lapse microscopy, Qu et al. demonstrated that MG63 osteoblast-like cells on modSLA surfaces began to form clusters as a precursor for noduli formation after 2 days of incubation, whereas cells on SLA still spread homogenously [114]. After 4 days of incubation, cells also began to form clusters on SLA, and after 9 days, modSLA still showed larger cell clusters compared to SLA [114]. When investigating human osteoblasts, minor morphological differences were found. After 6 h of seeding, human osteoblasts on modSLA showed increased spreading behavior by forming better-defined actin stress fibers in comparison to SLA [118]. After 24 h incubation, the cells on SLA had a more elongated structure, whereas osteoblasts on modSLA were smaller and rather roundish [119]. These studies suggest that bone-forming cells are in general stimulated to differentiate earlier on modSLA surfaces compared to the hydrophobic SLA surface and that this effect is cell type dependent.

Within the implant healing process, after recruitment, attachment, and proliferation, the cells undergo osteoblastic differentiation by producing osteoid, including matrix vesicles and growth factors (3–6 days). After that, the cells begin to calcify their matrix, indicated by increased alkaline phosphatase and phospholipase A_2 activity (6–14 days) [32, 35]. In this context, more differentiated and more active MG63-, MC3T3-E1 osteoblast-like cells, human osteoblast cells, human mesenchymal stem cells, and human periodontal ligament cells on modSLA in comparison to SLA have been reported, indicated by significant increases of factors that stimulate early and late osteogenic differentiation, like cell layer alkaline phosphatase (ALP), osteoprotegerin (OPG), type I collagen, osteopontin (OPN), and osteocalcin (OC) [2, 114, 117, 120, 121, 123, 125, 127, 128]. In addition to that, by producing significantly higher levels of local factors like prostaglandin E_2 (PGE_2), transforming growth factor-β1 (TGF-β1), phospholipase D, and protein kinase C (PKC), the cells seeded on modSLA surfaces also created a more osteogenic microenvironment when compared to cells seeded on SLA surfaces [2, 120, 121, 123]. In contrast to cell number, the addition of calcitriol ($1\alpha,25(OH)_2D_3$) caused further remarkable increases in the amount of ALP, OC, PGE_2, TGF-β1, and vascular endothelial growth factor-A (VEGF-A) production [2, 123]. Additionally, it has been shown that the differentiation of human mesenchymal stem cells into an osteoblastic phenotype was not only sensitive to surface microstructure but also to surface hydrophilicity [125]. Again, these results clearly indicate that the bone-forming cells begin to differentiate earlier and even more distinctively on modSLA compared to the SLA surface. This particular effect seems to be independent from the cell type.

After a cell differentiation period around inserted implants, the newly formed woven bone begins to be remodeled (21 days after initial implant placement), and this involves recruitment of osteoclasts that resorb the newly formed bone tissue [32, 35]. Osteoclasts are activated by a protein that is called receptor activator of nuclear factor kappa-B ligand (RANKL). This protein is produced by fibroblasts, T lymphocytes, B lymphocytes, and also osteoblasts and binds to the RANK receptor on the surface of mature osteoclasts or osteoclast precursors [129, 130]. Another protein called OPG is also produced by osteoblasts. It inhibits the differentiation of osteoclasts by blocking RANKL binding to its cellular receptor RANK [129]. Thus, bone formation occurs when the RANKL/OPG ratio decreases, whereas bone resorption occurs when the RANKL/OPG ratio increases [130]. It has been shown that the modSLA surface could directly influence the RANKL-RANK-OPG axis. An in vitro study investigated the mRNA gene expression for OPG and RANKL of human periodontal ligament cells that were seeded on modSLA and SLA surfaces [117]. After 5, 24 h, 3, and 5 days of investigation, no differences could be detected between both types of surfaces, indicating that bone cells are selectively activated on implant surfaces. Though, after 7 days of seeding, the authors demonstrated a significantly increased OPG gene expression and a significantly decreased RANKL gene expression on modSLA surfaces in comparison to SLA surfaces [117]. In addition to that, mouse bone marrow-derived macrophages showed a significantly reduced gene expression of osteoclastogenesis-related genes (TRAP, NFATc1, OSCAR, c-Fos) on modSLA surfaces compared to SLA surfaces [127]. Mature dendritic cells can also initiate T-cell activation and therefore influence the differentiation of osteoclasts [131]. It has been demonstrated that dendritic cells seeded on SLA surfaces promoted a more mature phenotype (based on surface marker expression, cytokine profiles, and cell morphology), whereas dendritic cells that were cultivated on modSLA surfaces promoted an inactive, immature phenotype that might indicate a noninflammatory biological peri-implant environment enhancing peri-implant bone formation [131]. These results suggest that the differentiation of osteoclasts is suppressed on modSLA surfaces, thus leading to decreased bone resorption and a further increased bone formation on modSLA implant surfaces in comparison to SLA surfaces within the bone remodeling processes.

ModSLA: Angiogenesis and Neovascularization

Besides osteoblastic and osteoclastic differentiation, further important factors that influence a successful osseointegration are peri-implant angiogenesis and neovascularization processes, predominantly initiated by endothelial cells but also involving other cell types [35, 132]. MG63 osteoblast-like cells seeded on modSLA implant surfaces demonstrated significantly increased production of growth factors that serve to initiate and control angiogenesis (VEGF-A, basic fibroblast growth factor (FGF-2), epidermal growth factor (EGF)) compared to cells seeded on SLA surfaces. Furthermore, these growth factors induced a significantly increased differentiation of human aortic endothelial cells (HAEC, indicated by endothelial tube formation and number of branch points) on modSLA surfaces compared to SLA surfaces. When investigating human osteoblasts, only significantly increased amounts of VEGF-A on modSLA in comparison to SLA surfaces could be demonstrated, whereas the increased amounts of other growth factors (see above) could not be detected [124]. Rausch-Fan et al. confirmed the significantly increased VEGF-A production of MG63 osteoblast-like cells and human osteoblasts on modSLA compared to SLA surfaces [123]. When investigating endothelial progenitor cells from goats, a remarkable increase of VEGF-A production was detected on modSLA compared to SLA surfaces; however, the results were not statistically significant [133]. In addition to that, human umbilical vascular endothelial cells (HUVECs) grown on modSLA demonstrated a significantly increased gene expression of angiogenesis-related factors (von Willebrand factor, thrombomodulin, endothelial cell protein C receptor) when compared to cells grown on SLA surfaces [134]. These results indicate that bone-forming cells as well as endothelial cells might provoke an earlier angiogenesis and an increased neovascularization on modSLA compared to SLA surfaces, thus probably enhancing the early peri-implant healing process around these hydrophilic implant surfaces.

ModSLA: Soft Tissue Healing

Not only bone tissue is a decisive factor for a successful implant healing process but also the peri-implant soft tissues [135] are important. In contrast to MG63 osteoblast-like cells and human osteoblasts, when investigating epithelial cells (oral squamous carcinoma cell line), an increase in initial cell attachment, proliferation rate, and cell spreading could be demonstrated on modSLA compared to SLA surfaces, but no differences in gene expression of functional factors that influence cytokine secretion were detected [136]. In addition to that, also human periodontal ligament cells seeded on modSLA surfaces demonstrated significantly increased proliferation rates after 24 h, 5, and 7 of days of incubation compared to cells seeded on SLA surfaces [117]. Thus, this increase in cell proliferation rate appears to be specific for non-bone-producing cells and may stimulate a more rapid soft tissue healing around implants with a modSLA surface.

ModSLA: Summary of In Vitro Studies

In summary, the results of in vitro studies demonstrate that modSLA surfaces in comparison to SLA surfaces increase the recruitment and migration of osteogenic cells to the implant surface in the very early healing period, indicated by increased platelet activation and an attenuated pro-inflammatory response of activated macrophages. After migration, only human osteoblasts showed a significantly increased cell attachment rate on modSLA compared to SLA surfaces within the first 48 h of investigation demonstrating a preferential selectioning of cell types for modSLA. Not only surface roughness but also an increased surface free energy induced a further significant decrease in the number of proliferated MG63 osteoblast-like cells and human osteoblasts on modSLA compared to SLA surfaces indicating that cells stop proliferation and rather increase differentiation, thus preparing for new bone. Only the proliferation of soft tissue cells (human periodontal ligament fibroblasts) was significantly increased on modSLA compared to SLA surfaces. Concerning cell morphology, no differences were observed between both types of surfaces; however, MG63 osteoblast-like and human osteoblast cells on modSLA surfaces showed a faster initial cell spreading behavior compared to cells seeded on SLA surfaces. After attachment and proliferation, all investigated types of osteogenic-related cells were significantly more differentiated and more active and created a more osteogenic environment on the modSLA surfaces compared to cells that were incubated on the SLA surfaces. In addition to that, modSLA surfaces promoted bone formation within the bone remodeling process by decreasing the RANKL/OPG ratio, thus inhibiting the differentiation of osteoclasts. Furthermore, in comparison to SLA, MG63 osteoblast-like cells and human osteoblasts seeded on modSLA surfaces also demonstrated significantly increased productions of growth factors that initiate and control angiogenesis and enhance the differentiation of endothelial cells that initiate neovascularization (Fig. 9.6). Besides osteogenic-related cells, increased surface free energy also directly influenced other soft tissue cells (epithelial cells) by increasing epithelial attachment, proliferation, and cell spreading on modSLA compared to SLA surfaces. Thus, the chemically active hydrophilic modSLA surface compared to the hydrophobic SLA surface promotes bone cell attachment and differentiation, blood vessel formation, and soft tissue proliferation.

In Vivo Studies

As osseointegration is a very complex process that involves a wide variety of different types of cells and in vitro protocols only allow investigating interactions of single cell types (e.g., osteoblasts), controlled in vivo models are clinically most relevant to study the osseous integration and culmination of cellular interactions of dental implants [52]. In addition, as implant restorations in the oral cavity always have to penetrate the soft tissues, the implant restoration-gingival tissues should provide an effective barrier function similar to dentogingival tissues to ensure the integrity of the integument. Based on this fact, it has been demonstrated that nonsubmerged dental implants

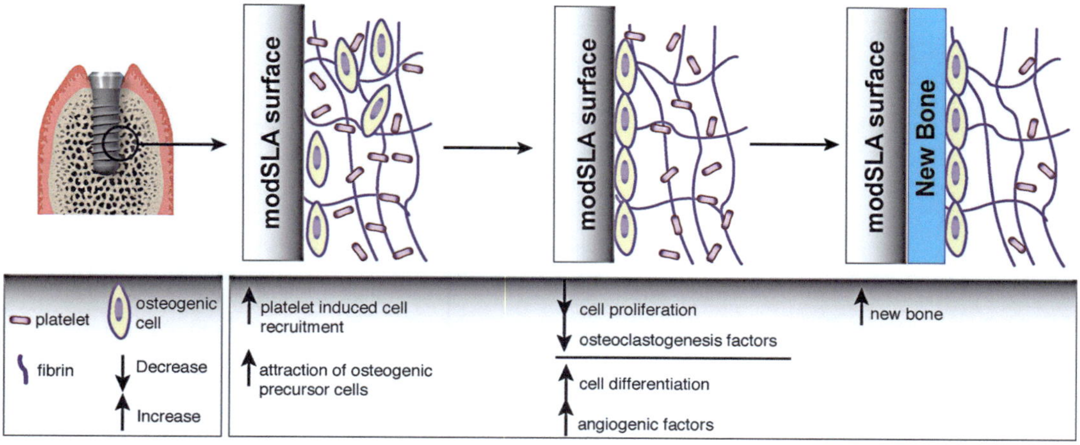

Fig. 9.6 Schematic diagram of enhanced peri-implant bone healing around modSLA implant surface

must successfully integrate with bone tissue as well as with connective tissue and epithelium at the time of implant placement [135, 137]. The following section presents preclinical in vivo studies investigating peri-implant bone integration and defect regeneration, as well as soft tissue integration around c.p. titanium and TiZr alloy implants with a modSLA surface that were performed using different animal models and different examination methods.

ModSLA: Bone Tissue Integration

Concerning bone tissue integration, it has been reported that implants with a modSLA surface showed a faster osseous healing within the initial osseointegration process in comparison to SLA surfaces [11, 52, 66, 132, 138–141]. Qualitative histological findings of preclinical studies performed in canines [132, 138] reported on modSLA implants that showed stabilized blood coagulums substituted by dense connective tissue with oriented collagen fibers after 1 and 4 days of healing, whereas SLA implants demonstrated partially collapsed blood clots substituted by granulation tissue and provisional connective tissue at the same time (Fig. 9.7).

By performing immunohistochemical staining in these studies, it was also demonstrated that after 1 day, initial neovascularization was initiated on both surfaces but after 4 and 7 days modSLA implants revealed more newly formed blood vessels surrounded by tiny trabeculae of woven bone compared to SLA implants [132, 138]. Furthermore, after 4 days, only the connective tissue adjacent to the modSLA surface already showed positive osteocalcin antigen reactions, indicating osteoblastic differentiation. After 14 days, newly formed bone tissue was more mature on modSLA compared to SLA, since on modSLA surfaces, parallel fibered woven bone was found that occasionally already showed formation of primary osteons [132, 138]. All these results demonstrate that bone formation is more rapid around implants with a modSLA surface compared to implants with an SLA surface beginning immediately on implant placement.

Within the course of the further integration period, these descriptive differences were no longer evident. Buser et al. and Bornstein et al. performed histological investigations of modSLA implants in miniature pigs and in canines. The authors could not demonstrate any qualitative differences after 2 and 4 weeks of investigation between both types of implants [11, 66]. Thus, the process of osseointegration is the same on both implant surfaces; however, the process occurs more rapidly on modSLA implants.

To quantify the histological findings, histomorphometrical evaluations were performed. Similar to the histological findings, it has been reported that modSLA implants showed a higher degree of osseous integration (indicated by

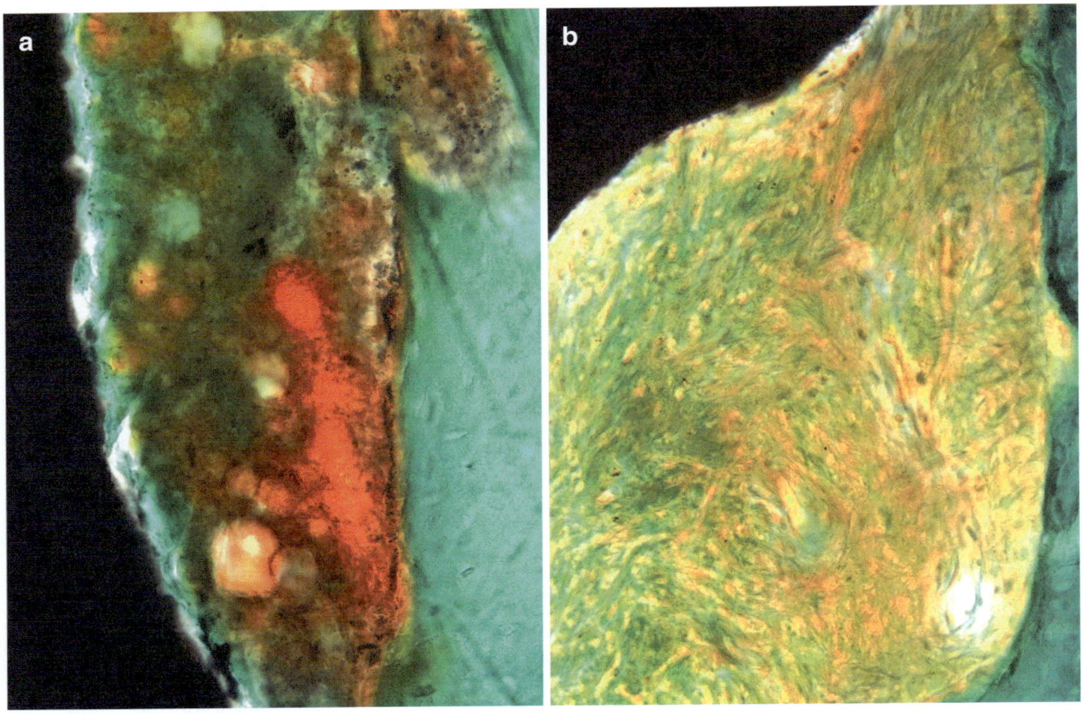

Fig. 9.7 Histological pictures (section stained with Masson-Goldner trichrome) showing wound healing procedures at 4 days after implant placement. (**a**) Partially collapsed blood clot substituted by granulation tissue and provisional connective tissue in direct environment of implant with SLA surface. (**b**) Stabilized blood coagulum substituted by dense connective tissue with oriented collagen fibers, partially running perpendicular to the modSLA implant surface (From Schwarz et al. [132]. Reprinted with permission from John Wiley and Sons)

increased bone-to-implant contact (BIC) and bone density (BD)) within the initial osseointegration process. Buser et al. who inserted experimental bone chamber implants (core diameter 2.7 mm, outer diameter 4.2 mm) in the maxillae of 6 miniature pigs performed the first study investigating this issue. The authors demonstrated statistically significantly increased mean BIC values for modSLA after 2 and 4 weeks of submerged, unloaded healing (49.3 %±7.49 and 81.9 1 %±3.59) in comparison to SLA (29.42 %±7.58 and 66.57 %±8.14) but not after 8 weeks (modSLA 78.47 %±11.14; SLA 75.45 %±7.66) [11]. Similar results were also reported in studies that used different animal models and comparable observation periods. It could be shown that unloaded modSLA implants used in canines, sheep, and human patients revealed remarkably increased BIC values at early healing periods compared to SLA implants [52, 66, 132, 138–141].

Initial osseointegration of modSLA implants was not only investigated in healthy bone but also in indications that showed compromised general health conditions. It was shown that modSLA enhanced the osseointegrative capacity of commercially available implants placed in the calvaria of diabetic pigs. Although there were no differences concerning BIC between both types of implants after 30 and 90 days in healthy animals, modSLA implants revealed significantly higher BIC values in diabetic animals after 90 days compared to SLA implants. The evaluation of BD showed significantly increased values for modSLA implants for healthy as well as for compromised pigs after both investigation time points [142]. These results again suggest that the modSLA surface results in more tissue differentiation to bone compared to the SLA surface, which also promotes bone formation but at a slightly delayed rate of formation.

Faster initial osseointegration for modSLA compared to SLA was also demonstrated by biomechanical investigations of the bone-implant interface. Torque-out testing of implants inserted in miniature pig maxillae demonstrated significantly increased removal torque-out and interfacial stiffness values for modSLA compared to SLA after 2, 4, and 8 weeks of healing [143]. Also pullout testing of titanium disks in another animal species, rabbits, showed significantly increased pullout values for modSLA in comparison to SLA after 4 and 8 weeks [103]. Moreover, nondestructive testing of the implant stability confirmed the faster initial osseous integration of modSLA compared to SLA implants. By performing electronic resonance frequency analysis (RFA, Ostell®, Integration Diagnostics AB, Savedalen, Sweden) measurements of implants inserted in sheep, modSLA implants showed significantly increased RFA values after 3 but not after 6 weeks in comparison to SLA implants. The same authors could not demonstrate any differences in removal torque-out testing between both types of implants after 6 weeks [140]. These results clearly indicate that modSLA implants show increased biomechanical stability compared to SLA implants in the initial healing period.

Besides histological and biomechanical investigational results, an accelerated osseointegration process for modSLA compared to SLA was also indicated by microarray and gene expression analysis of implants placed in human mandibles [144]. The authors could demonstrate that differences in functionally relevant gene expression begin to be evident after 7 days of integration, since the expression of several functionally important osteogenesis-, angiogenesis-, and neurogenesis-associated genes were overrepresented on cells or tissue grown on SLActive implant surfaces compared to SLA implant surfaces [144]. These results again suggest a faster initial osseointegration process for modSLA implants compared to SLA implants.

ModSLA: Bone Tissue Regeneration

As described above, the initial osseointegration process was investigated by placing implants into native bone tissue. Since the placement of an implant can sometimes be compromised by crestal bone defects due to limited bone volume, due to anatomic limitations during placement, or due to implant placement immediately after tooth extraction, the ability of an implant surface to promote osseous formation is of great importance. In different studies in canines, rabbits, and miniature pigs, it has been shown that modSLA implant surfaces provided reliable and effective new bone healing at acute and chronic lateral ridge defects and at coronal circumferential defects [141, 145–149]. Different types of guided bone regeneration (GBR) and different types of membranes were investigated adjacent to modSLA implants placed in canines [146, 147]. When compared to biphasic calcium phosphate (Bone Ceramic®, Straumann AG, Basel, Switzerland) or bovine-derived, collagen-coated (Bio-Oss®, Geistlich Biomaterials, Wolhusen, Switzerland) bone-grafting material, it was shown that initial new woven bone formation of crestal bone defects, surgically induced 4 weeks prior to implant and bone graft placement (width/depth 6 mm, height between 2 and 8 mm) or surgically induced directly following implant bed preparation (width 3 mm, depth 2 mm, height 4 mm), was more pronounced on the modSLA implant surface than on the graft particles. The authors in these latter studies concluded that a higher osteoconductivity for the modSLA surface existed than for the particular grafting material or technique [146, 147]. Furthermore, it has been demonstrated that GBR did not improve the outcome of vertical bone regeneration but tended to increase the bone formed on modSLA surfaces [147]. In addition to these studies, modSLA implants with a different overall shape (tapered effect design) that were placed into miniature pig mandibles immediately after tooth extraction without using any grafting procedures or membranes showed histologically and histomorphometrically successful osseointegration. Furthermore, the authors in this study demonstrated that the immediately loaded implants showed similar BIC values and identical crestal bone loss after 8 weeks of healing compared to implants that were loaded 4 weeks after placement

[149]. In comparison to SLA implants, modSLA implants showed significantly increased bone formation (indicated by new bone height, percent linear fill, BIC, area of new bone fill) of acute buccal dehiscence defects in canines (surgically induced following implant bed preparation, width 3 mm, depth 3 mm, height 3–4 mm) after 2, 4, 8, and 12 weeks of submerged and transgingival healing resulting in complete osseous filling of the previously created defects after 12 weeks only on modSLA implants [141, 145]. Regarding crestal circumferential bone defects (circumferential gap, width 0.5–1 mm, height 5 mm), it has also been shown that BIC and new bone fill were significantly increased after 2 and 4 weeks but not after 8 weeks on modSLA implants compared to SLA implants placed in canines [148]. Even when comparing both types of implants in rabbits with experimentally induced osteoporosis, modSLA significantly increased new bone healing (indicated by newly formed bone, newly formed mineralized bone, BIC) after 30 and 120 days of investigation compared to SLA [150]. Thus, the excellent osteoconductive properties of the modSLA implant surface were not only demonstrated around implants placed in bone defect areas but also when investigating peri-implant crestal bone levels in non-defect areas and in different animal models.

In another study, modSLA implants with either a machined collar (MC, $n=36$) or a modSLA collar (NMC, $n=36$) were placed in the mandibles of 6 canines. Both types of implants were prosthetically loaded after 21 days. After 3 and 12 months of loading, the histomorphometrical evaluation showed a mean crestal bone gain of 0.13 ± 0.37 and 0.13 ± 0.44 mm, respectively, for NMC implants, whereas MC implants revealed a mean bone loss of -0.32 ± 0.7 mm (3 months) and -0.79 ± 0.35 mm (6 months). The radiographic investigations also confirmed these results (3 months, NMC 0.29 ± 0.68 mm, MC -0.51 ± 1.1 mm; 12 months, NMC 0.11 ± 0.48 mm, MC -1.0 ± 0.37 mm). The differences after both investigation periods were statistically significant. The authors described the crestal bone gain as "creeping osseointegration" and related it not only to the absence of the machined collar but mainly to the excellent osteoconductive properties of the modSLA surface [151, 152]. These results taken together clearly indicate that new bone growth in defect or non-defect areas is faster and greater on the modSLA implant surface compared to the SLA implant surface or a machined surface. When using GBR procedures for defect regeneration, the modSLA surface itself enhances bone formation more distinctively than the additionally used xenogenic or alloplastic graft particles or membranes.

ModSLA: Soft Tissue Integration

As described above, integration of dental implant restorations, besides osseointegration, also necessitates successful connective tissue and epithelial integration [153, 154]. In different studies on canines, it has been shown that submerged and non-submerged modSLA implants showed superior soft tissue integration compared to SLA implants [138, 155, 156]. Investigating the connective tissue zone by placing implants with either a modSLA or SLA transmucosal part and, using submerged or transgingival healing protocols, the histological results after 14 and 28 days of unloaded healing showed a well-vascularized connective tissue in direct contact to the modSLA surfaces. Besides parallel fibers, the connective tissue also exhibited collagen fibers that have started to extend and run partially perpendicular to the modSLA implant surface. Within the connective tissue, no different zones were demonstrated. In contrast to that, on SLA surfaces the connective tissue could be divided into 2 different zones. The inner zone consisted of a dense connective tissue capsule with only parallel running collagen fibers that had no contact to the implant surface and rare blood vessel formation. Towards the periphery, that zone was surrounded by well-vascularized loose connective tissue formed of collagen fibers running in different directions [138, 155]. When investigating the attachment of the junctional epithelium to modSLA and SLA implants, using a non-submerged healing protocol, it was shown that after 14 days of healing, the epithelial cells were in close contact to the modSLA surface, whereas the junctional epithelium was generally separated by a gap from the SLA surface [138]. Using a similar study protocol, the same authors demonstrated that the above-described differences are still evident after 6 months of unloaded healing. Furthermore, it was reported that frequent clinical probing (3×, 4× prior to euthanasia) increased mean probing depths and disrupted epithelial and connective tissue attachment on both surfaces. Frequent probing even destroyed the perpendicular orientation of the collagen fibers on modSLA implants after 12 weeks of investigation [156]. Overall, these results on the soft tissues around modSLA implant surfaces indicate that the formation of the peri-implant connective tissue as well as the junctional epithelium is faster and more pronounced on the modSLA surface compared to the SLA surface, thus probably providing a more effective barrier against pathological bacterial intrusion.

ModSLA: Compared to Other Implant Surfaces

ModSLA implants have been mostly compared to SLA implants because, due to the identical geometrical design, the different results concerning osseous and soft tissue integration of both types of implants could be directly attributed to the different implant surface chemical properties. Thus, a direct comparison of implants with different surface structures and designs is less informative since differences cannot be attributed to just the surface chemistry as both surface chemistry and geometry are different. Nevertheless, modSLA implants have also been directly compared to implants with different geometrical and surface chemistry designs. In comparison to calcium phosphate nanoparticle-modified dual acid-etched (DCD/CaP) implants (Nanotite®, 3i implant innovations, Biomet 3i, Palm Beach Gardens, USA), modSLA implants showed no significant differences concerning BIC, first BIC, and amount of bone volume after 2, 4, and 8 weeks of unloaded healing when inserted in canine mandibles with sufficient native bone volume [157]; however, when the same types of implants were inserted in canines with buccal dehiscence-type defects that were created immediately following implant placement (compare above), modSLA implants revealed statistically significantly increased amounts of new bone height and BIC after 2 and 8 weeks of unloaded healing in comparison to DCD/CaP implants [158]. In another study, Gottlow et al. compared modSLA implants and titanium implants with an oxidized surface (TiUnite®, Nobel Biocare AB, Gothenburg, Sweden; OX) in rabbits after 10 days and 3 and 6 weeks of integration. ModSLA implants showed significantly increased removal torque-out values after 3 weeks and significantly increased interfacial shear strength values after 3 and 6 weeks compared to OX. Significantly increased BIC values were reported after 10 days for modSLA and after 6 weeks for OX implants [159]. These results suggest that, in comparison to other implant types, modSLA implants show at least comparable and in many cases better osseointegrative capacities than other types of implants.

ModSLA: On Particular TiZr Alloy Implants

As described above, the modSLA surface was not only produced on commercially pure titanium implants but also on implants that were made of a particular titanium-zirconium alloy. Qualitative histological findings of experimental studies in canines and in miniature pigs showed similar bone formation and bone remodeling processes for unloaded TiZr alloy and c.p. Ti implants with a modSLA surface within the first 8 weeks of integration [109, 160]. However, quantitative histomorphometrical investigations also reported on some delay in the initial osseous healing process for TiZr-modSLA implants compared to Ti-modSLA implants [11, 160, 161]. By inserting both types of implants (diameter, 3.3 mm; length, 8 mm) 3 mm above the bone level in the tibia of rabbits, the authors demonstrated significantly decreased new bone healing (indicated by linear bone fill, new vertical bone height, and vertical BIC) after 10 days of investigation for TiZr-modSLA implants compared to c.p. Ti-modSLA implants. After 20 and 30 days of healing, these results were not different (no statistically significant differences) [161]. Another study in miniature pigs also reported no differences for BIC values for TiZr implants with a modSLA surface after 1, 2, 4 and 8 weeks of unloaded healing compared to c.p. Ti implants with a modSLA surface, whereas the amount of bony ingrowth into the implants' groves was increased after 4 and 8 weeks for TiZr [109]. Slightly but not significantly increased BIC values for TiZr-modSLA implants in comparison to c.p. Ti-modSLA implants were reported for implants placed in rabbits after 3 and 6 weeks of healing [162] and for implants placed in canines after 2 and 8 weeks of healing, but not after 4 weeks [160]. One study in miniature pigs demonstrated significantly increased newly formed bone area within the chambers of experimentally designed bone chamber implants after 4 weeks of unloaded healing for TiZr-modSLA implants compared to c.p. Ti-modSLA implants; however, the additionally reported BIC values presented no significant differences between implant types [163]. When investigating vertical bone formation in combination with bone mineral proteins in miniature pigs, TiZr-modSLA and c.p. Ti-modSLA implants showed direct supracrestal bone growth of good quality and density [164]. These results suggest that bone tissue similarly adapts on the modSLA surface of TiZr implants as well as on c.p. titanium implants in the early healing period.

In contrast to the histomorphometrical investigations, biomechanical investigations of the bone-implant interface showed an accelerated osseointegration process for TiZr-modSLA implants compared to c.p. Ti-modSLA implants, by demonstrating statistically significantly increased removal torque-out values after 4 weeks of healing in miniature pigs [163] and after 3 and 6 weeks of healing in rabbits [162]. Additionally, a further study investigated the nanomechanical properties of TiZr-modSLA and c.p. Ti-modSLA implants that were inserted in miniature pigs by performing nanoindentation testing [165]. After 4 weeks of healing, the authors reported a similar elastic modulus and hardness of the newly formed bone in proximity of the implant surface for both types of implants [165]. These results again indicate that TiZr implants with a modSLA surface show similar or, in some cases, stronger bone tissue response than the c.p. titanium implants with a modSLA surface.

ModSLA: Summary of In Vivo Studies

In summary, regarding bone tissue formation, the histological, histomorphometrical, biomechanical, and gene expression investigations clearly indicate an accelerated osseous integration within the first 4 weeks of healing for implants with a modSLA surface in comparison to implants with an SLA surface in different animal models and under varying time points and conditions. Successful osseointegration was demonstrated for implants placed in healed sites as well as for implants placed directly after tooth extraction. When used in diabetic miniature pigs, unloaded modSLA implants showed significantly increased bone apposition compared to SLA implants after an investigation period of 3 months. ModSLA implants placed in osteoporotic rabbits revealed significantly increased bone regeneration after 30 and 120 days compared to SLA implants. Immediately and early loaded implants showed comparable BIC values and no significant differences between both loading protocols in regard to peri-implant crestal bone loss. Thus, the modSLA surface demonstrated excellent osteoconductive properties investigated in healthy or compromised animal models, and bone regeneration/formation could successfully be performed with or without grafting material or GBR procedures. Regarding the soft tissues around implants, the histological results also reported an accelerated integration for modSLA compared to SLA. Moreover, due to the perpendicular fibers starting from the modSLA surface, it could be concluded that connective tissue on the modSLA surface could provide a more effective barrier against the oral cavity and against pathological bacterial intrusion than the connective tissue on SLA implants. In comparison to other implant types, modSLA showed at least comparable and in many cases better osseointegrative properties; however, these results must be interpreted with caution due to the different implant geometries. TiZr implants with a modSLA surface showed similar osseointegrative capacities as c.p. Ti implants with a modSLA surface.

Clinical Studies

The SLA implant surface has been extensively clinically investigated, and the results concluded that implants with this surface topography can be successfully loaded after 6–12 weeks of integration depending on bone type with favorable survival and success rates up to and after 10 years of follow-up [5, 76, 87, 90] and as noted above. It has been stated "A further reduction of the healing period required to complete therapy is beneficial to patients, simplifies clinical procedures, and may improve the acceptance of implant therapy by patients" [166]. Since the results of the preclinical investigations indicated a faster osseointegration for modSLA in comparison to SLA (see above), the aims of some clinical studies were to investigate if the modSLA implants could be successfully loaded even earlier than SLA implants such as immediately loaded or loaded 21 days following placement. Additionally, these studies evaluated if the chemically active hydrophilic surface could show at least comparable survival and success rates when used in normal (sufficient bone volume, healthy patient) or in compromised (insufficient bone volume, patients with high general risk factors) indications. Furthermore, clinical (probing depths (PD)) and radiographic parameters (crestal bone changes) were investigated. As it was demonstrated that surface hydrophilicity and energy did not have any significant influence on supragingival plaque biofilm formation [167], further clinical parameters like modified sulcus bleeding index (mSBI) or modified plaque index were not included in this review. The following section presents findings and data from the current clinical investigations on modSLA implants with a tissue-level and bone-level design.

ModSLA: On c.p. Ti Tissue-Level Implants

The first prospective clinical study investigating implant stability within an early healing period of modSLA implants was performed by Oates et al. [168]. One modSLA and one SLA implant were randomly placed into the posterior mandible or maxilla of 31 patients (50 implants placed in the mandible and 12 implants in maxillary sextants). Electronic RFA to define the implant stability quotient (ISQ, Osstell®, Integration Diagnostics AB, Gothenburg, Sweden) was performed weekly over the first 6 weeks following implant placement. After 6 weeks of healing, all 62 study implants were successfully integrated and could be restored. Overall, RFA values for both implant types decreased within the first weeks of healing, but for implants placed in the mandible, a significant shift from decreasing to increasing stability occurred for the modSLA implants after 2 weeks and for SLA implants after 4 weeks, indicating an earlier transition from predominantly resorptive to predominantly formative bone metabolism for modSLA surfaces [168]. Further studies confirmed significantly increased RFA values for modSLA implants compared to SLA in investigations when implants were placed in mandibles and when RFA was performed electronically [169]. In additional studies, no significant ISQ differences between both types of implants were detected when RFA was performed magnetically (Osstell mentor®, Integration Diagnostics AB, Gothenburg, Sweden) [169–171] or when both implants were compared in diabetic patients [171]. For implants placed in the maxilla, only palatal-inserted orthodontic implants (Orthosystem®, Institut Straumann AG, Basel, Switzerland) with a modSLA surface showed significantly increased ISQ values after 12 weeks of healing compared to SLA implants (electronic RFA). Furthermore, it was reported that the transition point from decreasing to increasing ISQ values was obtained after 28 days for modSLA and after 35 days for SLA [172] supporting the study by Oates et al. [168]. These results, taken together, suggest that modSLA implants integrate faster compared to SLA implants in the early healing period, when investigating implant stability.

Based on the findings of the above-described studies, prospective clinical investigations were initiated in which modSLA implants were loaded in full occlusion after 21 days of healing. A multicenter study reported on 56 patients with partial edentulism in the posterior mandible or maxilla who received 89 implants. After 2 years of investigation, only 2 implants failed (after 21 days of integration), and another 2 implants ("spinners") could not be loaded after 21 days and required more healing time due to slight implant mobility during removal of the healing cap. A 2-year survival and success rate of 97.7 % was reported in this study for modSLA implants loaded after 21 days. Furthermore, the authors evaluated mean probing depths of 3.07 ± 0.11 and 3.21 ± 0.11 mm and a mean crestal bone loss of 0.23 and 0.2 mm, 1 and 2 years after implant placement, respectively [166]. As one part of the above-described multicenter study, Bornstein et al. presented data after 3 years of investigation for 39 out of the 56 patients who received 56 implants. In this patient population, within the first 6 months of healing, the modSLA implants showed steadily increasing ISQ values throughout the follow-up period. No implant loss occurred and only the 2 "spinners" were observed; thus, 3-year survival and success rate of 100 % was reported. The authors demonstrated a mean crestal bone loss of 0.24, 0.15, and 0.12 mm and PD values of 3.65 ± 0.1, 3.76 ± 0.11, and 3.53 ± 0.09 mm after 1, 2, and 3 years of healing, respectively. Furthermore, the authors compared the collected soft tissue and radiographic parameters with a historic control group of SLA implants that were loaded after 6 weeks. No differences were found concerning distance between implant shoulder and mucosal margin (DIM), distance between implant shoulder and first bone-implant contact (DIB) and mSBI, whereas the modSLA implants revealed significantly decreased mean PD (3.53 ± 0.09 mm) and decreased clinical attachment levels (CAL, 2.53 ± 0.07 mm) after 3 years compared to SLA. No numerical data concerning both parameters were provided for SLA implants [173, 174]. ModSLA implants, which did not fail to integrate but that necessitated extended healing time (due to rotation or sensitivity when an abutment was torqued to 35 Ncm) prior to prosthetic reconstruction, were also reported in a further prospective study. In this investigation, out of 35 implants inserted in the posterior maxilla of 35 patients by using bone-condensing implant site preparation, 6 implants could not be loaded after 21 days but after another 3–4 weeks. One year after implantation, all implants were successfully integrated and showed mean PD of 3.4 ± 1.0 mm and a mean crestal bone loss 0.22 ± 0.35 mm [175]. These results clearly indicate that modSLA implants can successfully be loaded after 21 days of healing.

A direct comparison of loaded modSLA and SLA implants in non-compromised patients using a split-mouth design has been performed in 1 study [176]. In 22 partially edentulous patients, a total of 96 implants (48× modSLA, 48× SLA) were placed in the anterior and posterior mandible or maxilla. Each patient received at least 1 modSLA and 1 SLA implant. In the mandible, implant loading was performed after 8 weeks and in the maxilla after 12 weeks. One modSLA implant was lost 3 weeks after placement; thus, a survival rate of 97.91 % and 100 % for modSLA and SLA was reported, respectively, for this study after 12 months of loading. Furthermore, the authors demonstrated no significant differences with regard to RFA values between both implant types, but a significantly decreased mean marginal bone loss for modSLA (0.18 ± 0.06 mm) compared to SLA (0.22 ± 0.07 mm) at the beginning of the loading period. No significant differences in marginal bone loss between both types of implants could be found after 12 months of loading (modSLA, 0.43 ± 0.11 mm; SLA, 0.46 ± 0.07 mm). In addition, PD also was significantly decreased for modSLA at the beginning of the loading period (modSLA, 2.56 ± 0.38 mm; SLA, 2.66 ± 0.32 mm), whereas SLA implants revealed significantly decreased PD values after 1 year of loading (modSLA, 3.2 ± 0.46 mm; SLA, 3.12 ± 0.56 mm) [176]. These results suggest that modSLA and SLA implants show comparable short-term survival rates when implants are loaded after 8 or 12 weeks [176].

Besides early and conventional loading, also immediate loading was investigated on modSLA implants. A multicenter study comparing modSLA implants that were restored immediately following implant placement (without occlusal contact) and modSLA implants that were provisionally restored, again without occlusal contact,

28–34 days following implant placement provided clinical data after 5 months and 1 and 3 years after implant placement [177–179]. In both groups, the implants were fully loaded with permanent restorations 20–23 weeks after placement. After 3 years, 239 partially edentulous patients who received 340 implants in the posterior maxilla or mandible could be evaluated. The authors demonstrated significant differences in mean crestal bone level loss after 5 months between immediately (0.81 ± 0.89 mm) or early (0.56 ± 0.73 mm) loaded implants (however, the immediately placed implants were initially placed more apically), whereas no further significant increase in bone loss occurred for both loading protocols between 5 and 36 months (immediate, 0.076 mm; early, 0.006 mm). Furthermore, no significant differences between both treatment groups were found on survival rate (immediate, 98 %; early, 97 %) after 1 year and on survival rate (immediate, 97.4 %; early, 96.7 %) and success rate (immediate, 96.9 %; early, 96.7 %) after 3 years [179]. Out of 11 implant failures that were reported in this multicenter trial, 10 failures (4 implants in immediate group, 6 implants in early group) occurred between day 7 and 82 after implant placement, before permanent loading could be performed [177]. One failure (immediate group) occurred after permanent loading, 458 days following placement [179].

Immediate loading has also been investigated in fully edentulous patients using a prospective case series. One hundred twenty-four patients received 2 bar-splinted modSLA implants, which were immediately loaded with implant-retained mandibular overdentures. Three out of the 248 implants were lost 3 weeks after placement. After an average evaluation period of 2 years (range between 12 and 40 months), the authors presented a survival rate of 98.8 % [180]. In another study, it was demonstrated that in 21 patients, in which no bone augmentation was performed prior to implant placement, the bone quality did not have any influence on crestal bone resorption or on survival rate of 137 immediately (24 h after implant placement) loaded modSLA implants. Thus, 1 year after placement, a survival rate of 100 % was reported [181]. These results indicate that modSLA implants can successfully be loaded immediately after placement in different bone types and in different indications; however, in comparison to early loading, the immediately loaded implants showed slightly increased crestal bone loss. Furthermore, it should be noted that all of the abovementioned studies included only patients according to strict inclusion and exclusion criteria (e.g., excellent oral hygiene, no medical risk patients, no previously or simultaneously performed bone augmentations) and strictly controlled study protocols. This should be considered when interpreting these results, relative to results expected in less well-controlled conditions such as in private practice.

In private practice, patient treatment according to a strictly defined study protocol with specified inclusion and exclusion criteria is hardly possible, since the decision on implant treatment (implant placement, loading protocol) most frequently is taken by the clinician according to the current situation and the patients' needs, and not according to a study protocol. In this context, Luongo et al. presented clinical data from a noninterventional study using 276 modSLA implants that were placed in 218 patients by private practitioners in 29 clinical centers [182]. Patients with risk factors like smoking, untreated gingivitis or periodontitis and bruxism, as well as patients who needed a simultaneous bone augmentation during implant placement were also included. The implants were loaded after 48 h up to 6 months after implantation, and the authors reported a 1-year survival and success rate of 98.2 %. All 5 implant failures in this study occurred before the implants could be permanently restored and when sinus floor bone augmentation was performed simultaneously with implant placement [182].

With regard to implant placement and sinus floor bone augmentations, in an additional study, 230 days after performance of sinus floor augmentation using Bone Ceramic® or Bio-Oss® on 11 patients, 62 modSLA implants were placed. One implant (Bio-Oss® group) was lost before functional loading and 1 implant was lost after

3 months of loading (Bone Ceramic® group). Thus, after 1 year of loading, an overall survival rate of 96.8 % was reported [183]. A further study investigated 27 patients and 42 modSLA implants that were placed simultaneously during internal sinus floor elevation using the osteotome sinus floor elevation technique. No implant failure was reported 2 years after implant placement. Forty implants were successfully loaded after only 6 weeks of healing and 2 implants could be loaded 6 months after placement [184]. In addition to that, short modSLA implants (length 6 mm) were investigated in cases with limited bone volume but without previously or simultaneously performed bone augmentation procedures [185]. A total of 40 modSLA implants (length 6 mm, 19 with a diameter of 4.1 mm, 21 with a diameter of 4.8 mm) were inserted in 35 patients. Thirty-eight out of the 40 implants demonstrated steadily increasing RFA values and could be loaded after 6 weeks of healing with single crowns, whereas 2 implants (4.1 mm) were lost before loading could be performed. Between implant placement and 2 years of loading, a survival rate of 95 % and a mean crestal bone loss of 0.75±0.71 mm were reported [185]. These results indicate that modSLA implants provide a very high survival and success predictability when used in patients with moderate risk factors, when used in combination with bone augmentation procedures, and when used in sites with anatomical limitations.

ModSLA implants have also been compared to SLA implants in compromised patients as well as in healthy patients. For example, Heberer et al. [186] reported on 102 implants (52 modSLA implants (test), 50 SLA implants (control)) that were placed in the maxilla and mandible of 20 irradiated patients. Test and control implant sites were randomly assigned according to a split-mouth design. In these 20 patients, a malignant tumor of the mandible was surgically removed followed by a radio-chemotherapy up to 72 Gy for a period of 6 weeks. All implants were placed after a minimum of 6 months following radio-chemotherapy. Implants in the mandible were loaded after 6 weeks and after 10 weeks in the maxilla. Two SLA implants were lost before loading; thus, after a mean investigation period of 14.4 months, the authors demonstrated success rates of 100 % and 96 % for modSLA and SLA implants, respectively, and slightly decreased crestal bone loss for modSLA (0.3 mm mesial and distal) in comparison to SLA (0.4 mm, mesial and distal). However, no significant differences between implants with an SLA and a modSLA surface were reported concerning probing depths [186]. A further study investigated 48 implants (24 modSLA implants, 24 SLA implants) that were placed in the posterior mandible of 24 patients with type 2 diabetes having poor glycemic control (HbA1c levels between 7.5 % and 11.4 %) according to a randomly assigned split-mouth protocol [171]. Magnetic RFA measurement revealed no significant differences between both types of implants within the first 16 weeks of integration. One SLA implant failed between week 4 and 6 [171]. These results again suggest that, when used in compromised patients, modSLA implants show a very high predictability of success and significantly less crestal bone loss in short-term healing compared to SLA implants, which also successfully integrate.

ModSLA: On c.p. Ti Bone-Level Implants

Since progressive loss of crestal bone can lead to implant complications and possibly failure, the crestal bone level is considered as one of the most decisive factors for implant success [187]. Thus, in recent years, various concepts have been developed to minimize crestal bone loss during functional loading. In this context, one treatment option is to use a smaller abutment diameter compared to the implant diameter, leading to a horizontal mismatch between abutment and implant (platform-switching) [188]. Therefore, 2-part modSLA implants with a platform-switching design (Bone Level SLActive® implant, Institut Straumann AG, Basel, Switzerland) were clinically investigated as well as tissue-level implants. A prospective multicenter study investigated modSLA bone-level implants that were placed in patients with healed single-tooth gaps in the anterior maxilla or mandible [189, 190]. Implants were either designated for submerged or transmucosal healing according to a randomly assigned protocol. GBR procedures were performed if needed. Between 8 and 12 weeks after placement, all implants were functionally loaded. Just prior to loading, the submerged implants were surgically exposed. After 1 year of loading, the authors presented data on 126 implants that showed PD values of 2.5 and 2.4 mm and crestal bone loss of 0.47 ± 0.64 and 0.48 ± 0.65 mm for submerged and transmucosal implants, respectively [189]. Three years after placement, clinical data was available for 106 implants, showing mean crestal bone loss of 0.68 ± 0.98 mm (submerged healing) and 0.58 ± 0.77 mm (transmucosal healing) and similar PD values between 2 and 2.5 mm [190]. None of the differences after 1 and 3 years were statistically significant. One transmucosal-healed modSLA implant was lost after functional loading, 6 months after placement; thus, 3-year survival rates of 100 % and 98.1 % were reported for submerged and transmucosal implants, respectively [189, 190].

In addition, a case series study was performed that investigated bone-level implants with a modSLA surface that were placed in the anterior maxilla of 20 patients with single-tooth gaps 4–8 weeks after tooth extraction [191–193]. To cover the peri-implant bone defect on the facial aspect of the implants, autogenous bone chips, deproteinized bovine bone mineral (Bio-Oss®, Geistlich Biomaterials, Wolhusen, Switzerland), and a porcine-derived collagen membrane (Bio-Gide®, Geistlich Biomaterials, Wolhusen, Switzerland) in combination with a submerged healing protocol were used. All implant sites were surgically reopened for abutment connection between 8 and 12 weeks after placement. Within 7 days after reopening, all implants were loaded. After 1, 3, and 6 years of investigation, the authors presented PD values of 4.43 ± 0.57, 4.00 ± 0.56, and 4.24 ± 0.49 mm and crestal bone loss of 0.18 ± 0.20, 0.18 ± 0.23, and 0.44 ± 0.24 mm, respectively. Six years after placement, none of the implants was lost [191–193]. These results suggest that bone-level modSLA implants with a platform-switching design show similar crestal bone resorption, PD values, and survival rates up to and after 6 years after placement compared to modSLA implants with a conventional tissue-level design.

ModSLA: On Particular TiZr Alloy Implants

As mentioned before (compare above), the production of a chemically active, highly hydrophilic sandblasted and acid-etched surface topography is not a unique manufacturing process that can be used only on commercially pure titanium but also on a specific titanium-zirconium alloy. Thus, clinical studies not only investigated c.p. titanium implants but also TiZr alloy implants with a reduced implant diameter (3.3 mm) and a chemically modified surface topography [194–198]. As some of the preclinical studies suggested that the healing process around TiZr implants with a modSLA surface might be slightly delayed compared to c.p. titanium modSLA implants (compare above), most of the prospective clinical studies reported on implant loading not immediately or 21 days after placement but after healing periods between 6 weeks and 12 months following implant placement [194–198]. Only 1 study reported on 1 patient who received 4 implants that were placed in an edentulous mandible and successfully loaded immediately after placement [194]. In all these studies, the reported survival and success rates ranged between 95.2 % and 100 % for loading periods up to and after 24 months [194–197]. All of the reported implant failures occurred within the early healing period before loading could be performed [195, 197, 198]. When investigating crestal bone loss, no differences between implants with a modSLA surface that were made either of TiZr or c.p. Ti could be demonstrated [196, 197]. These results clearly indicate that TiZr implants with a chemically active, hydrophilic SLA surface that are loaded between 6 weeks and 12 months after placement, show at least comparable survival and success rates up to and after 2 years of loading compared to c.p. Ti implants with a modSLA surface.

ModSLA: Summary of Clinical Studies

In summary, in regard to implant stability, it has been shown that modSLA implants relative to

SLA implants tend to have an earlier shift from decreasing to increasing values, but the results appear to be dependent on the RFA technique, bone quality, and implant location. Furthermore, it has been demonstrated that modSLA implants could be successfully loaded immediately or 21 days after implant placement resulting in survival rates of 95 % or more for investigation periods up to and after 3 years. Even implants that could not be loaded after 21 days due to implant mobility did not show increased failure rates when loaded after an additional 3–4 weeks of healing. In short-term healing, when conventionally loaded, modSLA implants compared to SLA implants showed similar survival rates. Within a short-time investigation period of 1 year, bone quality did not have any influence on implant survival and on peri-implant crestal bone loss. Also implant placement in combination with simultaneously or previously performed bone augmentation revealed successful clinical outcomes. ModSLA implants were also successfully placed in compromised patients and revealed minor (statistically not significant) advantages compared to SLA implants. In addition, immediately loaded modSLA implants showed slightly but statistically significantly increased crestal bone-level loss within the first 5 months of investigation compared to early-loaded modSLA implants. Interestingly, however, the immediately placed implants were generally seated more apically than the early-loaded implants. The reason for the increased bone loss is most likely caused by this fact. Bone-level modSLA implants with a platform-switching design showed similar crestal bone loss, PD values, and survival rates for up to and after 3 years of loading compared to modSLA implants with a tissue-level design. When investigating the healing protocol around bone-level implants with a modSLA surface, a submerged healing protocol showed nonsignificant but slightly increased crestal bone loss compared to a transgingival healing protocol. Furthermore, TiZr-modSLA implants that are loaded between 6 weeks and 12 months after placement, demonstrated similar clinical outcomes compared to c.p. Ti-modSLA implants for loading periods up to 2 years. These results taken together indicate that the TiZr-modSLA implants perform in a similar fashion as do c.p. Ti-modSLA implants but have the added advantage of being a much stronger material.

Concluding Remarks

Due to modifications in the manufacturing process (sandblasting and acid-etching, rinsing of implant under N_2 protection, storage in isotonic NaCl solution), a chemically activated and hydrophilic micro-rough titanium surface topography (like in its native, uncontaminated state) can be produced. Thus, clinically, it can be concluded from the chemical analysis studies that the Na and Cl solutions shield the hydroxylated dioxide chemically active layer from contamination with hydrocarbons and carbons from the atmosphere, preserving the surface chemistry and hydrophilicity and high surface free energy during the storage and placement of the implant. After implant placement, the sodium and chloride ions can easily dissociate from the surface creating a clean, chemically active hydrophilic dioxide layer that provides more hydroxylated groups to react with proteins, ions, sugars, and lipids that are present in the blood and tissue fluids that condition the implant's surface immediately after placement [2, 199]. This fact is very important especially for the initial osseointegration process since it could be shown that the hydroxylated groups from the TiO_2 layer react with phosphate and calcium from body fluids to create an apatite layer that is considered as the prerequisite for the bonding between the implant surface and the peri-implant bone tissue [200].

Overall, the in vitro, in vivo animal and human clinical studies reveal that the chemically active and hydrophilic modSLA implant surface results in faster bone and soft tissue apposition than the highly successful hydrophobic SLA implant surface. Both implant surfaces with identical surface geometries result in large amounts of bone-to-implant contact, high removal torque-out values, and a tight adhesion to the surrounding bone and soft tissue. The chemically active modSLA surface also provides an additional advantage in that the bone and soft tissue healing process is accelerated by the surface. This has been demonstrated at the molecular, cellular, and tissue levels.

During the osseous healing process, the initial primary mechanical stability of an implant provided by the cut native bone (primary bone contact) is gradually replaced by secondary biologic stability provided by the new bone formation on the implant surface and remodeled primary bone contact areas and is termed secondary bone contact [201, 202]. In detail, after placement, the implant surface is in direct contact (osseointegrated) with the surrounding bone tissue, leading to primary stability. Later on, the surrounding bone tissue, that is responsible for the primary implant stability, becomes resorbed by osteoclasts and is replaced by newly formed viable bone tissue plus new bone formation on an osteoconductive implant surface which together lead to secondary stability [201]. Thus, the time period when osteoclast activity has decreased primary stability and the newly remodeled and newly formed peri-implant bone tissue is not yet stable enough to provide sufficient secondary stability is the most critical phase for early implant failure. For human patients receiving titanium implants with a hydrophobic sandblasted and acid-etched surface, this critical time frame has been shown to occur generally between 2 and 3 weeks after implant placement [68, 202]. By using implants with the chemically activated and highly hydrophilic modSLA surface, this critical biological time frame can be further shortened (Figs. 9.8 and 9.9). This has also been confirmed by randomized controlled prospective human clinical investigations that showed an earlier transition from a relatively unstable presumably resorptive bone phase to a more stable presumably formative bone phase for implants with a modSLA surface compared to implants with a hydrophobic SLA surface [168–172]. This observation is not only relevant for early or immediate loading but might also increase the safety for patients with challenging conditions like bone grafts, certain conditions like osteoporosis, or diabetic patients.

Besides biological activities, also patient compliance (overloading of implants, poor oral hygiene, smoking, bruxism, noxious habits, etc.) can directly interfere with the implant healing period and thus increase the risk of implant failure. This places the implant at risk in the patient due to the longer healing times where the less stable period is extended. In contrast, the accelerated bone healing around implants with more osteoconductive implant surfaces (compared to machined surfaces) such as the SLA surface or the chemically active hydrophilic sandblasted and acid-etched surface, indicated by increased BIC and removal torque-out values, can decrease the "danger zone," in which the patients can interfere with the implant healing period and therefore decrease the chance for implant failure and patient tooth replacement morbidity (Fig. 9.10).

For commercially pure titanium implants with the modSLA surface and a special

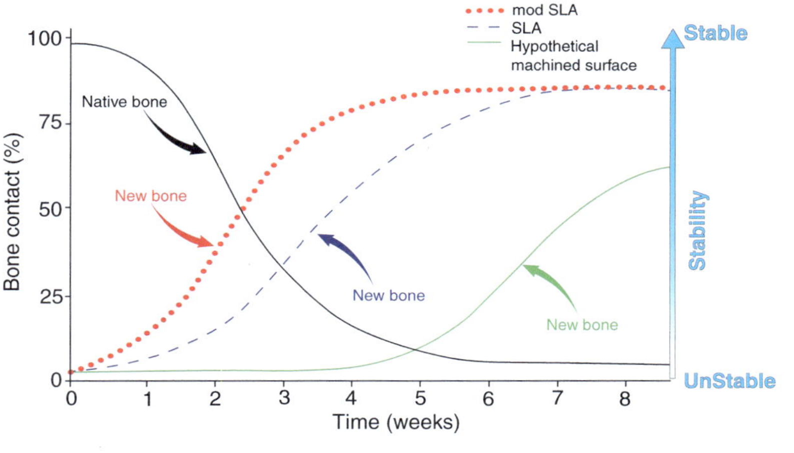

Fig. 9.8 Transition from primary stability to secondary stability. Earlier transition (left shift of the curve) around titanium implants with modSLA surface compared to implants with SLA surface or a machined surface (Graph modified according to Raghavendra et al. [202])

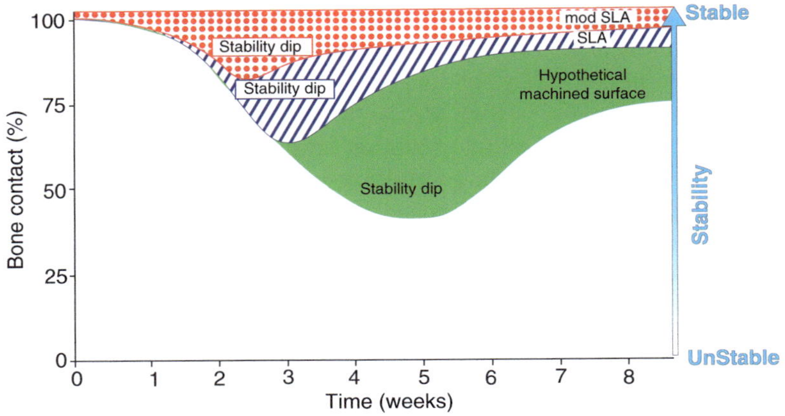

Fig. 9.9 Earlier transition from primary stability to secondary stability (Fig. 9.7) leads to a reduced loss of implant stability within the osseous healing period around implants with a modSLA surface compared to implants with an SLA or a machined surface topography

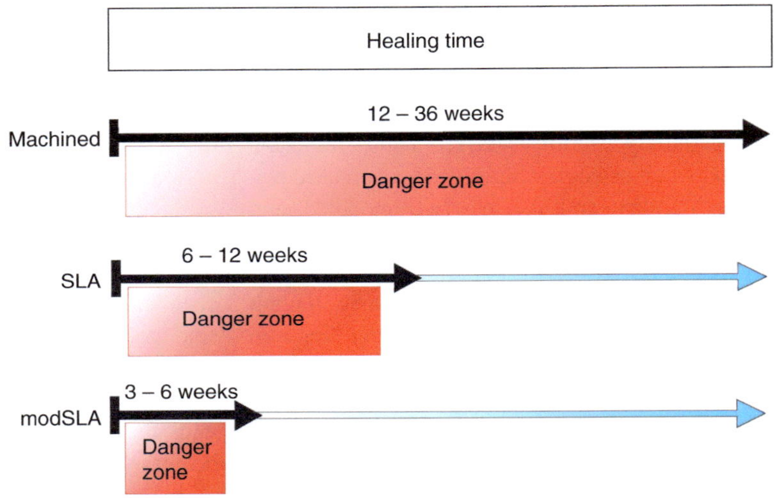

Fig. 9.10 Accelerated implant healing decreases risk due to patient interference in the healing period (decreased "danger zone")

titanium-zirconium alloy implants with their increased strength and with the modSLA surface, the survival rates ranged between 95.2 % and 100 %, between 95 % and 97.7 %, and between 96.7 % and 100 % for investigation periods of 1, 2, and 3 years, respectively [166, 173, 175, 176, 178–180, 183, 185, 189, 190, 194–198], in regard to reported success rates for implants with a modSLA surface at corresponding time intervals, the outcomes ranged between 95.2 % and 100 %, between 97.7 % and 100 %, and between 96.7 % and 100 %, respectively [166, 173, 179, 182, 186, 194, 195, 197, 198]. These results are similar to the reported findings on survival (range between 96.1 % and 99.56 %) and success rates (range between 99.12 % and 99.56 %) for implants with the SLA surface up to and after 3 years of investigation [76, 87, 203].

Implants with a hydrophobic SLA surface have been available for longer periods of time, and these implants also have very high survival and success rates for longer investigation periods. For example, Buser et al. presented survival and success rates of 98.8 % and 97 % for implants with a hydrophobic SLA surface for an investigation period of 10 years [5].

With regard to implant failures, few implant failures with a modSLA surface were lost before loading could be performed [166, 173, 174, 176, 182, 183, 185, 195, 197, 198], only 2 studies (2 implants) reported late failures after prosthetic restoration [183, 189]. Similar observations were demonstrated for implants with the hydrophobic SLA surface, since most of the observed failures occurred prior to loading of the implants [55, 90, 92, 203]. Additionally, for implants with a modSLA surface, out of the 19 failures (excluding studies investigating immediate loading), 7 failures were associated with previously (2 implants) or simultaneously performed (5 implants) sinus floor bone augmentations [182, 183]. However, 5 of these failures were reported in a noninterventional study, performed by private practitioners without specific defined inclusion and exclusion criteria, which also included higher-risk patients [182]. Therefore, even under more at risk, less-controlled conditions, both the SLA implants and the implants with the modSLA surface performed with high survival and success rates. Under more controlled clinical trials, with defined inclusion and exclusion criteria, investigating implants with a modSLA surface that were placed in combination with previously or simultaneously performed sinus floor elevations, only 2 failures were reported (previously performed bone augmentation) out of 104 investigated implants [183, 184]. These results are in agreement with findings of a controlled clinical trial, with defined inclusion and exclusion criteria, on implants with a hydrophobic SLA surface that were placed in combination with sinus floor bone augmentations [70]. Within an investigation period of 2 years, the authors observed 1 implant failure out of 48 simultaneously placed implants; however, no implant failure occurred out of 135 implants, when implants were placed after mean healing period of 4.9 months following the bone augmentation procedures [70]. Thus, the success and survival rates of SLA implants and modSLA implants are very high and few failures have been reported. In addition, when failures do occur, they are mostly associated with early healing period.

The mean values for crestal bone loss for early and conventionally loaded tissue-level implants with a modSLA surface ranged between 0.15 and 0.63 mm, between 0.2 and 0.75 mm, and between 0.2 and 0.57 mm after 1, 2, and 3 years of investigation, respectively [166, 173–176, 178, 179, 181, 183, 185, 186, 195–197]. The mean probing depths ranged between 0.08 and 3.76 mm for investigation periods between 1 and 3 years [166, 173–176, 179, 183, 186, 195, 198]. Similar results were demonstrated for conventionally loaded tissue-level implants with a hydrophobic SLA surface for loading periods up to and after 3 years (crestal bone loss: 0.33–0.68 mm) [92, 203]; however, in contrast to that, slightly increased clinical probing depth values (2.20–4.47 mm) were reported for the SLA implants [76, 92, 203].

These results clearly indicate that early implant loading after 21 days of healing as well as immediate implant loading (directly after placement) of implants with a modSLA surface can be performed with high success and survival rates and that these implants with a hydrophilic sandblasted and acid-etched surface show similar survival and success rates for investigation periods up to and after 3 years compared to implants with a hydrophobic sandblasted and acid-etched surface. With regard to clinical and radiographic parameters, in general, both types of surfaces (SLA and modSLA) show comparable results and can therefore be considered as similar. Thus, both surfaces, the chemically active and hydrophilic as well as the hydrophobic sandblasted and acid-etched implant surface, can be used in the clinical daily routine, providing a very reliable treatment option for every type of patient and indication that allows for implant placement. An accelerated initial bone healing of the chemically active and highly hydrophilic modSLA surface allows for a faster loading protocol, compared to implants with the hydrophobic SLA surface, without compromising the overall survival and success rates. Furthermore, the modSLA surface can be created on a special alloy of titanium and zirconium that allows for similarly high survival and success rates and, in addition, provides greater material strength. These innovations in surface technology and material composition represent significant advancements in the field of implant dentistry and, most importantly, for tooth replacement and patient care.

Acknowledgment The authors gratefully acknowledge Dr. Michael Hotze and Dr. Simon Berner (Institut Straumann AG, Basel, Switzerland) for support and proofreading the text, for providing images, and for their valuable comments with regard to the content.

References

1. Albrektsson T, Branemark PI, Hansson HA, Lindstrom J. Osseointegrated titanium implants. Requirements for ensuring a long-lasting, direct bone-to-implant anchorage in man. Acta Orthop Scand. 1981;52(2):155–70.
2. Zhao G, Schwartz Z, Wieland M, Rupp F, Geis-Gerstorfer J, Cochran DL, et al. High surface energy enhances cell response to titanium substrate microstructure. J Biomed Mater Res A. 2005;74(1):49–58.
3. Buser D, Schenk RK, Steinemann S, Fiorellini JP, Fox CH, Stich H. Influence of surface characteristics on bone integration of titanium implants. A histomorphometric study in miniature pigs. J Biomed Mater Res. 1991;25(7):889–902.
4. Buser D, Nydegger T, Oxland T, Cochran DL, Schenk RK, Hirt HP, et al. Interface shear strength of titanium implants with a sandblasted and acid-etched surface: a biomechanical study in the maxilla of miniature pigs. J Biomed Mater Res. 1999;45(2):75–83.
5. Buser D, Janner SF, Wittneben JG, Bragger U, Ramseier CA, Salvi GE. 10-year survival and success rates of 511 titanium implants with a sandblasted and acid-etched surface: a retrospective study in 303 partially edentulous patients. Clin Implant Dent Relat Res. 2012;14(6):839–51.
6. Zhang EW, Wang YB, Shuai KG, Gao F, Bai YJ, Cheng Y, et al. In vitro and in vivo evaluation of SLA titanium surfaces with further alkali or hydrogen peroxide and heat treatment. Biomed Mater. 2011; 6(2):025001.
7. Funato A, Yamada M, Ogawa T. Success rate, healing time, and implant stability of photofunctionalized dental implants. Int J Oral Maxillofac Implants. 2013;28(5):1261–71.
8. Att W, Ogawa T. Biological aging of implant surfaces and their restoration with ultraviolet light treatment: a novel understanding of osseointegration. Int J Oral Maxillofac Implants. 2012;27(4):753–61.
9. Tugulu S, Lowe K, Scharnweber D, Schlottig F. Preparation of superhydrophilic microrough titanium implant surfaces by alkali treatment. J Mater Sci Mater Med. 2010;21(10):2751–63.
10. Stadlinger B, Lode AT, Eckelt U, Range U, Schlottig F, Hefti T, et al. Surface-conditioned dental implants: an animal study on bone formation. J Clin Periodontol. 2009;36(10):882–91.
11. Buser D, Broggini N, Wieland M, Schenk RK, Denzer AJ, Cochran DL, et al. Enhanced bone apposition to a chemically modified SLA titanium surface. J Dent Res. 2004;83(7):529–33.
12. Rupp F, Scheideler L, Olshanska N, de Wild M, Wieland M, Geis-Gerstorfer J. Enhancing surface free energy and hydrophilicity through chemical modification of microstructured titanium implant surfaces. J Biomed Mater Res A. 2006;76(2):323–34.
13. Grandin HM, Berner S, Dard M. A review of Titanium Zirconium (TiZr) alloys for use in endosseous dental implants. Materials. 2012;5(8):1348–60.
14. Buser D, Nydegger T, Hirt HP, Cochran DL, Nolte LP. Removal torque values of titanium implants in the maxilla of miniature pigs. Int J Oral Maxillofac Implants. 1998;13(5):611–9.
15. Martin JY, Schwartz Z, Hummert TW, Schraub DM, Simpson J, Lankford Jr J, et al. Effect of titanium surface roughness on proliferation, differentiation, and protein synthesis of human osteoblast-like cells (MG63). J Biomed Mater Res. 1995;29(3):389–401.
16. Cochran DL, Nummikoski PV, Higginbottom FL, Hermann JS, Makins SR, Buser D. Evaluation of an endosseous titanium implant with a sandblasted and acid-etched surface in the canine mandible: radiographic results. Clin Oral Implants Res. 1996;7(3):240–52.
17. Lossdorfer S, Schwartz Z, Wang L, Lohmann CH, Turner JD, Wieland M, et al. Microrough implant surface topographies increase osteogenesis by reducing osteoclast formation and activity. J Biomed Mater Res A. 2004;70(3):361–9.
18. Wennerberg A, Albrektsson T. Suggested guidelines for the topographic evaluation of implant surfaces. Int J Oral Maxillofac Implants. 2000;15(3):331–44.
19. Sammons RL, Lumbikanonda N, Gross M, Cantzler P. Comparison of osteoblast spreading on microstructured dental implant surfaces and cell behaviour in an explant model of osseointegration. A scanning electron microscopic study. Clin Oral Implants Res. 2005;16(6):657–66.
20. Taborelli M, Jobin M, Francois P, Vaudaux P, Tonetti M, Szmukler-Moncler S, et al. Influence of surface treatments developed for oral implants on the physical and biological properties of titanium. (I) surface characterization. Clin Oral Implants Res. 1997;8(3): 208–16.
21. Szmukler-Moncler S, Bischof M, Nedir R, Ermrich M. Titanium hydride and hydrogen concentration in acid-etched commercially pure titanium and titanium alloy implants: a comparative analysis of five implant systems. Clin Oral Implants Res. 2010;21(9):944–50.
22. Szmukler-Moncler S, Simpson JP. Physicochemical characterization of a titanium textured surface prepared by sandblasting and acid etching. Transactions of the 5th World Biomaterials congress, 29 May–2 June, Toronto; 1996. p. 837.
23. Perrin D, Szmukler-Moncler S, Echikou C, Pointaire P, Bernard JP. Bone response to alteration of surface topography and surface composition of sandblasted and acid etched (SLA) implants. Clin Oral Implants Res. 2002;13(5):465–9.
24. Szmukler-Moncler S, Perrin D, Ahossi V, Magnin G, Bernard JP. Biological properties of acid etched titanium implants: effect of sandblasting on bone

anchorage. J Biomed Mater Res B Appl Biomater. 2004;68(2):149–59.
25. Kang BS, Sul YT, Oh SJ, Lee HJ, Albrektsson T. XPS, AES and SEM analysis of recent dental implants. Acta Biomater. 2009;5(6):2222–9.
26. Gahlert M, Burtscher D, Grunert I, Kniha H, Steinhauser E. Failure analysis of fractured dental zirconia implants. Clin Oral Implants Res. 2012;23(3): 287–93.
27. Osman RB, Ma S, Duncan W, De Silva RK, Siddiqi A, Swain MV. Fractured zirconia implants and related implant designs: scanning electron microscopy analysis. Clin Oral Implants Res. 2013;24(5):592–7.
28. Gahlert M, Rohling S, Wieland M, Sprecher CM, Kniha H, Milz S. Osseointegration of zirconia and titanium dental implants: a histological and histomorphometrical study in the maxilla of pigs. Clin Oral Implants Res. 2009;20(11):1247–53.
29. Gahlert M, Rohling S, Wieland M, Eichhorn S, Kuchenhoff H, Kniha H. A comparison study of the osseointegration of zirconia and titanium dental implants. A biomechanical evaluation in the maxilla of pigs. Clin Implant Dent Relat Res. 2010;12(4):297–305.
30. Gahlert M, Roehling S, Sprecher CM, Kniha H, Milz S, Bormann K. In vivo performance of zirconia and titanium implants: a histomorphometric study in mini pig maxillae. Clin Oral Implants Res. 2012;23(3):281–6.
31. Bormann KH, Gellrich NC, Kniha H, Dard M, Wieland M, Gahlert M. Biomechanical evaluation of a microstructured zirconia implant by a removal torque comparison with a standard Ti-SLA implant. Clin Oral Implants Res. 2012;23(10):1210–6.
32. Schwartz Z, Boyan BD. Underlying mechanisms at the bone-biomaterial interface. J Cell Biochem. 1994;56(3):340–7.
33. Kieswetter K, Schwartz Z, Dean DD, Boyan BD. The role of implant surface characteristics in the healing of bone. Crit Rev Oral Biol Med Off Publ Am Assoc Oral Biologist. 1996;7(4):329–45.
34. Baschong W, Jaquiery C, Martin I, Lambrecht TJ. Surface-induced modulation of human mesenchymal progenitor cells. An in vitro model for early implant integration. Schweiz Monatsschr Zahnmed. 2007;117(9):906–10.
35. Davies JE. Understanding peri-implant endosseous healing. J Dent Educ. 2003;67(8):932–49.
36. Marco F, Milena F, Gianluca G, Vittoria O. Peri-implant osteogenesis in health and osteoporosis. Micron. 2005;36(7–8):630–44.
37. Orsini G, Assenza B, Scarano A, Piattelli M, Piattelli A. Surface analysis of machined versus sandblasted and acid-etched titanium implants. Int J Oral Maxillofac Implants. 2000;15(6):779–84.
38. Zinger O, Anselme K, Denzer A, Habersetzer P, Wieland M, Jeanfils J, et al. Time-dependent morphology and adhesion of osteoblastic cells on titanium model surfaces featuring scale-resolved topography. Biomaterials. 2004;25(14):2695–711.
39. Bowers KT, Keller JC, Randolph BA, Wick DG, Michaels CM. Optimization of surface micromorphology for enhanced osteoblast responses in vitro. Int J Oral Maxillofac Implants. 1992;7(3):302–10.
40. Schwartz Z, Lohmann CH, Oefinger J, Bonewald LF, Dean DD, Boyan BD. Implant surface characteristics modulate differentiation behavior of cells in the osteoblastic lineage. Adv Dent Res. 1999;13:38–48.
41. Boyan BD, Batzer R, Kieswetter K, Liu Y, Cochran DL, Szmuckler-Moncler S, et al. Titanium surface roughness alters responsiveness of MG63 osteoblast-like cells to 1 alpha,25-(OH)2D3. J Biomed Mater Res. 1998;39(1):77–85.
42. Martin JY, Dean DD, Cochran DL, Simpson J, Boyan BD, Schwartz Z. Proliferation, differentiation, and protein synthesis of human osteoblast-like cells (MG63) cultured on previously used titanium surfaces. Clin Oral Implants Res. 1996;7(1):27–37.
43. Kieswetter K, Schwartz Z, Hummert TW, Cochran DL, Simpson J, Dean DD, et al. Surface roughness modulates the local production of growth factors and cytokines by osteoblast-like MG-63 cells. J Biomed Mater Res. 1996;32(1):55–63.
44. Lohmann CH, Bonewald LF, Sisk MA, Sylvia VL, Cochran DL, Dean DD, et al. Maturation state determines the response of osteogenic cells to surface roughness and 1,25-dihydroxyvitamin D3. J Bone Miner Res. 2000;15(6):1169–80.
45. Schwartz Z, Lohmann CH, Sisk M, Cochran DL, Sylvia VL, Simpson J, et al. Local factor production by MG63 osteoblast-like cells in response to surface roughness and 1,25-(OH)2D3 is mediated via protein kinase C- and protein kinase A-dependent pathways. Biomaterials. 2001;22(7):731–41.
46. Ogawa T, Nishimura I. Different bone integration profiles of turned and acid-etched implants associated with modulated expression of extracellular matrix genes. Int J Oral Maxillofac Implants. 2003;18(2): 200–10.
47. Brinkmann J, Hefti T, Schlottig F, Spencer ND, Hall H. Response of osteoclasts to titanium surfaces with increasing surface roughness: an in vitro study. Biointerphases. 2012;7(1–4):34.
48. Thomas KA, Cook SD. An evaluation of variables influencing implant fixation by direct bone apposition. J Biomed Mater Res. 1985;19(8):875–901.
49. Carlsson L, Rostlund T, Albrektsson B, Albrektsson T. Removal torques for polished and rough titanium implants. Int J Oral Maxillofac Implants. 1988;3(1): 21–4.
50. Cochran DL, Schenk RK, Lussi A, Higginbottom FL, Buser D. Bone response to unloaded and loaded titanium implants with a sandblasted and acid-etched surface: a histometric study in the canine mandible. J Biomed Mater Res. 1998;40(1):1–11.
51. Li D, Ferguson SJ, Beutler T, Cochran DL, Sittig C, Hirt HP, et al. Biomechanical comparison of the sandblasted and acid-etched and the machined and acid-etched titanium surface for dental implants. J Biomed Mater Res. 2002;60(2):325–32.
52. Lang NP, Salvi GE, Huynh-Ba G, Ivanovski S, Donos N, Bosshardt DD. Early osseointegration to hydro-

philic and hydrophobic implant surfaces in humans. Clin Oral Implants Res. 2011;22(4):349–56.
53. Roccuzzo M, Aglietta M, Bunino M, Bonino L. Early loading of sandblasted and acid-etched implants: a randomized-controlled double-blind split-mouth study. Five-year results. Clin Oral Implants Res. 2008;19(2):148–52.
54. Wong M, Eulenberger J, Schenk R, Hunziker E. Effect of surface topology on the osseointegration of implant materials in trabecular bone. J Biomed Mater Res. 1995;29(12):1567–75.
55. Arlin ML. Survival and success of sandblasted, large-grit, acid-etched and titanium plasma-sprayed implants: a retrospective study. Journal. 2007;73(9):821.
56. Carmagnola D, Abati S, Addis A, Ferrieri G, Chiapasco M, Romeo E, et al. Time sequence of bone healing around two implant systems in minipigs: preliminary histologic results. Int J Periodontics Restorative Dent. 2009;29(5):549–55.
57. Botticelli D, Berglundh T, Buser D, Lindhe J. Appositional bone formation in marginal defects at implants. Clin Oral Implants Res. 2003;14(1):1–9.
58. Botticelli D, Berglundh T, Persson LG, Lindhe J. Bone regeneration at implants with turned or rough surfaces in self-contained defects. An experimental study in the dog. J Clin Periodontol. 2005;32(5):448–55.
59. Botticelli D, Berglundh T, Lindhe J. The influence of a biomaterial on the closure of a marginal hard tissue defect adjacent to implants. An experimental study in the dog. Clin Oral Implants Res. 2004;15(3):285–92.
60. Botticelli D, Berglundh T, Lindhe J. Resolution of bone defects of varying dimension and configuration in the marginal portion of the peri-implant bone. An experimental study in the dog. J Clin Periodontol. 2004;31(4):309–17.
61. Botticelli D, Berglundh T, Buser D, Lindhe J. The jumping distance revisited: an experimental study in the dog. Clin Oral Implants Res. 2003;14(1):35–42.
62. Freilich M, Shafer D, Wei M, Kompalli R, Adams D, Kuhn L. Implant system for guiding a new layer of bone. Computed microtomography and histomorphometric analysis in the rabbit mandible. Clin Oral Implants Res. 2009;20(2):201–7.
63. Carmagnola D, Abati S, Celestino S, Chiapasco M, Bosshardt D, Lang NP. Oral implants placed in bone defects treated with Bio-Oss, Ostim-Paste or PerioGlas: an experimental study in the rabbit tibiae. Clin Oral Implants Res. 2008;19(12):1246–53.
64. de Vicente JC, Recio O, Martin-Villa L, Junquera LM, Lopez-Arranz JS. Histomorphometric evaluation of guided bone regeneration around implants with SLA surface: an experimental study in beagle dogs. Int J Oral Maxillofac Surg. 2006;35(11):1047–53.
65. Retzepi M, Lewis MP, Donos N. Effect of diabetes and metabolic control on de novo bone formation following guided bone regeneration. Clin Oral Implants Res. 2010;21(1):71–9.
66. Bornstein MM, Valderrama P, Jones AA, Wilson TG, Seibl R, Cochran DL. Bone apposition around two different sandblasted and acid-etched titanium implant surfaces: a histomorphometric study in canine mandibles. Clin Oral Implants Res. 2008;19(3):233–41.
67. Botticelli D, Berglundh T, Lindhe J. Hard-tissue alterations following immediate implant placement in extraction sites. J Clin Periodontol. 2004;31(10):820–8.
68. Barewal RM, Oates TW, Meredith N, Cochran DL. Resonance frequency measurement of implant stability in vivo on implants with a sandblasted and acid-etched surface. Int J Oral Maxillofac Implants. 2003;18(5):641–51.
69. Pinholt EM. Branemark and ITI dental implants in the human bone-grafted maxilla: a comparative evaluation. Clin Oral Implants Res. 2003;14(5):584–92.
70. Stricker A, Voss PJ, Gutwald R, Schramm A, Schmelzeisen R. Maxillary sinus floor augmention with autogenous bone grafts to enable placement of SLA-surfaced implants: preliminary results after 15–40 months. Clin Oral Implants Res. 2003;14(2):207–12.
71. Cochran DL, Buser D, ten Bruggenkate CM, Weingart D, Taylor TM, Bernard JP, et al. The use of reduced healing times on ITI implants with a sandblasted and acid-etched (SLA) surface: early results from clinical trials on ITI SLA implants. Clin Oral Implants Res. 2002;13(2):144–53.
72. Bornstein MM, Lussi A, Schmid B, Belser UC, Buser D. Early loading of nonsubmerged titanium implants with a sandblasted and acid-etched (SLA) surface: 3-year results of a prospective study in partially edentulous patients. Int J Oral Maxillofac Implants. 2003;18(5):659–66.
73. Buser D, Belser UC, Lang NP. The original one-stage dental implant system and its clinical application. Periodontology 2000. 1998;17:106–18.
74. Roccuzzo M, Wilson T. A prospective study evaluating a protocol for 6 weeks' loading of SLA implants in the posterior maxilla: one year results. Clin Oral Implants Res. 2002;13(5):502–7.
75. Cochran DL. The scientific basis for and clinical experiences with Straumann implants including the ITI dental implant system: a consensus report. Clin Oral Implants Res. 2000;11 Suppl 1:33–58.
76. Bornstein MM, Schmid B, Belser UC, Lussi A, Buser D. Early loading of non-submerged titanium implants with a sandblasted and acid-etched surface. 5-year results of a prospective study in partially edentulous patients. Clin Oral Implants Res. 2005;16(6):631–8.
77. Salvi GE, Gallini G, Lang NP. Early loading (2 or 6 weeks) of sandblasted and acid-etched (SLA) ITI implants in the posterior mandible. A 1-year randomized controlled clinical trial. Clin Oral Implants Res. 2004;15(2):142–9.
78. Quinlan P, Nummikoski P, Schenk R, Cagna D, Mellonig J, Higginbottom F, et al. Immediate and

early loading of SLA ITI single-tooth implants: an in vivo study. Int J Oral Maxillofac Implants. 2005;20(3):360–70.
79. Cornelini R, Cangini F, Covani U, Barone A, Buser D. Immediate restoration of single-tooth implants in mandibular molar sites: a 12-month preliminary report. Int J Oral Maxillofac Implants. 2004;19(6):855–60.
80. Bergkvist G, Sahlholm S, Karlsson U, Nilner K, Lindh C. Immediately loaded implants supporting fixed prostheses in the edentulous maxilla: a preliminary clinical and radiologic report. Int J Oral Maxillofac Implants. 2005;20(3):399–405.
81. Luongo G, Di Raimondo R, Filippini P, Gualini F, Paoleschi C. Early loading of sandblasted, acid-etched implants in the posterior maxilla and mandible: a 1-year follow-up report from a multicenter 3-year prospective study. Int J Oral Maxillofac Implants. 2005;20(1):84–91.
82. Tortamano P, Orii TC, Yamanochi J, Nakamae AE, Guarnieri Tde C. Outcomes of fixed prostheses supported by immediately loaded endosseous implants. Int J Oral Maxillofac Implants. 2006;21(1):63–70.
83. Fischer K, Stenberg T. Three-year data from a randomized, controlled study of early loading of single-stage dental implants supporting maxillary full-arch prostheses. Int J Oral Maxillofac Implants. 2006;21(2):245–52.
84. Stricker A, Gutwald R, Schmelzeisen R, Gellrich NG. Immediate loading of 2 interforaminal dental implants supporting an overdenture: clinical and radiographic results after 24 months. Int J Oral Maxillofac Implants. 2004;19(6):868–72.
85. Boyan BD, Bonewald LF, Paschalis EP, Lohmann CH, Rosser J, Cochran DL, et al. Osteoblast-mediated mineral deposition in culture is dependent on surface microtopography. Calcif Tissue Int. 2002;71(6):519–29.
86. Cochran DL. A comparison of endosseous dental implant surfaces. J Periodontol. 1999;70(12):1523–39.
87. Cochran D, Oates T, Morton D, Jones A, Buser D, Peters F. Clinical field trial examining an implant with a sand-blasted, acid-etched surface. J Periodontol. 2007;78(6):974–82.
88. Roccuzzo M, Bonino L, Dalmasso P, Aglietta M. Long-term results of a three arms prospective cohort study on implants in periodontally compromised patients: 10-year data around sandblasted and acid-etched (SLA) surface. Clin Oral Implants Res. 2014;25(10):1105–12.
89. Fischer K, Stenberg T. Prospective 10-year cohort study based on a randomized controlled trial (RCT) on implant-supported full-arch maxillary prostheses. Part 1: sandblasted and acid-etched implants and mucosal tissue. Clin Implant Dent Relat Res. 2012;14(6):808–15.
90. Cochran DL, Jackson JM, Bernard JP, ten Bruggenkate CM, Buser D, Taylor TD, et al. A 5-year prospective multicenter study of early loaded titanium implants with a sandblasted and acid-etched surface. Int J Oral Maxillofac Implants. 2011;26(6):1324–32.
91. Dam HG, Najm SA, Nurdin N, Bischof M, Finkelman M, Nedir R. A 5- to 6-year radiological evaluation of titanium plasma sprayed/sandblasted and acid-etched implants: results from private practice. Clin Oral Implants Res. 2014;25(2):e159–65.
92. Lethaus B, Kalber J, Petrin G, Brandstatter A, Weingart D. Early loading of sandblasted and acid-etched titanium implants in the edentulous mandible: a prospective 5-year study. Int J Oral Maxillofac Implants. 2011;26(4):887–92.
93. Baker D, London RM, O'Neal R. Rate of pull-out strength gain of dual-etched titanium implants: a comparative study in rabbits. Int J Oral Maxillofac Implants. 1999;14(5):722–8.
94. Cochran DL, Jackson JM, Jones AA, Jones JD, Kaiser DA, Taylor TD, et al. A 5-year prospective multicenter clinical trial of non-submerged dental implants with a titanium plasma-sprayed surface in 200 patients. J Periodontol. 2011;82(7):990–9.
95. van Steenberghe D, Jacobs R, Desnyder M, Maffei G, Quirynen M. The relative impact of local and endogenous patient-related factors on implant failure up to the abutment stage. Clin Oral Implants Res. 2002;13(6):617–22.
96. Wennerberg A, Albrektsson T. Effects of titanium surface topography on bone integration: a systematic review. Clin Oral Implants Res. 2009;20 Suppl 4:172–84.
97. Kasemo B. Biocompatibility of titanium implants: surface science aspects. J Prosthet Dent. 1983;49(6):832–7.
98. Kasemo B, Lausmaa J. Biomaterial and implant surfaces: a surface science approach. Int J Oral Maxillofac Implants. 1988;3(4):247–59.
99. Kilpadi DV, Lemons JE. Surface energy characterization of unalloyed titanium implants. J Biomed Mater Res. 1994;28(12):1419–25.
100. Baier RE, Meyer AE, Natiella JR, Natiella RR, Carter JM. Surface properties determine bioadhesive outcomes: methods and results. J Biomed Mater Res. 1984;18(4):337–55.
101. Schrader ME. On adhesion of biological substances to low energy solid surfaces. J Colloid Interface Sci. 1982;88(1):296–7.
102. Boehm HP. Acidic and basic properties of hydroxylated metal oxide surfaces. Discuss Faraday Soc. 1971;52:264–75.
103. Wennerberg A, Jimbo R, Stubinger S, Obrecht M, Dard M, Berner S. Nanostructures and hydrophilicity influence osseointegration: a biomechanical study in the rabbit tibia. Clin Oral Implants Res. 2014;25(9):1041–50.
104. Dohan Ehrenfest DM, Vazquez L, Park YJ, Sammartino G, Bernard JP. Identification card and codification of the chemical and morphological characteristics of 14 dental implant surfaces. J Oral Implantol. 2011;37(5):525–42.
105. Sittig C, Textor M, Spencer ND, Wieland M, Vallotton PH. Surface characterization of implant

materials c.p. Ti, Ti-6Al-7Nb and Ti-6Al-4V with different pretreatments. J Mater Sci Mater Med. 1999;10(1):35–46.
106. Jamieson JC. Crystal structures of titanium, zirconium, and hafnium at high pressures. Science. 1963;140(3562):72–3.
107. Frank MJ, Walter MS, Lyngstadaas SP, Wintermantel E, Haugen HJ. Hydrogen content in titanium and a titanium-zirconium alloy after acid etching. Mater Sci Eng C Mater Biol Appl. 2013;33(3):1282–8.
108. Kobayashi E, Matsumoto S, Doi H, Yoneyama T, Hamanaka H. Mechanical properties of the binary titanium-zirconium alloys and their potential for biomedical materials. J Biomed Mater Res. 1995;29(8):943–50.
109. Saulacic N, Bosshardt DD, Bornstein MM, Berner S, Buser D. Bone apposition to a titanium-zirconium alloy implant, as compared to two other titanium-containing implants. Eur Cell Mater. 2012;23:273–86; discussion 286–8.
110. Davies JE. In vitro modeling of the bone/implant interface. Anat Rec. 1996;245(2):426–45.
111. Hong J, Kurt S, Thor A. A hydrophilic dental implant surface exhibit thrombogenic properties in vitro. Clin Implant Dent Relat Res. 2013;15(1):105–12.
112. Hamlet S, Alfarsi M, George R, Ivanovski S. The effect of hydrophilic titanium surface modification on macrophage inflammatory cytokine gene expression. Clin Oral Implants Res. 2012;23(5):584–90.
113. Alfarsi MA, Hamlet SM, Ivanovski S. Titanium surface hydrophilicity modulates the human macrophage inflammatory cytokine response. J Biomed Mater Res A. 2014;102A:60–7.
114. Qu Z, Rausch-Fan X, Wieland M, Matejka M, Schedle A. The initial attachment and subsequent behavior regulation of osteoblasts by dental implant surface modification. J Biomed Mater Res A. 2007;82(3):658–68.
115. Mamalis AA, Silvestros SS. Analysis of osteoblastic gene expression in the early human mesenchymal cell response to a chemically modified implant surface: an in vitro study. Clin Oral Implants Res. 2011;22(5):530–7.
116. Wall I, Donos N, Carlqvist K, Jones F, Brett P. Modified titanium surfaces promote accelerated osteogenic differentiation of mesenchymal stromal cells in vitro. Bone. 2009;45(1):17–26.
117. Mamalis AA, Markopoulou C, Vrotsos I, Koutsilirieris M. Chemical modification of an implant surface increases osteogenesis and simultaneously reduces osteoclastogenesis: an in vitro study. Clin Oral Implants Res. 2011;22(6):619–26.
118. Lai HC, Zhuang LF, Liu X, Wieland M, Zhang ZY. The influence of surface energy on early adherent events of osteoblast on titanium substrates. J Biomed Mater Res A. 2010;93(1):289–96.
119. Klein MO, Bijelic A, Ziebart T, Koch F, Kammerer PW, Wieland M, et al. Submicron scale-structured hydrophilic titanium surfaces promote early osteogenic gene response for cell adhesion and cell differentiation. Clin Implant Dent Relat Res. 2013;15(2):166–75.
120. Zhao G, Raines AL, Wieland M, Schwartz Z, Boyan BD. Requirement for both micron- and submicron scale structure for synergistic responses of osteoblasts to substrate surface energy and topography. Biomaterials. 2007;28(18):2821–9.
121. Fang M, Olivares-Navarrete R, Wieland M, Cochran DL, Boyan BD, Schwartz Z. The role of phospholipase D in osteoblast response to titanium surface microstructure. J Biomed Mater Res A. 2010;93(3):897–909.
122. Zhang Y, Andrukhov O, Berner S, Matejka M, Wieland M, Rausch-Fan X, et al. Osteogenic properties of hydrophilic and hydrophobic titanium surfaces evaluated with osteoblast-like cells (MG63) in coculture with human umbilical vein endothelial cells (HUVEC). Dent Mater: Off Publ Acad Dent Mater. 2010;26(11):1043–51.
123. Rausch-fan X, Qu Z, Wieland M, Matejka M, Schedle A. Differentiation and cytokine synthesis of human alveolar osteoblasts compared to osteoblast-like cells (MG63) in response to titanium surfaces. Dent Mater: Off Publ Acad Dent Mater. 2008;24(1):102–10.
124. Raines AL, Olivares-Navarrete R, Wieland M, Cochran DL, Schwartz Z, Boyan BD. Regulation of angiogenesis during osseointegration by titanium surface microstructure and energy. Biomaterials. 2010;31(18):4909–17.
125. Olivares-Navarrete R, Hyzy SL, Hutton DL, Erdman CP, Wieland M, Boyan BD, et al. Direct and indirect effects of microstructured titanium substrates on the induction of mesenchymal stem cell differentiation towards the osteoblast lineage. Biomaterials. 2010;31(10):2728–35.
126. Stein GS, Lian JB, Owen TA. Relationship of cell growth to the regulation of tissue-specific gene expression during osteoblast differentiation. FASEB J: Off Publ Fed Am Soc Exp Biol. 1990;4(13):3111–23.
127. Bang SM, Moon HJ, Kwon YD, Yoo JY, Pae A, Kwon IK. Osteoblastic and osteoclastic differentiation on SLA and hydrophilic modified SLA titanium surfaces. Clin Oral Implants Res. 2014;25(7):831–7.
128. Masaki C, Schneider GB, Zaharias R, Seabold D, Stanford C. Effects of implant surface microtopography on osteoblast gene expression. Clin Oral Implants Res. 2005;16(6):650–6.
129. Boyle WJ, Simonet WS, Lacey DL. Osteoclast differentiation and activation. Nature. 2003;423(6937):337–42.
130. Cochran DL. Inflammation and bone loss in periodontal disease. J Periodontol. 2008;79(8 Suppl):1569–76.
131. Kou PM, Schwartz Z, Boyan BD, Babensee JE. Dendritic cell responses to surface properties of clinical titanium surfaces. Acta Biomater. 2011;7(3):1354–63.

132. Schwarz F, Herten M, Sager M, Wieland M, Dard M, Becker J. Histological and immunohistochemical analysis of initial and early osseous integration at chemically modified and conventional SLA titanium implants: preliminary results of a pilot study in dogs. Clin Oral Implants Res. 2007;18(4):481–8.
133. Ziebart T, Schnell A, Walter C, Kammerer PW, Pabst A, Lehmann KM, et al. Interactions between endothelial progenitor cells (EPC) and titanium implant surfaces. Clin Oral Investig. 2013;17(1):301–9.
134. An N, Schedle A, Wieland M, Andrukhov O, Matejka M, Rausch-Fan X. Proliferation, behavior, and cytokine gene expression of human umbilical vascular endothelial cells in response to different titanium surfaces. J Biomed Mater Res A. 2010;93(1):364–72.
135. Cochran DL, Hermann JS, Schenk RK, Higginbottom FL, Buser D. Biologic width around titanium implants. A histometric analysis of the implanto-gingival junction around unloaded and loaded nonsubmerged implants in the canine mandible. J Periodontol. 1997;68(2):186–98.
136. An N, Rausch-fan X, Wieland M, Matejka M, Andrukhov O, Schedle A. Initial attachment, subsequent cell proliferation/viability and gene expression of epithelial cells related to attachment and wound healing in response to different titanium surfaces. Dent Mater: Off Publ Acad Dent Mater. 2012;28(12):1207–14.
137. Schroeder A, van der Zypen E, Stich H, Sutter F. The reactions of bone, connective tissue, and epithelium to endosteal implants with titanium-sprayed surfaces. J Maxillofac Surg. 1981;9(1):15–25.
138. Schwarz F, Ferrari D, Herten M, Mihatovic I, Wieland M, Sager M, et al. Effects of surface hydrophilicity and microtopography on early stages of soft and hard tissue integration at non-submerged titanium implants: an immunohistochemical study in dogs. J Periodontol. 2007;78(11):2171–84.
139. Bosshardt DD, Salvi GE, Huynh-Ba G, Ivanovski S, Donos N, Lang NP. The role of bone debris in early healing adjacent to hydrophilic and hydrophobic implant surfaces in man. Clin Oral Implants Res. 2011;22(4):357–64.
140. Abdel-Haq J, Karabuda CZ, Arisan V, Mutlu Z, Kurkcu M. Osseointegration and stability of a modified sand-blasted acid-etched implant: an experimental pilot study in sheep. Clin Oral Implants Res. 2011;22(3):265–74.
141. Schwarz F, Herten M, Sager M, Wieland M, Dard M, Becker J. Bone regeneration in dehiscence-type defects at chemically modified (SLActive) and conventional SLA titanium implants: a pilot study in dogs. J Clin Periodontol. 2007;34(1):78–86.
142. Schlegel KA, Prechtl C, Most T, Seidl C, Lutz R, von Wilmowsky C. Osseointegration of SLActive implants in diabetic pigs. Clin Oral Implants Res. 2013;24(2):128–34.
143. Ferguson SJ, Broggini N, Wieland M, de Wild M, Rupp F, Geis-Gerstorfer J, et al. Biomechanical evaluation of the interfacial strength of a chemically modified sandblasted and acid-etched titanium surface. J Biomed Mater Res A. 2006;78(2):291–7.
144. Donos N, Hamlet S, Lang NP, Salvi GE, Huynh-Ba G, Bosshardt DD, et al. Gene expression profile of osseointegration of a hydrophilic compared with a hydrophobic microrough implant surface. Clin Oral Implants Res. 2011;22(4):365–72.
145. Schwarz F, Sager M, Ferrari D, Herten M, Wieland M, Becker J. Bone regeneration in dehiscence-type defects at non-submerged and submerged chemically modified (SLActive) and conventional SLA titanium implants: an immunohistochemical study in dogs. J Clin Periodontol. 2008;35(1):64–75.
146. Schwarz F, Rothamel D, Herten M, Wustefeld M, Sager M, Ferrari D, et al. Immunohistochemical characterization of guided bone regeneration at a dehiscence-type defect using different barrier membranes: an experimental study in dogs. Clin Oral Implants Res. 2008;19(4):402–15.
147. Schwarz F, Jung RE, Fienitz T, Wieland M, Becker J, Sager M. Impact of guided bone regeneration and defect dimension on wound healing at chemically modified hydrophilic titanium implant surfaces: an experimental study in dogs. J Clin Periodontol. 2010;37(5):474–85.
148. Lai HC, Zhuang LF, Zhang ZY, Wieland M, Liu X. Bone apposition around two different sandblasted, large-grit and acid-etched implant surfaces at sites with coronal circumferential defects: an experimental study in dogs. Clin Oral Implants Res. 2009;20(3):247–53.
149. Linares A, Mardas N, Dard M, Donos N. Effect of immediate or delayed loading following immediate placement of implants with a modified surface. Clin Oral Implants Res. 2011;22(1):38–46.
150. Mardas N, Schwarz F, Petrie A, Hakimi AR, Donos N. The effect of SLActive surface in guided bone formation in osteoporotic-like conditions. Clin Oral Implants Res. 2011;22(4):406–15.
151. Valderrama P, Jones AA, Wilson Jr TG, Higginbottom F, Schoolfield JD, Jung RE, et al. Bone changes around early loaded chemically modified sandblasted and acid-etched surfaced implants with and without a machined collar: a radiographic and resonance frequency analysis in the canine mandible. Int J Oral Maxillofac Implants. 2010;25(3):548–57.
152. Valderrama P, Bornstein MM, Jones AA, Wilson TG, Higginbottom FL, Cochran DL. Effects of implant design on marginal bone changes around early loaded, chemically modified, sandblasted acid-etched-surfaced implants: a histologic analysis in dogs. J Periodontol. 2011;82(7):1025–34.
153. Hermann JS, Buser D, Schenk RK, Schoolfield JD, Cochran DL. Biologic width around one- and two-piece titanium implants. Clin Oral Implants Res. 2001;12(6):559–71.
154. Hermann JS, Buser D, Schenk RK, Higginbottom FL, Cochran DL. Biologic width around titanium implants. A physiologically formed and stable

dimension over time. Clin Oral Implants Res. 2000;11(1):1–11.
155. Schwarz F, Herten M, Sager M, Wieland M, Dard M, Becker J. Histological and immunohistochemical analysis of initial and early subepithelial connective tissue attachment at chemically modified and conventional SLA titanium implants. A pilot study in dogs. Clin Oral Inv. 2007;11(3):245–55.
156. Schwarz F, Mihatovic I, Ferrari D, Wieland M, Becker J. Influence of frequent clinical probing during the healing phase on healthy peri-implant soft tissue formed at different titanium implant surfaces: a histomorphometrical study in dogs. J Clin Periodontol. 2010;37(6):551–62.
157. Al-Hamdan K, Al-Moaber SH, Junker R, Jansen JA. Effect of implant surface properties on peri-implant bone healing: a histological and histomorphometric study in dogs. Clin Oral Implants Res. 2011;22(4):399–405.
158. Schwarz F, Sager M, Kadelka I, Ferrari D, Becker J. Influence of titanium implant surface characteristics on bone regeneration in dehiscence-type defects: an experimental study in dogs. J Clin Periodontol. 2010;37(5):466–73.
159. Gottlow J, Barkarmo S, Sennerby L. An experimental comparison of two different clinically used implant designs and surfaces. Clin Implant Dent Relat Res. 2012;14 Suppl 1:e204–12.
160. Thoma DS, Jones AA, Dard M, Grize L, Obrecht M, Cochran DL. Tissue integration of a new titanium-zirconium dental implant: a comparative histologic and radiographic study in the canine. J Periodontol. 2011;82(10):1453–61.
161. Kammerer PW, Palarie V, Schiegnitz E, Hagmann S, Alshihri A, Al-Nawas B. Vertical osteoconductivity and early bone formation of titanium-zirconium and titanium implants in a subperiosteal rabbit animal model. Clin Oral Implants Res. 2014;25(7):774–80.
162. Wen B, Zhu F, Li Z, Zhang P, Lin X, Dard M. The osseointegration behavior of titanium-zirconium implants in ovariectomized rabbits. Clin Oral Implants Res. 2014;25(7):819–25.
163. Gottlow J, Dard M, Kjellson F, Obrecht M, Sennerby L. Evaluation of a new titanium-zirconium dental implant: a biomechanical and histological comparative study in the mini pig. Clin Implant Dent Relat Res. 2012;14(4):538–45.
164. Freilich M, Wen B, Shafer D, Schleier P, Dard M, Pendrys D, et al. Implant-guided vertical bone growth in the mini-pig. Clin Oral Implants Res. 2012;23(6):751–7.
165. Anchieta RB, Baldassarri M, Guastaldi F, Tovar N, Janal MN, Gottlow J, et al. Mechanical property assessment of bone healing around a titanium-zirconium alloy dental implant. Clin Implant Dent Relat Res. 2013;volume*(number*):1–7. Epub.
166. Morton D, Bornstein MM, Wittneben JG, Martin WC, Ruskin JD, Hart CN, et al. Early loading after 21 days of healing of nonsubmerged titanium implants with a chemically modified sandblasted and acid-etched surface: two-year results of a prospective two-center study. Clin Implant Dent Relat Res. 2010;12(1):9–17.
167. Schwarz F, Sculean A, Wieland M, Horn N, Nuesry E, Bube C, et al. Effects of hydrophilicity and microtopography of titanium implant surfaces on initial supragingival plaque biofilm formation. A pilot study. Mund-, Kiefer- und Gesichtschirurgie MKG. 2007;11(6):333–8.
168. Oates TW, Valderrama P, Bischof M, Nedir R, Jones A, Simpson J, et al. Enhanced implant stability with a chemically modified SLA surface: a randomized pilot study. Int J Oral Maxillofac Implants. 2007;22(5):755–60.
169. Valderrama P, Oates TW, Jones AA, Simpson J, Schoolfield JD, Cochran DL. Evaluation of two different resonance frequency devices to detect implant stability: a clinical trial. J Periodontol. 2007;78(2):262–72.
170. Han J, Lulic M, Lang NP. Factors influencing resonance frequency analysis assessed by Osstell mentor during implant tissue integration: II. Implant surface modifications and implant diameter. Clin Oral Implants Res. 2010;21(6):605–11.
171. Khandelwal N, Oates TW, Vargas A, Alexander PP, Schoolfield JD, Alex McMahan C. Conventional SLA and chemically modified SLA implants in patients with poorly controlled type 2 diabetes mellitus–a randomized controlled trial. Clin Oral Implants Res. 2013;24(1):13–9.
172. Schatzle M, Mannchen R, Balbach U, Hammerle CH, Toutenburg H, Jung RE. Stability change of chemically modified sandblasted/acid-etched titanium palatal implants. A randomized-controlled clinical trial. Clin Oral Implants Res. 2009;20(5):489–95.
173. Bornstein MM, Wittneben JG, Bragger U, Buser D. Early loading at 21 days of non-submerged titanium implants with a chemically modified sandblasted and acid-etched surface: 3-year results of a prospective study in the posterior mandible. J Periodontol. 2010;81(6):809–18.
174. Bornstein MM, Hart CN, Halbritter SA, Morton D, Buser D. Early loading of nonsubmerged titanium implants with a chemically modified sand-blasted and acid-etched surface: 6-month results of a prospective case series study in the posterior mandible focusing on peri-implant crestal bone changes and implant stability quotient (ISQ) values. Clin Implant Dent Relat Res. 2009;11(4):338–47.
175. Roccuzzo M, Wilson Jr TG. A prospective study of 3 weeks' loading of chemically modified titanium implants in the maxillary molar region: 1-year results. Int J Oral Maxillofac Implants. 2009;24(1):65–72.
176. Karabuda ZC, Abdel-Haq J, Arisan V. Stability, marginal bone loss and survival of standard and modified sand-blasted, acid-etched implants in bilateral edentulous spaces: a prospective 15-month evaluation. Clin Oral Implants Res. 2011;22(8):840–9.

177. Zollner A, Ganeles J, Korostoff J, Guerra F, Krafft T, Bragger U. Immediate and early non-occlusal loading of Straumann implants with a chemically modified surface (SLActive) in the posterior mandible and maxilla: interim results from a prospective multicenter randomized-controlled study. Clin Oral Implants Res. 2008;19(5):442–50.
178. Ganeles J, Zollner A, Jackowski J, ten Bruggenkate C, Beagle J, Guerra F. Immediate and early loading of Straumann implants with a chemically modified surface (SLActive) in the posterior mandible and maxilla: 1-year results from a prospective multicenter study. Clin Oral Implants Res. 2008;19(11):1119–28.
179. Nicolau P, Korostoff J, Ganeles J, Jackowski J, Krafft T, Neves M, et al. Immediate and early loading of chemically modified implants in posterior jaws: 3-year results from a prospective randomized multicenter study. Clin Implant Dent Relat Res. 2013;15(4):600–12.
180. Stoker GT, Wismeijer D. Immediate loading of two implants with a mandibular implant-retained overdenture: a new treatment protocol. Clin Implant Dent Relat Res. 2011;13(4):255–61.
181. Bergkvist G, Koh KJ, Sahlholm S, Klintstrom E, Lindh C. Bone density at implant sites and its relationship to assessment of bone quality and treatment outcome. Int J Oral Maxillofac Implants. 2010;25(2):321–8.
182. Luongo G, Oteri G. A noninterventional study documenting use and success of implants with a new chemically modified titanium surface in daily dental practice. J Oral Implantol. 2010;36(4):305–14.
183. Lindgren C, Mordenfeld A, Hallman M. A prospective 1-year clinical and radiographic study of implants placed after maxillary sinus floor augmentation with synthetic biphasic calcium phosphate or deproteinized bovine bone. Clin Implant Dent Relat Res. 2012;14(1):41–50.
184. Markovic A, Colic S, Drazic R, Gacic B, Todorovic A, Stajcic Z. Resonance frequency analysis as a reliable criterion for early loading of sandblasted/acid-etched active surface implants placed by the osteotome sinus floor elevation technique. Int J Oral Maxillofac Implants. 2011;26(4):718–24.
185. Rossi F, Ricci E, Marchetti C, Lang NP, Botticelli D. Early loading of single crowns supported by 6-mm-long implants with a moderately rough surface: a prospective 2-year follow-up cohort study. Clin Oral Implants Res. 2010;21(9):937–43.
186. Heberer S, Kilic S, Hossamo J, Raguse JD, Nelson K. Rehabilitation of irradiated patients with modified and conventional sandblasted acid-etched implants: preliminary results of a split-mouth study. Clin Oral Implants Res. 2011;22(5):546–51.
187. Albrektsson T, Zarb G, Worthington P, Eriksson AR. The long-term efficacy of currently used dental implants: a review and proposed criteria of success. Int J Oral Maxillofac Implants. 1986;1(1):11–25.
188. Lazzara RJ, Porter SS. Platform switching: a new concept in implant dentistry for controlling postrestorative crestal bone levels. Int J Periodontics Restorative Dent. 2006;26(1):9–17.
189. Hammerle CH, Jung RE, Sanz M, Chen S, Martin WC, Jackowski J, et al. Submerged and transmucosal healing yield the same clinical outcomes with two-piece implants in the anterior maxilla and mandible: interim 1-year results of a randomized, controlled clinical trial. Clin Oral Implants Res. 2012;23(2):211–9.
190. Sanz M, Ivanoff CJ, Weingart D, Wiltfang J, Gahlert M, Cordaro L, et al. Clinical and radiologic outcomes after submerged and transmucosal implant placement with two-piece implants in the anterior maxilla and mandible: 3-year results of a randomized controlled clinical trial. Clin Implant Dent Relat Res. 2013;volume*(number*):1–13. Epub.
191. Buser D, Halbritter S, Hart C, Bornstein MM, Grutter L, Chappuis V, et al. Early implant placement with simultaneous guided bone regeneration following single-tooth extraction in the esthetic zone: 12-month results of a prospective study with 20 consecutive patients. J Periodontol. 2009;80(1):152–62.
192. Buser D, Wittneben J, Bornstein MM, Grutter L, Chappuis V, Belser UC. Stability of contour augmentation and esthetic outcomes of implant-supported single crowns in the esthetic zone: 3-year results of a prospective study with early implant placement postextraction. J Periodontol. 2011;82(3):342–9.
193. Buser D, Chappuis V, Kuchler U, Bornstein MM, Wittneben JG, Buser R, et al. Long-term stability of early implant placement with contour augmentation. J Dent Res. 2013;92(12 Suppl):176S–82.
194. Chiapasco M, Casentini P, Zaniboni M, Corsi E, Anello T. Titanium-zirconium alloy narrow-diameter implants (Straumann Roxolid((R))) for the rehabilitation of horizontally deficient edentulous ridges: prospective study on 18 consecutive patients. Clin Oral Implants Res. 2012;23(10):1136–41.
195. Barter S, Stone P, Bragger U. A pilot study to evaluate the success and survival rate of titanium-zirconium implants in partially edentulous patients: results after 24 months of follow-up. Clin Oral Implants Res. 2012;23(7):873–81.
196. Benic GI, Gallucci GO, Mokti M, Hammerle CH, Weber HP, Jung RE. Titanium-zirconium narrow-diameter versus titanium regular-diameter implants for anterior and premolar single crowns: 1-year results of a randomized controlled clinical study. J Clin Periodontol. 2013;40(11):1052–61.
197. Al-Nawas B, Bragger U, Meijer HJ, Naert I, Persson R, Perucchi A, et al. A double-blind randomized controlled trial (RCT) of Titanium-13Zirconium versus Titanium Grade IV small-diameter bone level implants in edentulous mandibles–results from a 1-year observation period. Clin Implant Dent Relat Res. 2012;14(6):896–904.
198. Tolentino L, Sukekava F, Seabra M, Lima LA, Garcez-Filho J, Araujo MG. Success and survival

rates of narrow diameter implants made of titanium-zirconium alloy in the posterior region of the jaws – results from a 1-year follow-up. Clin Oral Implants Res. 2014;25(2):137–41.

199. Schwarz F, Wieland M, Schwartz Z, Zhao G, Rupp F, Geis-Gerstorfer J, et al. Potential of chemically modified hydrophilic surface characteristics to support tissue integration of titanium dental implants. J Biomed Mater Res B Appl Biomater. 2009;88(2):544–57.

200. Li P, Ohtsuki C, Kokubo T, Nakanishi K, Soga N, de Groot K. The role of hydrated silica, titania, and alumina in inducing apatite on implants. J Biomed Mater Res. 1994;28(1):7–15.

201. Berglundh T, Abrahamsson I, Lang NP, Lindhe J. De novo alveolar bone formation adjacent to endosseous implants. Clin Oral Implants Res. 2003;14(3):251–62.

202. Raghavendra S, Wood MC, Taylor TD. Early wound healing around endosseous implants: a review of the literature. Int J Oral Maxillofac Implants. 2005;20(3):425–31.

203. Bornstein MM, Harnisch H, Lussi A, Buser D. Clinical performance of wide-body implants with a sandblasted and acid-etched (SLA) surface: results of a 3-year follow-up study in a referral clinic. Int J Oral Maxillofac Implants. 2007;22(4):631–8.

Anodized Surface and Its Clinical Performance

10

Kiyoshi Koyano, Ikiru Atsuta, and Yohei Jinno

Abstract

Many implant surfaces and surface-modification techniques have been examined, and anodized surface on dental implant has been in continued clinical use and has demonstrated good stability during the healing phase. This proof has provided the basis for treatment modality of immediate function.

In this chapter, the evidences based on the clinical and basic study reporting the success of osseointegrated implants regarding anodized surface will be reviewed. An understanding of the current evidence may facilitate the most appropriate utilization of this important dental resource.

What Is an Anodized Implant?

Introduction

Osseointegration was discovered by Brånemark, and he and his colleagues pioneered clinical treatments with dental implants [1]. Pure titanium and titanium alloys are the standard materials for dental implants, because of their mechanical strength and biocompatibility. The first generation of clinical implants was machined, with a smooth surface texture. Since then, the importance of implant surface textures for osseointegration has become appreciated, and research into development of second-generation dental implants has been performed internationally. Many different implant surfaces and surface-modification techniques have been examined, including sandblasting, acid etching, and anodizing, laser-modified micro- and nanostructured surfaces, calcium phosphate coatings on titanium implants, and plasma spraying. In many of these studies, surface roughness has been recognized as critical for osseointegration [2].

In this chapter, we focus on anodized surfaces. In air at room temperature, the surface of titanium is covered by an oxide layer, which is 1.5–10 nm thick [3]. The oxide layer has a low level of electronic conductivity, high thermodynamic stability, and low ion-formation tendency, and

K. Koyano, DDS, PhD (✉)
Section of Implant and Rehabilitative Dentistry,
Division of Oral Rehabilitation,
Faculty of Dental Science, Kyushu University,
3-1-1 Maidashi, Higashi-ku, Fukuoka 812-8582, Japan
e-mail: koyano@dent.kyushu-u.ac.jp

I. Atsuta, DDS, PhD • Y. Jinno, DDS, PhD
Section of Implant and Rehabilitative Dentistry,
Division of Oral Rehabilitation, Kyushu University,
Fukuoka, Japan

A. Wennerberg et al. (eds.), *Implant Surfaces and their Biological and Clinical Impact*,
DOI 10.1007/978-3-662-45379-7_10, © Springer-Verlag Berlin Heidelberg 2015

Table 10.1 Reports of experimentally anodized implant

Treatment		Reference	Number of quotation (PubMed in 3.12.2014)
Calcium	Sodium p-glycerophosphate and calcium acetate	Ishizawa et al. [7]	221
	Calcium glycerophosphate	Suh et al. [8]	62
	Calcium acetate and calcium glycerophosphate	Li et al. [9]	73
	Calcium acetate and calcium glycerophosphate	Laurindo et al. [10]	–
Sulfuric acid	Sulfuric acid	Veleten et al. [11]	127
	Sulfuric acid	Zhao et al. [12]	94
	Sulfuric acid	Peterson et al. [13]	–
	Sulfuric acid	El-wassefy et al. [14]	–
Phosphoric acid	Phosphoric acid, hydrogen fluoride, and sulfuric acid		
	Phosphoric acid and sodium fluoride	Hieda et al. [15]	–
Hydrogen fluoride	Hydrogen fluoride	Puckett et al. [16]	108
	Hydrogen fluoride		–
	Hydrogen fluoride		–
Sodium hydroxide	Sodium hydroxide, calcium hydroxide, phosphoric acid, and acetic acid	Sul et al. [4]	255
	Sodium hydroxide		–

these properties explain the excellent biocompatibility of titanium implants [4]. When a positive voltage is applied to a piece of titanium immersed in an electrolyte, anodic oxidation of Ti occurs to form a TiO_2 layer on the surface [5]. It has been reported that bone formation around implants is promoted by this surface modification and that the bone formation also depends upon the oxide layer thickness and surface topography [6]. Therefore, knowledge of the chemical and physical properties of titanium oxide layers on titanium and titanium alloys is important for the reaction of cells in contact with biomaterials made of titanium and titanium alloys, and various surface treatments (Table 10.1).

On behalf of anodized surfaces, the TiUnite surface was introduced in 2000 by Nobel Biocare. The TiUnite surface is an anodized surface, which presents with good osseointegration [17]. The TiUnite surface features a moderately rough, thickened titanium oxide crystalline layer with phosphorus content. During anodizing, the gas included in the titanium oxide layer of the implant is discharged, pores are formed, and it is believed that the surface area is increased.

The ceramic-like properties and micropores of TiUnite ensure high osteoconductivity and fast anchorage of newly formed bone compared with the turned surface [18]. The negatively charged TiUnite surface attracts blood proteins and inactive platelets immediately after implant insertion. Simultaneously, fibrils from the fibrin meshwork become visible. The platelets begin to swell and form pseudopodia. By releasing adenosine diphosphate (ADP), they become sticky and clump together to close the injured blood vessels at the wound edges and stop the bleeding. The newly formed fibrin matrix allows the blood to clot. Activated platelets become embedded in the matrix and release granules full of enzymes as well as growth factors needed for wound healing and bone formation. Blood cells, activated platelets, and fibrin form a blood clot that adheres to the moderately rough TiUnite surface. It is crucial for contact osteogenesis that the blood clot remains attached to the surface [19]. Neutrophils and, later, macrophages remove the blood clot during the first 2 days of wound healing, enabling a provisional matrix to occupy the wound area. Osteogenic cells stream to the TiUnite surface and migrate – using their pseudopodia and the open pores as attachment points – to the bone-formation front, where they transform into osteoblasts. Newly formed bone spreads over the osteoconductive TiUnite surface and forms a thin band of woven bone deposited directly on and along the surface. This thin bone layer will grow by further bone apposition and become lamellar bone. Bone-forming osteoblasts attach to the TiUnite surface with their pseudopodia and cover the orifices of the open pores [20]. They start to secrete the collagen matrix of woven bone directly into the pores and move away from the surface, forming the collagenous bone matrix that will eventually mineralize.

Numerous in vitro examinations have been carried out, and various properties such as the surface energy, variation in surface texture at the nanolevel, increase in infiltration, and chemical stability have been reported [21, 22]. Despite these in vitro studies, no definite clarification has been made regarding the biological basis for the acceleration of osseointegration which is recognized in vivo.

TiUnite Surface After Implant Insertion

When the implant is placed in the jaw bone, the inserted portion of the TiUnite surface is polished by the bone. This results in a several-micron-thick smear layer composed of bone debris and blood, which has osteoinductive potential because of the presence of growth factors needed for bone formation [23]. However, since this smear layer covers the implant surface, it may be argued that the properties of the TiUnite surface itself do not have any remarkable influence on either the initial wound healing or the subsequent bone formation. The macro design of the implant, the degree of surface roughness, and the drilling protocol are considered to influence the existence and amount of the smear layer. When the diameter in a cervical section in the extraction socket is greater than the implant diameter, no smear layer occurs over the implant surface. However, the TiUnite surface implant still accelerates the bone-healing process, compared to nontreated titanium surfaces, even in the absence of a smear layer; this implies that the surface properties of the implant itself also improve healing [23].

TiUnite Surface and Integration to Surrounding Tissue

The observations described in the section above clarified the biological basis for osseointegration and in particular explain the high predictability of osseointegration of implants with TiUnite surfaces. The TiUnite surface is well studied and also has a very long clinical history in the field of implant dentistry.

Direct adhesion between titanium implant surface and surrounding soft tissue is said to be promoted when the epithelium in the periphery of the implant attaches to the surface through the hemidesmosome. Cellular soft tissue adhesion behaves similarly to soft tissue around a natural tooth [24]. Research into the implant surface originally focused on promotion of osseointegration, and TiUnite surface processing was only applied to the part of the implant intended to be embedded inside the bone. However, in recent years, sealing of the peripheral edge via direct adhesion to implant surfaces by fibrous and epithelial cells is desired [25], and use of implants with TiUnite surface treatment on the top section of the implant has also begun.

Reports About TiUnite

Changes Between Turned and TiUnite Surfaces

Many in vivo and in vitro studies involving the surface properties of oxidized implants have overlooked the fact that the electrochemical-microarc oxidation (MAO) process used for oxidized implants not only alters surface roughness but also changes the surface chemistry, pore configuration (pore size, density, morphology), and crystal structure of TiO_2 [25, 26]. These studies found that when the initial implant stability values were very

Table 10.2 Survival rate of All-on-4

Reference	Location of implantation (number)	Follow-up time		
		1 year	5 year	10 year
Malo et al. [35]	In the mandible (980 implants)			94.8
Malo et al. [36]	In the maxilla (968)		98.0	
	In the maxilla (136)		100	
Agliardi et al. [43]	In the maxilla/mandible (692)		98.4/99.7	
	In the maxilla/mandible (1,001)		97.1/98.0	
Malo et al. [36]	In the maxilla/mandible (227)		97.7/94.8	
Francetti et al. [38]	In the maxilla/mandible (196)		100/100	
Galindo et al. [39]	In the mandible (731)	99.9		
Pomares et al. [40]	In the maxilla/mandible (195)	98.0		

high, the degree of osseointegration increased only slightly or sometimes even decreased at early healing times, while when the implant stability at placement was lower, the subsequent stability increased rapidly over time [25]. From a biological perspective, this discrepancy could be explained in part by the fact that dissimilarities in bone properties (density, volume, thickness, architecture, and associated modeling/remodeling) between experimental animals (rabbit, dog, goat, pig, and sheep) and between different bones in humans (mandible, maxilla, anterior, and posterior area) have a strong impact on the various measurements.

In the first clinical studies reporting the success of osseointegrated implants, the survival rates of Brånemark implants (Nobel Biocare, Gothenburg, Sweden) were 86 % in the mandible and 78 % in the maxilla after 15 years of function in completely edentulous arches [27]. The survival rates of this implant system have improved in recent years, after the surface of the Brånemark implant system was changed from a turned surface to the TiUnite surface. As discussed above, this surface is characterized by many open pores in the low micrometer range [28], which are thought to improve the bone-to-titanium surface contact. The survival rate for the TiUnite surface implants was shown to be higher (98.6 %) than that for Brånemark implants with turned surfaces (92.1 %) [29]. The overall survival rate of the TiUnite implants in this study compares favorably with previous reports.

Why do turned and TiUnite implants produce such different results in clinical studies? In the clinical field, each dentist might have subjective thoughts on the relationship between the risk of implantitis and the type of implant surface. Charalampakis et al. [30] showed that, following ligature placement (to induce plaque formation) and subsequent ligature removal 10 weeks after placement, the total bacterial load increased over time for each of the groups in their study (tooth, implant with turned surface, and TiUnite implant) [30]. The TiUnite implants with enhanced surface characteristics (micropores obtained via electrochemical oxidation) were introduced by Nobel Biocare to accelerate the osseointegration process. Several studies have indeed clearly confirmed this accelerated healing and bone-to-implant contact [28, 31, 32]. Therefore, TiUnite implants showed a clear decrease in early failure, especially in areas with poor bone density such as the maxilla [33, 34]. Nobel Biocare's new treatment concept, All-on-4™, has been studied by many groups (Table 10.2). This concept uses two axial implants in the anterior region and two tilted posterior implants as has been published by Malo et al. with cumulative survival rates well above 92.2 %. This concept based on only four implants per arch is able to provide an edentulous arch with an immediate function fixed aesthetic provisional prosthesis [41–43]. However, it has been suggested that the higher incidence of retrograde peri-implantitis for TiUnite implants can also be explained by faster osseointegration [44]. When the turned implants come into contact with a granuloma or endodontic pathology, they will soon be completely surrounded by granulation tissue; however, the TiUnite surface implants will not have the same fate, because of the accelerated bone apposition. As such, the coronal part of the TiUnite implant still integrates before the fibrous encapsulation can reach this area. Although this hypothesis still needs to be proven by further research, it is consistent with some experimental observations.

Short-Term Clinical Findings

Preclinical studies show that the speed of osseointegration is enhanced for TiUnite-coated implants compared with the turned surfaces implants. This effect was measured as an increase in bone-to-implant contact at a given time point. In fact, the surface properties of TiUnite stimulate bone growth directly on its surface. Compared with turned surfaces, clinical findings demonstrate that the drop in initial stability during the healing phase was significantly reduced with implants featuring TiUnite [45]. The benefit of this observation is that the risk over the first 6 months is significantly reduced. Bone formation follows the contours of the threads of the implant even during the early phase of healing.

This yields higher maintained initial stability than that offered by implants with a machined surface. During its first 5 years on the market, more than 84 scientific publications documenting in vitro investigations as well as preclinical and clinical studies have been generated. These support the clinical success of TiUnite implants in two-stage procedures as well as for immediate loading protocols, and for all types of bone qualities.

Long-Term Clinical Findings

Of the 84 publications, five recently published studies demonstrate the long-term stability of TiUnite [46, 47]. In these, more than 550 TiUnite implants of different designs demonstrated a cumulative survival rate of 94–100 %. Follow-up periods were at least 2 years, and implants were inserted in both immediate function and two-stage protocols. The report by Glauser et al. is a 5-year follow-up of immediately loaded TiUnite implants in regions of soft bone finalized in 2007, which confirms the long-term stability of TiUnite implants [47]. What is more, TiUnite stability had cleared by clinical reports over a period of 10 year by Ostman et al. and Degidi et al. [48, 49].

In these publications, which demonstrated an implant survival of more 97 %, it was shown that TiUnite implants are clinically stable over the 10-year period. In other words, no drop in the clinical stability, as measured by resonance frequency analysis (RFA), was observed. Furthermore, these reports show that bone levels around TiUnite implants remain stable for long term. Albrektsson et al. concluded on their paper that TiUnite implants do result in somewhat greater first year crestal bone loss than the other modern implants, but as observed in a recent paper, TiUnite develops a steady-state situation with respect to further bone loss with good clinical long-term results with maintained bone levels [50].

Representative Dental Implants Used in Clinical Research

Is the success rate of TiUnite implants different from those of other dental implants? Polizzi et al. [51] reported that the treatment outcome for implants with TiUnite surfaces was entirely different from that observed for other implant types [51]. Two TiUnite implants were lost after surgical treatment of peri-implantitis, and radiographic and histological analyses of remaining sites revealed that continuous bone loss occurred and that large inflammatory lesions persisted in the peri-implant soft tissues. However, the longer-term findings from Polizzi's study confirm the favorable results that were previously mentioned and those subsequently published by other authors [44, 52]. In 2004, Cornelini and colleagues reported on the immediate restoration of 30 unsplinted transmucosal International Team Implantology (ITI) solid implants with a sand-blasted, acid-etched surface (Straumann Institute, Waldenburg, Switzerland) in mandibular molar sites [53]. In that study, only one implant was lost during the 1-year follow-up period, resulting in a 96.7 % survival rate after 12 months. They concluded that, in the molar mandibular area with good implant primary stability, this protocol of immediate restoration can be safe and successful.

In 2007, Rao and Benzi published a report on single, mandibular first-molar implants (Replace Select Tapered TiUnite) placed with flapless

Table 10.3 Survival rate of TiUnite and the other type implants

Reference	Type of implants (number)		Follow-up time		
			1 year	5 year	10 year
	Straumann (6 mm)(642 implants)		98.6		
	ITI implant (1,268)			98	
Filippi et al. [56]	SLActive (Pt:759; imp:1,355)		98.5		
Vanlioglu et al. [57]	Straumann (177)			97.7	
Akoglu et al. [58]	ITI (24)			100	
	Astra (24)			100	
	SwissPlus (24)			100	
	Straumann			93.75	
Gotfredsen et al. [59]	Astra			100	
Lekholm et al. [60]	Branemark (461)	Man	93	90	
		Max	94	94	
Ostman et al. [49]	Branemark (121)				99.2
Degidi et al. [48]	Branemark (210)				97.3
	Branemark (136)				98.5
Mura et al. [37]	Branemark (79)			100	
	Branemark (310)			99.4	
Jung et al. [61]	Branemark (112)		96.4		

guided surgery and immediately loaded with pre-manufactured individualized abutments and crowns [54]. All 51 tapered implants placed were stable and functioning after 1 year, providing a 100 % survival rate.

More recently, Schincaglia and colleagues published the findings from a randomized controlled study comparing immediate versus delayed loading of wide-body implants (TiUnite Wide Platform MK III) supporting single-unit restorations in the molar area [55]. No implants were lost in the delayed group (0 %), whereas one implant failed (6.7 %) in the immediate loading group after 1-year follow-up. In this study, the radiographic bone level change observed after 12 months of loading was statistically significantly less for immediate loading implants than for implants with delayed loading (Table 10.2).

In conclusion, because there are many differences in variables like patient selection criteria, type of one-stage surgical approach (flap elevation or flapless), and type of immediate restorations delivered (screw-retained or cemented, standardized or individualized restorative components), it is difficult to directly compare all these studies.

Future Evolution of TiUnite Implants

Extended TiUnite on NobelDirect®, Speedy and Groovy Implant Types

Introduced in 2004, the one-piece implant, NobelDirect, was the first to benefit from extension of the TiUnite surface to contact the soft tissue. Histological analyses from preclinical studies have revealed an affinity to bone formation within and along a groove incorporated at the implant thread along the length of the intraosseous portion. The Speedy and Groovy implant lines were launched in 2005. A 100-μm groove was introduced on these implants, to further enhance the speed of osseointegration, and the TiUnite surface was extended to the collar of the implant. In five ongoing studies sponsored by Nobel Biocare, implants with the TiUnite surface extending to the soft tissue are being reviewed (Table 10.3). The current, cumulative survival rate for these studies is in the range 96.8–100 %. For 256 implants in 137 patients, stable bone levels are reported at 1-year follow-up. Continuous, stable bone levels have been confirmed over 3 years in a follow-up of 99 implants in 53 patients. A 2-year follow-up from one of these studies on NobelDirect was recently published, and the reported implant survival rate was 98.8 % [62]. The bone levels were stable between 1 and 3 years, and the authors concluded that: "Within the limits of this study, the stable marginal bone level and soft tissue health support the hypothesis that the one-piece implant evaluated has the ability to preserve both hard and soft tissue."

Conclusion

TiUnite is a pure titanium oxide surface coating developed into an osteoconductive biomaterial through an anodic oxidation process. TiUnite builds on the tradition of the machined titanium implant surface, but offers improved results. Since its introduction in 2000, the TiUnite surface has been in continued clinical use and has demonstrated good stability during the healing phase. This proof has provided the basis for treatment modality of immediate function. Now, 10-year clinical documentation has been published demonstrating high long-term clinical stability and stable marginal bone levels. On NobelDirect, Speedy, and Groovy implants, the TiUnite surface has been extended to the coronal part of the implant. Published 2-year data on NobelDirect show stable bone levels and recently compiled 3-year data show continued stability.

References

1. Brånemark PI, Adell R, Albrektsson T, Lekholm U, Lundkvist S, Rockler B. Osseointegrated titanium fixtures in the treatment of edentulousness. Biomaterials. 1983;4:25–8.
2. Albrektsson T. Direct bone anchorage of dental implants. J Prosthet Dent. 1983;50:255–61.
3. Kasemo B. Biocompatibility of titanium implants: surface science aspects. J Prosthet Dent. 1983;49:832–7.
4. Sul YT, Johansson CB, Jeong Y, Albrektsson T. The electrochemical oxide growth behaviour on titanium in acid and alkaline electrolytes. Med Eng Phys. 2001;23:329–46.
5. Choi JW, Heo SJ, Koak JY, Kim SK, Lim YJ, Kim SH, et al. Biological responses of anodized titanium implants under different current voltages. J Oral Rehabil. 2006;33:889–97.
6. Larsson C, Thomsen P, Lausmaa J, Rodahl M, Kasemo B, Ericson LE. Bone response to surface modified titanium implants: studies on electropolished implants with different oxide thicknesses and morphology. Biomaterials. 1994;15:1062–74.
7. Ishizawa H, Ogino M. Formation and characterization of anodic titanium oxide films containing Ca and P. J Biomed Mater Res. 1995;29:65–72.
8. Suh JY, Jang BC, Zhu X, Ong JL, Kim K. Effect of hydrothermally treated anodic oxide films on osteoblast attachment and proliferation. Biomaterials. 2003;24:347–55.
9. Li Y, Lee IS, Cui FZ, Choi SH. The biocompatibility of nanostructured calcium phosphate coated on micro-arc oxidized titanium. Biomaterials. 2008;29:2025–32.
10. Laurindo CA, Torres RD, Mali SA, Gilbert JL, Soares P. Incorporation of Ca and P on anodized titanium surface: Effect of high current density. Mater Sci Eng C Mater Biol Appl. 2014;37:223–31.
11. Velten D, Biehl V, Aubertin F, Valeske B, Possart W, Breme J. Preparation of TiO(2) layers on cp-Ti and Ti6Al4V by thermal and anodic oxidation and by sol-gel coating techniques and their characterization. J Biomed Mater Res. 2002;59:18–28.
12. Zhao G, Zinger O, Schwartz Z, Wieland M, Landolt D, Boyan BD. Osteoblast-like cells are sensitive to submicron-scale surface structure. Clin Oral Implants Res. 2006;17:258–64.
13. Peterson AM, Pilz-Allen C, Kolesnikova T, Mohwald H, Shchukin D. Growth factor release from polyelectrolyte-coated titanium for implant applications. ACS Appl Mater Interfaces. 2014;6:1866–71.
14. El-wassefy NA, Hammouda IM, Habib AN, El-awady GY, Marzook HA. Assessment of anodized titanium implants bioactivity. Clin Oral Implants Res. 2014;25:e1–9.
15. Hieda J, Niinomi M, Nakai M, Cho K, Mohri T, Hanawa T. Adhesive strength of medical polymer on anodic oxide nanostructures fabricated on biomedical beta-type titanium alloy. Mater Sci Eng C Mater Biol Appl. 2014;36:244–51.
16. Puckett SD, Taylor E, Raimondo T, Webster TJ. The relationship between the nanostructure of titanium surfaces and bacterial attachment. Biomaterials. 2010;31:706–13.
17. Zechner W, Tangl S, Furst G, Tepper G, Thams U, Mailath G, et al. Osseous healing characteristics of three different implant types. Clin Oral Implants Res. 2003;14:150–7.
18. Schupbach P, Glauser R, Rocci A, Martignoni M, Sennerby L, Lundgren A, et al. The human bone-oxidized titanium implant interface: a light microscopic, scanning electron microscopic, back-scatter scanning electron microscopic, and energy-dispersive x-ray study of clinically retrieved dental implants. Clin Implant Dent Relat Res. 2005;7 Suppl 1:S36–43.
19. Vanegas-Acosta JC, Garzon-Alvarado DA, Lancellotti V. Numerical investigation into blood clotting at the bone-dental implant interface in the presence of an electrical stimulus. Comput Biol Med. 2013;43:2079–88.

20. Kohal RJ, Bachle M, Att W, Chaar S, Altmann B, Renz A, et al. Osteoblast and bone tissue response to surface modified zirconia and titanium implant materials. Dent Mater. 2013;29:763–76.
21. Liu R, Lei T, Dusevich V, Yao X, Liu Y, Walker MP, et al. Surface characteristics and cell adhesion: a comparative study of four commercial dental implants. J Prosthodont. 2013;22:641–51.
22. Choi JY, Lee HJ, Jang JU, Yeo IS. Comparison between bioactive fluoride modified and bioinert anodically oxidized implant surfaces in early bone response using rabbit tibia model. Implant Dent. 2012;21:124–8.
23. Tabassum A, Walboomers F, Wolke JG, Meijer GJ, Jansen JA. The influence of surface roughness on the displacement of osteogenic bone particles during placement of titanium screw-type implants. Clin Implant Dent Relat Res. 2011;13:269–78.
24. Schupbach P, Glauser R. The defense architecture of the human periimplant mucosa: a histological study. J Prosthet Dent. 2007;97:S15–25.
25. Sul YT, Johansson C, Albrektsson T. Which surface properties enhance bone response to implants? Comparison of oxidized magnesium, TiUnite, and osseotite implant surfaces. Int J Prosthodont. 2006;19:319–28.
26. Zhang R, Liu Y, Yan K, Chen L, Chen XR, Li P, et al. Anti-inflammatory and immunomodulatory mechanisms of mesenchymal stem cell transplantation in experimental traumatic brain injury. J Neuroinflammation. 2013;10:106.
27. Adell R, Lekholm U. On osseointegration – a response. N Y State Dent J. 1987;53:8–9.
28. Sawase T, Wennerberg A, Hallgren C, Albrektsson T, Baba K. Chemical and topographical surface analysis of five different implant abutments. Clin Oral Implants Res. 2000;11:44–50.
29. Baqain ZH, Moqbel WY, Sawair FA. Early dental implant failure: risk factors. Br J Oral Maxillofac Surg. 2012;50:239–43.
30. Charalampakis G, Abrahamsson I, Carcuac O, Dahlen G, Berglundh T. Microbiota in experimental periodontitis and peri-implantitis in dogs. Clin Oral Implants Res. 2014;25(9):1094–8.
31. Gottlow J, Sennerby L, Rosengren A, Flynn M. An experimental evaluation of a new craniofacial implant using the rabbit tibia model: part I. Histologic findings. Otol Neurotol. 2010;31:832–9.
32. Friberg B, Jisander S, Widmark G, Lundgren A, Ivanoff CJ, Sennerby L, et al. One-year prospective three-center study comparing the outcome of a "soft bone implant" (prototype Mk IV) and the standard Branemark implant. Clin Implant Dent Relat Res. 2003;5:71–7.
33. Balshi TJ, Wolfinger GJ, Pryszlak MC, Balshi SF. Facial and oral reconstruction following trauma and failed chin implant: a case report. Implant Dent. 2005;14:221–6.
34. Balshi SF, Wolfinger GJ, Balshi TJ. Analysis of 164 titanium oxide-surface implants in completely edentulous arches for fixed prosthesis anchorage using the pterygomaxillary region. Int J Oral Maxillofac Implants. 2005;20:946–52.
35. Malo P, de Araujo Nobre M, Lopes A, Moss SM, Molina GJ. A longitudinal study of the survival of All-on-4 implants in the mandible with up to 10 years of follow-up. J Am Dent Assoc. 2011;142:310–20.
36. Malo P, de Araujo Nobre M, Lopes A, Francischone C, Rigolizzo M. "All-on-4" immediate-function concept for completely edentulous maxillae: a clinical report on the medium (3 years) and long-term (5 years) outcomes. Clin Implant Dent Relat Res. 2012;14 Suppl 1:e139–50.
37. Mura P. Immediate loading of tapered implants placed in postextraction sockets: retrospective analysis of the 5-year clinical outcome. Clin Implant Dent Relat Res. 2012;14:565–74.
38. Francetti L, Romeo D, Corbella S, Taschieri S, Del Fabbro M. Bone level changes around axial and tilted implants in full-arch fixed immediate restorations. Interim results of a prospective study. Clin Implant Dent Relat Res. 2012;14:646–54.
39. Galindo DF, Butura CC. Immediately loaded mandibular fixed implant prostheses using the all-on-four protocol: a report of 183 consecutively treated patients with 1 year of function in definitive prostheses. Int J Oral Maxillofac Implants. 2012;27:628–33.
40. Pomares C. A retrospective study of edentulous patients rehabilitated according to the 'all-on-four' or the 'all-on-six' immediate function concept using flapless computer-guided implant surgery. Eur J Oral Implantol. 2010;3:155–63.
41. Khatami AH, Smith CR. "All-on-four" immediate function concept and clinical report of treatment of an edentulous mandible with a fixed complete denture and milled titanium framework. J Prosthodont. 2008;17:47–51.
42. Malo P, Nobre Mde A, Petersson U, Wigren S. A pilot study of complete edentulous rehabilitation with immediate function using a new implant design: case series. Clin Implant Dent Relat Res. 2006;8:223–32.
43. Agliardi E, Panigatti S, Clerico M, Villa C, Malo P. Immediate rehabilitation of the edentulous jaws with full fixed prostheses supported by four implants: interim results of a single cohort prospective study. Clin Oral Implants Res. 2010;21:459–65.
44. Calandriello R, Tomatis M. Immediate occlusal loading of single lower molars using Branemark System(R) Wide Platform TiUnite implants: a 5-year follow-up report of a prospective clinical multicenter study. Clin Implant Dent Relat Res. 2011;13:311–8.
45. Glauser R, Ree A, Lundgren A, Gottlow J, Hammerle CH, Scharer P. Immediate occlusal loading of Branemark implants applied in various jawbone regions: a prospective, 1-year clinical study. Clin Implant Dent Relat Res. 2001;3:204–13.
46. Degidi M, Scarano A, Iezzi G, Piattelli A. Histologic analysis of an immediately loaded implant retrieved after 2 months. J Oral Implantol. 2005;31:247–54.

47. Glauser R, Zembic A, Ruhstaller P, Windisch S. Five-year results of implants with an oxidized surface placed predominantly in soft quality bone and subjected to immediate occlusal loading. J Prosthet Dent. 2007;97:S59–68.
48. Degidi M, Nardi D, Piattelli A. 10-year follow-up of immediately loaded implants with TiUnite porous anodized surface. Clin Implant Dent Relat Res. 2012;14:828–38.
49. Ostman PO, Hellman M, Sennerby L. Ten years later. Results from a prospective single-centre clinical study on 121 oxidized (TiUnite) Branemark implants in 46 patients. Clin Implant Dent Relat Res. 2012;14:852–60.
50. Albrektsson T, Buser D, Sennerby L. Crestal bone loss and oral implants. Clin Implant Dent Relat Res. 2012;14:783–91.
51. Polizzi G, Gualini F, Friberg B. A two-center retrospective analysis of long-term clinical and radiologic data of TiUnite and turned implants placed in the same mouth. Int J Prosthodont. 2013;26:350–8.
52. Calandriello R, Tomatis M, Vallone R, Rangert B, Gottlow J. Immediate occlusal loading of single lower molars using Branemark System Wide-Platform TiUnite implants: an interim report of a prospective open-ended clinical multicenter study. Clin Implant Dent Relat Res. 2003;5 Suppl 1:74–80.
53. Cornelini R, Cangini F, Covani U, Barone A, Buser D. Immediate restoration of single-tooth implants in mandibular molar sites: a 12-month preliminary report. Int J Oral Maxillofac Implants. 2004;19:855–60.
54. Rao W, Benzi R. Single mandibular first molar implants with flapless guided surgery and immediate function: preliminary clinical and radiographic results of a prospective study. J Prosthet Dent. 2007;97:S3–14.
55. Schincaglia GP, Marzola R, Giovanni GF, Chiara CS, Scotti R. Replacement of mandibular molars with single-unit restorations supported by wide-body implants: immediate versus delayed loading. A randomized controlled study. Int J Oral Maxillofac Implants. 2008;23:474–80.
56. Filippi A, Higginbottom FL, Lambrecht T, Levin BP, Meier JL, Rosen PS, et al. A prospective noninterventional study to document implant success and survival of the Straumann Bone Level SLActive dental implant in daily dental practice. Quintessence Int. 2013;44:499–512.
57. Vanlioglu B, Ozkan Y, Kulak-Ozkan Y. Retrospective analysis of prosthetic complications of implant-supported fixed partial dentures after an observation period of 5 to 10 years. Int J Oral Maxillofac Implants. 2013;28:1300–4.
58. Akoglu B, Ucankale M, Ozkan Y, Kulak-Ozkan Y. Five-year treatment outcomes with three brands of implants supporting mandibular overdentures. Int J Oral Maxillofac Implants. 2011;26:188–94.
59. Gotfredsen K. A 5-year prospective study of single-tooth replacements supported by the Astra Tech implant: a pilot study. Clin Implant Dent Relat Res. 2004;6:1–8.
60. Lekholm U, Gunne J, Henry P, Higuchi K, Linden U, Bergstrom C, et al. Survival of the Branemark implant in partially edentulous jaws: a 10-year prospective multicenter study. Int J Oral Maxillofac Implants. 1999;14:639–45.
61. Jung UW, Choi JY, Kim CS, Cho KS, Chai JK, Kim CK, et al. Evaluation of mandibular posterior single implants with two different surfaces: a 5-year comparative study. J Periodontol. 2008;79:1857–63.
62. Zembic A, Bosch A, Jung RE, Hammerle CH, Sailer I. Five-year results of a randomized controlled clinical trial comparing zirconia and titanium abutments supporting single-implant crowns in canine and posterior regions. Clin Oral Implants Res. 2013;24:384–90.

Implant Coatings and Its Application in Clinical Reality

11

Klaus Gotfredsen

Abstract

Even though dental implants are highly successful, there are still clinical situations where new developments in implant coatings could improve implant stabilization, bone formation, and long-term implant performance. Significant improvements were obtained when the surface topography of the implants were changed from smooth to a moderately rough surface, and in the future we expect that inorganic or organic nanocoatings could improve the clinical outcome also in compromised bone sites. Various bioactive coatings have been tested in vitro and in vivo, and the biological knowledge increases, but still no evidence exist that nanocoatings are able to significantly improve clinical outcome.

Introduction

The implementation of osseointegrated implants in oral health care has been a great success and the most important innovation for clinical dentistry for decades. Replacing missing teeth with osseointegrated titanium implants has improved Oral Health–Related Quality of Life (OHRQoL) for a great number of patients [1]. The original concepts of osseointegration focused on the host bone, the surgical and prosthetic procedures, and the biocompatibility and macro- and microdesign of the implants [2]. Research projects still elaborate these areas, and especially the host bone, and its relation to the general health of the patient seems to be of outmost importance for the clinical outcome of implant treatment although randomized clinical trials within the subject area are few [3]. The topography of the implant surface, which can be changed by coating procedures, has proven to be of major importance for the clinical outcome [4, 5].

A great variety of clinical situation exists where implant-supported reconstructions could improve OHRQoL for the patient, and some of these cases are more challenging than others. Patients with compromised bone sites caused by reduced bone quality, e.g., low bone healing and repair capacity, may demonstrate slow bone regeneration and inappropriate bone strength, and patients with low bone quantity will have low volume of mineralized bone for implant stabilization and anchorage (Fig. 11.1). Such clinical situations will influence the structural and

K. Gotfredsen, PhD, DDS
Department of Odontology, Faculty of Health and Medical Sciences, University of Copenhagen, 20 Noerre Allé, DK-2200 Copenhagen N, Denmark
e-mail: klg@sund.ku.dk

A. Wennerberg et al. (eds.), *Implant Surfaces and their Biological and Clinical Impact*,
DOI 10.1007/978-3-662-45379-7_11, © Springer-Verlag Berlin Heidelberg 2015

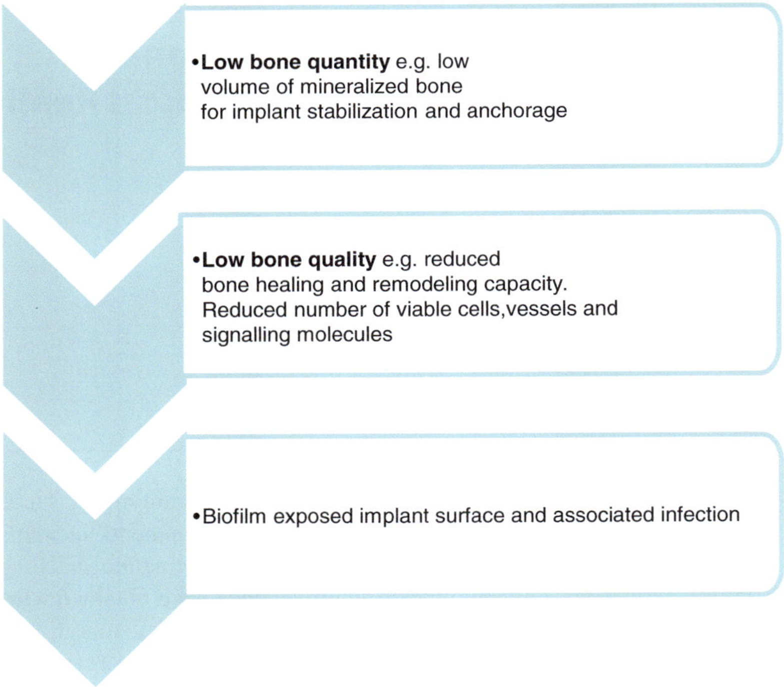

Fig. 11.1 Clinical situations with compromised alveolar bone sites

functional connection between ordered living bone and the surface of a load-carrying implant, and surface modifications of implants are done to improve osseointegration in compromised bone sites. The coating may inhibit bone resorption or enhance bone formation at the implant surface, and it may accelerate bone regeneration [6].

During the last decades great interest has been shown for biofilm formation on exposed implant surfaces and its sequelae [7]. Especially, the influence of the surface characteristics for developing peri-implantitis has been examined in animal studies, where significant differences between implant surface modifications have been found [8]. Thus, critical clinical situations arise when implant surface coatings originally designed to accelerate and improve bone healing become exposed to oral biofilm and increase the risk for peri-implant inflammation and bone destruction (Fig. 11.1).

Macro-, Micro-, and Nanocoatings

Basically, surface modification can be performed by subtractive techniques, e.g., acid etching, oxidation, and blasting procedures, resulting in a plastic deformation of the surface, or by additive techniques, resulting in depositions of the surface. The latter is called a coating, and this may affect chemical inertness, surface energy, hydrophilicity, cell adhesion, and resistance to infections. Coatings can have different thickness and roughness. A few decades ago coatings within orthopedics and implant dentistry were macro- and microcoatings, e.g., titanium plasma-spray coatings and hydroxyapatite coatings, with coating thicknesses 30 μm and upwards [9]. This period was succeeded with implant surface modifications using a microscale surface topography, described with a great number of surface characterizing height, space, and hybrid parameters with the average height deviation from a mean plane (Sa-value) as the most frequently describing surface roughness parameter. Thus, surfaces were divided into smooth (Sa = 0.0–0.4 μm), minimally rough (Sa = 0.5–1.0 μm), moderately rough (Sa = 1.0–2.0 μm), and rough (Sa >2 μm). The change from smooth to moderately rough implant surfaces improved the clinical outcome of implant therapy significantly [4]. Today most dental implants have moderately rough implant surfaces, and an increasing number of companies

Table 11.1 Examples of nanocoatings used for dental implants

Chemical group	Chemical subgroup	Substance/molecule/fluid	References
Inorganic	Element (periodic table)	Diamond	[12]
		Fluoride	[13]
		Silver	[14]
		Calcium phosphate	[14–16]
		Zinc	[14]
		Titanium	[17]
Organic	Protein	Collagen I	[18]
		Elastin	[6]
		Fibronectin	[19]
		Laminin	[20]
		Osteopontin	[21]
		Bone sialoprotein	[22]
	Growth factors	BMP-2, BMP-4, BMP-7	[6, 16, 23]
	Peptides	RGD	[24]
		Parathyroid hormone	[25]
		Antimicrobial Gl13K	[26]
	Polysaccharides	Hyaluronic acid	[27]
		Chondroitin 4-sulfate	[28]
		Chitosan	[27]
		Pectins	[6]
	Drugs	Bisphosphonate	[29]
		Simvastatin	[30]
		Strontium ranelate	[31]

add nanocoatings, where the thickness of the coating is measured on a nanoscale (1–100 nm). In contrast to the moderately rough implant surface modifications, no clear evidence exists that nanocoatings will improve the clinical outcome of implant therapy. This will also be difficult as the 5- and 10-year survival rates of implants with moderately rough surface are reported to be better than 97 % [4, 10]. Thus, nanocoatings or new surface modifications will primary be indicated for compromised bone sites or cases with a need for accelerated bone healing.

Most nanocoatings are characterized as bioactive. This has been defined as a surface which elicits biological activity on the surrounding tissue [11]. A biochemical bonding between implant surfaces and surrounding tissue is aimed in contrast to only microstructured surfaces, where the interface results in a physical bonding depending on the surface topography at the micrometer level. It is, however, important to realize that by changing one surface property other surface properties, chemical and physical, will consequently be affected. The chemical strategies with nanocoatings focus on interface bonding using inorganic and/or organic molecules [6] (Table 11.1).

Inorganic Coatings

Titanium plasma coating is one of the most well-known surface modifications used in implant dentistry. It was adopted from the orthopedic field and had a coating thickness between 30 and 40 μm. An arc flame temperature of 15–20,000 °C and a gas jet velocity more than 3,000 m/s characterized the coating technique called titanium plasma spraying (TPS). The titanium powder grain size was 0.05–0.1 mm and resulted in a very rough implant surface [9]. It could be characterized as a porous surface with approximately ten times greater surface area than the titanium surface without coating [17]. Experimental studies with the TPS surface demonstrated osseointegration, and clinical studies reported good

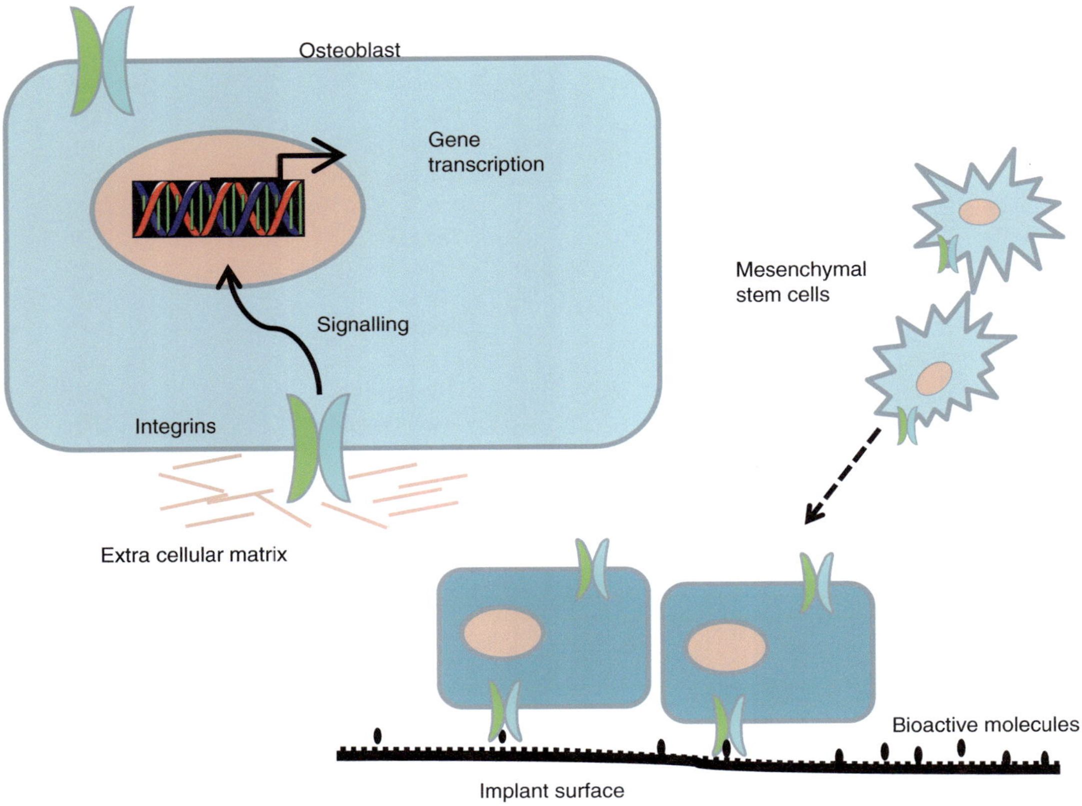

Fig. 11.2 Cells with targeting integrins to promote bone formation at implant surfaces coated with bioactive molecules

survival rates even in clinical cases with low bone quantity [32]. However, peri-implant infections adjacent to the biofilm exposed implant surface were also reported [33] and abandoned the surface coating.

Coating of medical implants with calcium phosphates (CaP) including hydroxyapatite (HA) has been done for several decades to increase the biocompatibility of the implant and enhance peri-implant bone formation [15]. Originally, the HA coatings were plasma sprayed by high temperature at the implant surface, resulting in a very thick and rough coating. In clinical reality adhesion failure and cracking were reported on the thick HA coatings [34] and in dentistry also peri-implantitis. By using new physical deposition and wet-chemical techniques, very thin CaP coatings <100 nm have been developed, and the requirements to HA coatings have been described in details [14]. Numerous studies have been performed with CaP nanocoatings, and most in vitro experiments have shown an enhanced osteoblast-like cell adhesion, proliferation, and differentiation indicating an accelerated and increased bone formation [14]. CaP coatings have frequently been used as carrier for organic molecules. Various bioactive molecules that promote bone regeneration in vitro have been incorporated into CaP coatings [14]. The adhesion of bioactive molecules or drugs at implant surfaces may modulate integrin binding and subsequent cellular response (Fig. 11.2). Thus, several examples of proteins, e.g., BMP-2, albumin, and amelogenin, incorporated into the latticework of CaP have been described, and CaP implants have been immersed into solutions with antimicrobial agents [35]. Although exciting theories for osteoconduction of CaP nanocoatings have been described and a vast number of promising in vitro and animal studies exist, the exact mechanism behind the biological response of CaP coatings is still unclear. It has also been reported that CaP nanocoating does not favor in vitro osteogenesis [36], and a recent well-controlled in vivo study in dogs could not either confirm that CaP nanocoatings improve early bone integration [37].

An attractive issue is cosubstitution of CaPs with metal ions, which are present as trace elements in bone. Several ions such as fluoride, strontium, zinc, silver, and even nanoparticle diamond [12] have exerted stimulatory effects on osteoblast-like cell activities in vitro both as additive to CaPs and as solely nanocoatings [14]. From a clinical point of view, it is interesting that an antibacterial effect of several metals, e.g., zinc and silver ions, has been reported [14]. However, no in vivo studies have until now examined the impact of the antibacterial effect on implant outcome.

Fluoride has been analyzed in several in vitro and in vivo studies described in a former chapter of this book, and the research has been translated to a dental implant system with success, although no randomized controlled trials (RCT) have demonstrated better outcome with fluoride-coated implant than other titanium implants [38]. The studies comparing fluoride-coated implants with non-fluoride-coated implants suffer from the fact that the surface topography of the test and control implants was unequal. Thus, the positive influence reported on fluoride-coated surfaces may be more related to the changed surface topography than the chemical effect of the fluoride.

Organic Coatings

Proteins mainly represent organic nanocoatings, but also glycoproteins and polysaccharides have obtained increased attention as bioactive molecules. Surface modifications with carbohydrates are easy to obtain and inexpensive and can be tailored with many compositions and structures. Osteoblasts with integrins recognize and adhere directly or indirectly through adhesive proteins to surfaces coated with polysaccharides, and a number of studies have indicated that different polysaccharides especially pectins are able to increase the hydrophilicity of surfaces and enhance the mineralized matrix formation of osteoblastic cells [6]. In vivo studies confirming the in vitro reports are, however, still not published, and although pectins have a number of advantages as nanocoatings compared to proteins, e.g., persist at the surface for longer time, with antibacterial effect, and much cheaper, the ideal tailored polysaccharide for bone implants still remains to be developed.

The potential of bone proteins as biomimetic agents have been well documented in cell cultures and animal models. Bone morphogenic proteins (BMPs) have shown significant enhancement of osseointegration [23], but especially the high cost of BMPs and the release profiles have limited their clinical use. Fibronectin, laminin, osteopontin, bone sialoprotein, elastin, and collagen as well as RGD peptides are other proteins used for biochemical modification of dental implant surfaces [6]. The cells are bonded to the proteins through different integrin receptors in the cell membrane (Fig. 11.2). Although studies have demonstrated positive effects of several proteins, a great number of challenges exist – concentration to be used, longevity of the coating, and the serious adverse effects caused by increased cellular activity. The risk of angioma formation following uncontrolled delivery of vascular endothelial growth factor has been described [39]. Adverse effects have to be properly examined before bioactive growth factors and biomimetic agents can be clinically applied.

From an academic point of view, it is also interesting that drugs as bisphosphonates (BPs), strontium ranelate, hormone therapy, and monoclonal antibodies that bind RANKL used in the treatment of osteoporosis and other bone diseases will cause increased bone density and mineralized bone-to-implant contact [40]. Most medical therapies for osteoporosis primarily inhibit bone resorption and reduce bone remodeling. However, parathyroid hormone has the potential to enhance skeletal microarchitecture [25]. Nevertheless, agents influencing the balance between bone resorption and formation can result in a higher bone density. The antiresorptive agents also illustrate that a high bone density or bone-to-implant contact is not equal to successful clinical outcome as a number of case reports for patient treated with high doses of bisphosphonates have caused osteonecrosis of the jaw after surgical procedures [41].

Relation Between Methods and Clinical Reality

When new implant surface coatings are introduced, a great variety of methods are used to document the efficacy of the coating. Before clinical human studies are initiated, biomechanical, histological, microradiographic, and molecular analyses are performed in controlled studies using coated implants, plates, or disks.

Biomechanical tests are used to evaluate the strength of the attachment between bone and implant surface. Push out and removal torque tests have been used intensively in animal studies to examine shear forces, but also pull out test for measuring tensile forces is a measure for attachment strength [42]. Biomechanical tests are important from a clinical point of view, but are quite coarse and mainly depending on the surface topography at the micrometer level. Thus, when bioactive surface modifications are tested, the surface topography should not be changed at the micrometer scale, as this would imply a risk for misinterpretation of the chemical effect. Studies with nanocoatings have also frequently indicated that the sensitivity of biomechanical tests of nanoscale surface changes is low [43] and other analyses, e.g., molecular analysis, may be more sensitive. On the other hand it can be argued that if standardized biomechanical and histological tests don't show significant benefits of a new surface modification, it has little clinical relevance.

Histological and histomorphometric methods are widely used techniques for grading osseointegration. This is obvious as osseointegration was defined as direct contact between bone and implant surface at the light microscopic level [2]. Although the definition does not state the proportion of bone in contact with the implant surface, the fraction of implant surface length in contact with mineralized bone, called bone-to-implant contact (BIC), is the most frequently used variable in histomorphometric analyses of dental implants. A great variety of histomorphological techniques have been used in animal studies, and very few methods have fulfilled stereological principles resulting in high bias and misinterpretation [44]. Usually one or two 2-dimensional sections are evaluated and wrongly extrapolated to 3D without any knowledge of stereology. When two-four sections are evaluated adjacent to one implant, a great variation in BIC has been registered in-between sections [44]. This intra-implant variation may be greater than the difference between implants in the same animal or even between implants placed in different animals [44]. Furthermore, no studies have yet proven a minimum BIC percentage for successful outcome, and it can be argued that a BIC percentage of 60 % versus 80 % does not have any clinical relevance. It may be that implant surfaces with 60 % BIC will be more successful than surfaces with 80 % BIC. No evidence exists for an optimal BIC or peri-implant bone density, and an early classification of bone quality by Lekholm and Zarb indicated that a too high bone density might have even negative effect on implant success rates [45].

The use of microcomputer tomography (μ-CT) can be a beneficial tool for evaluation of bone morphology and microstructure including BIC as a supplement to histology. The great advantage of μ-CT compared to histology is the three-dimensional evaluation of osseointegration and bone density. However this technique has limitations such as difficulties in obtaining optimal image quality and to discriminate between degrees of mineralization. Micro-CT is an interesting methodology, which still has to be examined for feasibility, reliability, and accuracy. Recently μ-CT has been used for reliability testing of cone-beam computer tomography (CBCT), which is highly clinically relevant [46]. CBCT as diagnostic tool allows objective quantification of bone density and can be very helpful in clinical dentistry, but the usefulness will still be limited because of the ionizing radiation and the costs.

A great number of authors have claimed that a simulated body solution (SBF) is a useful in vitro method in predicting in vivo bone-bonding activity or bioactivity [47]. SBF is a noncellular, protein-free solution with ion concentration almost equal to human blood plasma. The nucleating capacity of an implant coating can be evaluated by immersing it in SBF, and a clear correlation between apatite formation in SBF models and none bioactivity in vivo has been described [47]. On the other hand it has been argued that the precipitation of apatite on a surface will always happen, when SBF are supersaturated towards apatite crystals, because the system is metastable and will only become thermodynamic stable by forming apatite crystals. It is just a matter of time [48]. Thus, there are still discussions on the validity of the SBF method, and it is not a method, which can be used for predicting clinical outcome of an implant's coating, but can be applicable for initial in vitro screening of coatings.

Molecular biological methods have reached increased attention, and numerous in vitro studies have been performed with a high range of biomarkers. Real-time reverse transcription polymerase chain reaction (RT-PCR), enzyme-linked immunosorbent assay (ELISA), and a great number of assays, e.g., dsDNA assay, BCA assay, Wst-1 assay, and Alizarin red S assay, have been applied to study organic nanocoatings. The gene expression assays for RT-PCR are numerous with specie assays for collagen I; alkaline phosphatase; osteocalcin; osteopontin; osteoblast transcription factor (runt-related gen 2); receptor activator for nuclear factor KB ligand; bone morphogenetic proteins 2, 4, and 7; interleukin-1, interleukin-6, and interleukin-10; angiopoietins 1 and 2; and vascular endothelial growth factor as the most frequently used biomarkers describing up- and downregulated expression of genes. Although it has been claimed that some of the biomarkers are more predictive of osseointegration than others [42], the interface biology is so complex that simple correlation and regression analyses have to be interpreted with caution. The molecular analyses require considerable knowledge, and to evaluate osteoblastic differentiation, the cell cultures should be evaluated at different time points, which hamper more time observations of the same sample. Furthermore biochemical assay procedures require many reagents and complex equipment, which indicate not only high costs but also risk of bias.

The theoretical and especially molecular biological backgrounds for the nanocoatings are intriguing, and when molecular biological analyses are used, nanocoatings are usually interpreted to have a positive effect on bone healing and osseointegration. However, this is in contrast to clinical realities, where only few nanocoatings have proven to have a positive effect on bone healing and osseointegration [37, 49].

A great variety of other methods have been used to characterize and evaluate coatings, and new equipment and methods are continuously developed for screening the bone-bonding ability of surface coatings. Recently, a fluorescent primary osteoblast culture system, allowing noninvasive serial observation and quantification of osteoblastic proliferation and differentiation in vitro, was introduced [50]. This is very interesting from an academic point of view, but we have to realize that we cannot translate such bench science conducted in vitro, directly to clinical practice.

Thus, large animal experiments are still the most valid method for predicting outcomes in humans, and in vitro screening studies should still be succeeded by animal experiments before clinical trials are initiated.

Future

Currently used dental implant systems have developed implants with bioactive surfaces fabricated with various techniques, and although most companies claim increased bone apposition to their nanocoated implant surface, strong evidence for improved clinical outcome is missing. The optimal implant surface is yet to be developed, and it can be questioned whether an optimal implant surface exists as clinical situations have different needs [44]. Extensive empirical knowledge about implant coating is published, but the knowledge is still very fragmented, and we do not yet fully understand all biological processes at the interface. We will require further knowledge about interface biology including molecular and cellular processes, and new equipment and analytical tools will help us in acquiring the knowledge necessary for developing optimal properties of the implant surface. The development will continue, and in the future we expect that implant coatings are designed, which can enhance the biological performance of dental implants in compromised bone sites.

References

1. Thomason JM, Heydecke G, Feine JS, Ellis JS. How do patients perceive the benefit of reconstructive dentistry with regard to oral health-related quality of life and patient satisfaction? A systematic review. Clin Oral Implants Res. 2007;18 Suppl 3:168–88.
2. Albrektsson T, Branemark PI, Hansson HA, Lindstrom J. Osseointegrated titanium implants. Requirements for ensuring a long-lasting, direct bone-to-implant anchorage in man. Acta Orthop Scand. 1981;52:155–70.
3. Diz P, Scully C, Sanz M. Dental implants in the medically compromised patient. J Dent. 2013;41: 195–206.
4. Jemt T, Stenport V, Friberg B. Implant treatment with fixed prostheses in the edentulous maxilla. Part 1: implants and biologic response in two patient cohorts restored between 1986 and 1987 and 15 years later. Int J Prosthodont. 2011;24:345–55.
5. Albrektsson T, Sennerby L, Wennerberg A. State of the art of oral implants. Periodontol 2000. 2008;47: 15–26.
6. Gurzawska K, Svava R, Jorgensen NR, Gotfredsen K. Nanocoating of titanium implant surfaces with organic molecules. Polysaccharides including glycosaminoglycans. J Biomed Nanotechnol. 2012;8:1012–24.
7. Subramani K, Jung RE, Molenberg A, Hammerle CH. Biofilm on dental implants: a review of the literature. Int J Oral Maxillofac Implants. 2009;24:616–26.
8. Albouy JP, Abrahamsson I, Persson LG, Berglundh T. Implant surface characteristics influence the outcome of treatment of peri-implantitis: an experimental study in dogs. J Clin Periodontol. 2011;38:58–64.
9. Wennerberg A, Albrektsson T. On implant surfaces: a review of current knowledge and opinions. Int J Oral Maxillofac Implants. 2010;25:63–74.
10. Gotfredsen K. A 10-year prospective study of single tooth implants placed in the anterior maxilla. Clin Implant Dent Relat Res. 2012;14:80–7.
11. Williams. The Williams dictionary of biomaterials. Liverpool: Liverpool University Press; 1999.
12. Lechleitner T, Klauser F, Seppi T, Lechner J, Jennings P, Perco P, et al. The surface properties of nanocrystalline diamond and nanoparticulate diamond powder and their suitability as cell growth support surfaces. Biomaterials. 2008;29:4275–84.
13. Ellingsen JE, Johansson CB, Wennerberg A, Holmen A. Improved retention and bone-to-implant contact with fluoride-modified titanium implants. Int J Oral Maxillofac Implants. 2004;19:659–66.
14. Surmenev RA, Surmeneva MA, Ivanova AA. Significance of calcium phosphate coatings for the enhancement of new bone osteogenesis – a review. Acta Biomate. 2014;10:557–79. doi: 10.1016/j.actbio.2013.10.036.
15. de Groot K, Wolke JG, Jansen JA. Calcium phosphate coatings for medical implants. Proc Inst Mech Eng H. 1998;212:137–47.
16. Ishibe T, Goto T, Kodama T, Miyazaki T, Kobayashi S, Takahashi T. Bone formation on apatite-coated titanium with incorporated BMP-2/heparin in vivo. Oral Surg Oral Med Oral Pathol Oral Radiol Endod. 2009;108:867–75.
17. Buser D, Schenk RK, Steinemann S, Fiorellini JP, Fox CH, Stich H. Influence of surface characteristics on bone integration of titanium implants. A histomorphometric study in miniature pigs. J Biomed Mater Res. 1991;25:889–902.
18. Sverzut AT, Crippa GE, Morra M, de Oliveira PT, Beloti MM, Rosa AL. Effects of type I collagen coating on titanium osseointegration: histomorphometric, cellular and molecular analyses. Biomed Mater. 2012;7:035007.
19. Jimbo R, Sawase T, Shibata Y, Hirata K, Hishikawa Y, Tanaka Y, et al. Enhanced osseointegration by the chemotactic activity of plasma fibronectin for cellular fibronectin positive cells. Biomaterials. 2007;28:3469–77.
20. Bougas K, Jimbo R, Vandeweghe S, Hayashi M, Bryington M, Kozai Y, et al. Bone apposition to laminin-1 coated implants: histologic and 3D evaluation. Int J Oral Maxillofac Surg. 2013;42:677–82.
21. Jensen T, Baas J, Dolathshahi-Pirouz A, Jacobsen T, Singh G, Nygaard JV, et al. Osteopontin functionalization of hydroxyapatite nanoparticles in a PDLLA matrix promotes bone formation. J Biomed Mater Res A. 2011;99:94–101.
22. Chatakun P, Nunez-Toldra R, Diaz Lopez EJ, Gil-Recio C, Martinez-Sarra E, Hernandez-Alfaro F, et al. The effect of five proteins on stem cells used for osteoblast differentiation and proliferation: a current review of the literature. Cell Mol Life Sci. 2014;71:113–42.
23. Wikesjo UM, Huang YH, Xiropaidis AV, Sorensen RG, Rohrer MD, Prasad HS, et al. Bone formation at recombinant human bone morphogenetic protein-2-coated titanium implants in the posterior maxilla (Type IV bone) in non-human primates. J Clin Periodontol. 2008;35:992–1000.
24. Schliephake H, Scharnweber D, Dard M, Sewing A, Aref A, Roessler S. Functionalization of dental

implant surfaces using adhesion molecules. J Biomed Mater Res B Appl Biomater. 2005;73:88–96.
25. Yu X, Wang L, Jiang X, Rowe D, Wei M. Biomimetic CaP coating incorporated with parathyroid hormone improves the osseointegration of titanium implant. J Mater Sci Mater Med. 2012;23:2177–86.
26. Holmberg KV, Abdolhosseini M, Li Y, Chen X, Gorr SU, Aparicio C. Bio-inspired stable antimicrobial peptide coatings for dental applications. Acta Biomater. 2013;9:8224–31.
27. Chua PH, Neoh KG, Kang ET, Wang W. Surface functionalization of titanium with hyaluronic acid/chitosan polyelectrolyte multilayers and RGD for promoting osteoblast functions and inhibiting bacterial adhesion. Biomaterials. 2008;29:1412–21.
28. Stadlinger B, Pilling E, Huhle M, Mai R, Bierbaum S, Scharnweber D, et al. Evaluation of osseointegration of dental implants coated with collagen, chondroitin sulphate and BMP-4: an animal study. Int J Oral Maxillofac Surg. 2008;37:54–9.
29. Abtahi J, Agholme F, Sandberg O, Aspenberg P. Effect of local vs. systemic bisphosphonate delivery on dental implant fixation in a model of osteonecrosis of the jaw. J Dent Res. 2013;92:279–83.
30. Walter MS, Frank MJ, Rubert M, Monjo M, Lyngstadaas SP, Haugen HJ. Simvastatin-activated implant surface promotes osteoblast differentiation in vitro. J Biomater Appl. 2014;28:897–908.
31. Frank MJ, Walter MS, Tiainen H, Rubert M, Monjo M, Lyngstadaas SP, et al. Coating of metal implant materials with strontium. J Mater Sci Mater Med. 2013;24:2537–48.
32. Roccuzzo M, Bunino M, Prioglio F, Bianchi SD. Early loading of sandblasted and acid-etched (SLA) implants: a prospective split-mouth comparative study. Clin Oral Implants Res. 2001;12:572–8.
33. Astrand P, Anzen B, Karlsson U, Sahlholm S, Svardstrom P, Hellem S. Nonsubmerged implants in the treatment of the edentulous upper jaw: a prospective clinical and radiographic study of ITI implants – results after 1 year. Clin Implant Dent Relat Res. 2000;2:166–74.
34. Palmquist A, Omar OM, Esposito M, Lausmaa J, Thomsen P. Titanium oral implants: surface characteristics, interface biology and clinical outcome. J R Soc Interface. 2010;7 Suppl 5:S515–27.
35. Moradian-Oldak J, Wen HB, Schneider GB, Stanford CM. Tissue engineering strategies for the future generation of dental implants. Periodontol 2000. 2006;41:157–76.
36. Moura CC, Souza MA, Dechichi P, Zanetta-Barbosa D, Teixeira CC, Coelho PG. The effect of a nanothickness coating on rough titanium substrate in the osteogenic properties of human bone cells. J Biomed Mater Res A. 2010;94:103–11.
37. Abrahamsson I, Linder E, Larsson L, Berglundh T. Deposition of nanometer scaled calcium-phosphate crystals to implants with a dual acid-etched surface does not improve early tissue integration. Clin Oral Implants Res. 2013;24:57–62.
38. Esposito M, Grusovin MG, Willings M, Coulthard P, Worthington HV. The effectiveness of immediate, early, and conventional loading of dental implants: a Cochrane systematic review of randomized controlled clinical trials. Int J Oral Maxillofac Implants. 2007;22:893–904.
39. Carmeliet P, Jain RK. Angiogenesis in cancer and other diseases. Nature. 2000;407:249–57.
40. Otomo-Corgel J. Osteoporosis and osteopenia: implications for periodontal and implant therapy. Periodontol 2000. 2012;59:111–39.
41. King AE, Umland EM. Osteonecrosis of the jaw in patients receiving intravenous or oral bisphosphonates. Pharmacotherapy. 2008;28:667–77.
42. Monjo M, Ramis JM, Ronold HJ, Taxt-Lamolle SF, Ellingsen JE, Lyngstadaas SP. Correlation between molecular signals and bone bonding to titanium implants. Clin Oral Implants Res. 2013;24:1035–43.
43. Svanborg LM, Andersson M, Wennerberg A. Surface characterization of commercial oral implants on the nanometer level. J Biomed Mater Res B Appl Biomater. 2010;92:462–9.
44. Balatsouka D, Gotfredsen K, Gundersen HJ. Evaluation of bone-to-implant contact and bone density adjacent to titanium implants using a stereological technique on ground sections. Image Anal Stereol. 2006;25:12.
45. Truhlar RS, Farish SE, Scheitler LE, Morris HF, Ochi S. Bone quality and implant design-related outcomes through stage II surgical uncovering of spectra-system root form implants. J Oral Maxillofac Surg. 1997;55:46–54.
46. Gonzalez-Garcia R, Monje F. The reliability of cone-beam computed tomography to assess bone density at dental implant recipient sites: a histomorphometric analysis by micro-CT. Clin Oral Implants Res. 2013;24:871–9.
47. Kokubo T, Takadama H. How useful is SBF in predicting in vivo bone bioactivity? Biomaterials. 2006;27:2907–15.
48. Bohner M, Lemaitre J. Can bioactivity be tested in vitro with SBF solution? Biomaterials. 2009;30:2175–9.
49. Esposito M, Dojcinovic I, Germon L, Levy N, Curno R, Buchini S, et al. Safety and efficacy of a biomimetic monolayer of permanently bound multiphosphonic acid molecules on dental implants: 1 year post-loading results from a pilot quadruple-blinded randomised controlled trial. Eur J Oral Implantol. 2013;6:227–36.
50. Tsukanaka M, Yamamoto K, Fujibayashi S, Pattanayak DK, Matsushita T, Kokubo T, et al. Evaluation of bioactivity of alkali- and heat-treated titanium using fluorescent mouse osteoblasts. J Bone Miner Metab. 2013. [Epub ahead of print].

Orthodontic Implants and Orthodontic Implant Surfaces

12

Anna Westerlund

Abstract

Orthodontic implants as anchorage device has brought new dimensions to orthodontic treatment planning and biomechanics. Treatments that were previously not possible can now be accomplished successfully not only in children and adolescent but also in adults.

The chapter covers evaluated concepts of orthodontic implant: anchorage, origin, nomenclature, and applications. Parameters affecting success rates including patient-related factors, implant-related factors, and factors related to clinical procedures are discussed more in detail. Particular attention has been paid to parameters related to implant materials and implant surface. These parameters have not been fully evaluated since it is claimed that osseointegration is of secondary importance because of the temporary nature of these implants. It could be concluded that in order to develop the concept of orthodontic implants all parameters need to be considered. Orthodontic implants would favor from having their surfaces modified for proper osseointegration. This would increase not only the success rate during favorable conditions but also maintain the success rate when compensating for other parameters being compromised in the clinical situation. Moreover, to be able to optimize on orthodontic implant parameters in general, all independent variables need to be controlled. In most studies so far, there are scatters of variables, making it impossible to draw any evidence-based scientific conclusion.

Background

Orthodontic Anchorage

Anchorage is central in orthodontics and a major concern in treatment planning. Orthodontic anchorage is needed to resist and minimize the movement of certain teeth (the reactive unit)

A. Westerlund, DDS, PhD
Department of Orthodontics, Sahigrenska Academy, University of Gothenburg,
450, Gothenburg 405 30, Sweden
e-mail: anna.westerlund@odontologi.gu.se

A. Wennerberg et al. (eds.), *Implant Surfaces and their Biological and Clinical Impact*,
DOI 10.1007/978-3-662-45379-7_12, © Springer-Verlag Berlin Heidelberg 2015

while carrying out the desired movement of other teeth (the active unit). The basic principle is Newton's third law: for every action there is an equal and opposite reaction. Different intra- and extraoral techniques are used to increase anchorage. Traditional approaches, including extraoral traction (EOT) and lingual arches, have several drawbacks. They are often bulky and ineffective and depend on patient cooperation. Orthodontic implants make it possible to overcome these problems, and in addition they offer possibilities of anchorage where there are few teeth and reduced periodontal support. Furthermore, the potential to perform orthodontic treatments with orthopedic effects that were not previously possible without surgical interventions is also evolving and has gained a lot of attention.

Development of the Concept

In 1945, Gainsforth and Higley proposed the possibility of orthodontic anchorage provided via bone [1]. They used Vitallium screws and stainless steel wires in dog ramus to distalize canines. Although tooth movement was accomplished, an effective force could only be maintained for 1 month due to failure of the implants. Three decades later, Linkow presented the mandibular blade-type implants for orthodontic anchorage [2]. This anchorage was used to attach class II elastics while retracting maxillary incisors in a patient. In the early 1980s, there was an increased interest in using screw-shaped implants as a source of anchorage. Several studies have thoroughly tested the concept in animal models in a variety of applications of tooth movement and transversal palatal expansion [3–5]. Creekmore and Eklund were pioneers in using screw-shaped implants as orthodontic anchorage in patients. They placed Vitallium screws in anterior nasal spine to intrude maxillary incisors to correct a deep bite [6]. In 1984, Roberts and co-workers were among the first to evaluate the effect of orthodontic forces to restorative commercially pure (cp) titanium prosthodontic implants [7]. During this period, Roberts used these implants for various applications including protracting molars in a dog model [8]. Similarly, Linder Aronsson used them to support space closure in a monkey model (1990) [9], and Smalley (1988) used the infrazygomaticus implants to protract the entire maxilla [10]. In 1988, Ödman and co-workers presented case reports regarding treatment of space opening, extrusion, distalization, and pre-prosthodontic tooth movement [11]. Higuchi and co-workers in 1991 retracted and protracted upper and lower teeth using implants in the mandible [12]. These traditional prosthodontic implants offered rigid anchorage; however, these methods prove to have several disadvantages including extended flap surgery and long healing periods. Furthermore, as a result of their size and design, they provide limited possibilities for placement in the inter-radicular areas. In addition, they are difficult to remove.

By the 1990s, tailored implants for orthodontics were being used. In 1995, Block and Hoffman introduced the palate as an anchorage device location with the concept of disc-shaped onplants [13]. These are however not commonly used anymore. In 1996, Wehrbein and co-workers used the palate for the screw-shaped palatal implants [14, 15]. The orthodontic implants have their origin not only from the osseointegrated prosthodontic implants but also from the mechanical retained maxillofacial surgical screws and plating kits. In 1985, Jenner and Fitzpatrick introduced the plate system for orthodontic use [16]. The concept was further developed by Umemory, Sugawara, and co-workers with the skeletal anchorage system (SAS) [17, 18]. In 1997, Kanomi and co-workers introduced the mini-implants or "mini-screws" having a diameter of 1.2 mm [19]. Now more than 50 various brands are known worldwide. Most of the leading orthodontists still classify the orthodontic implants according to their origin, i.e., osseointegrated implants or mechanically retained surgical screws (Fig. 12.1). This classification is however questionable and will be further discussed.

Nomenclature

There is no general agreement on the nomenclature for this type of anchorage device. The names are based either on size (mini and micro), design (screw and plate), site of location (palatal and retromolar), or combinations thereof. Screw-shaped implants especially are named in more as 30 vari-

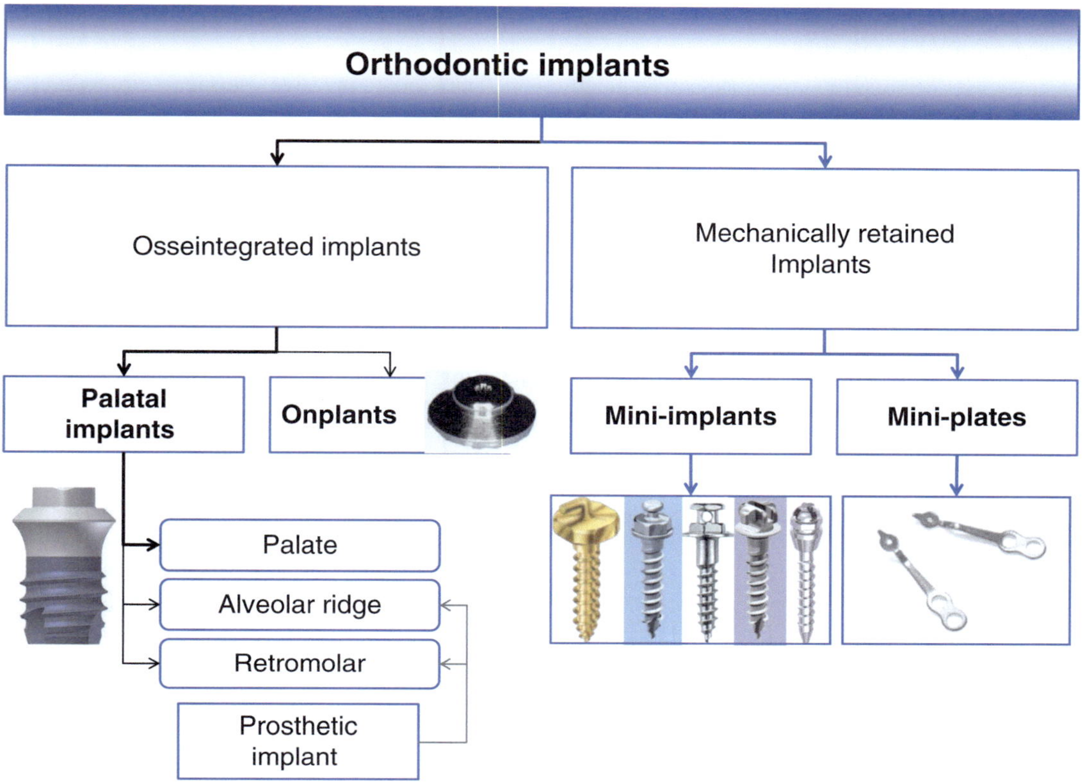

Fig. 12.1 Traditional classification of orthodontic implants (Courtesy T. Lietz)

ations including mini-implant, mini-screw, micro-implant, and micro-screw [20]. The most used term is mini-implant. The term "micro" is not appropriate because the size of the screws is in the range of millimeters. These devices could be referred to as "mini" particularly compared to prosthodontic restorative implants as the diameter usually does not exceed 2 mm. The term "implant" is discussed in the light of different regulatory guidelines regarding classification of medical devices. These differences are important to consider when launching a product. Because the orthodontic implants are removed after use, they are not considered as "implants" according to the general ISO implant body definition (2.150, ISO 1942:2010 Dentistry – vocabulary): "[an implant] . . . . . .primary single component or portion of a dental implant which is intended to remain within the tissues." However, the term orthodontic implant is included in the standard. Moreover, according to the Food and Drug Administration (FDA) in the USA and the European medical device regulatory within EU, an implant is "a device that is placed into a surgically or naturally formed cavity of the human body and is intended to remain there for a period of more than 30 days". Because orthodontic implants always are used more than 30 days, they are according to this definition considered as "implants."

Another frequently and popular term used for the various kinds of orthodontic implants are "temporary anchorage device." This term, however, could be misleading because it is not accurate enough. Traditional anchorage appliances, including EOT and lingual arches, could also be referred to as temporary anchorage devices (TADs). Furthermore, and as discussed earlier temporary means less than 30 days, so the designation as such is not appropriate. Moreover, for nonspecialists, "palatal implants" could be mixed up with mini-implants placed in the palate medially or paramedially. These concerns and the fact that companies and scientists want to launch unique products with unique brand names will most probably make it difficult to agree on nomenclature. However, the suggested correct term for all these devices are orthodontic implants; subsequently, they can be classified according to design (plates, screws, or discs) and position. The nomenclature, however, needs to be further discussed. In this chapter, the most common terms for the orthodontic implants will be used (Fig. 12.1).

- Palatal implant – placed mainly on the anterior palate
- Onplant – placed only on the anterior palate
- Mini-implant – placed inter-radicular in the mandible and maxilla and also in the palate
- Mini-plate – placed on the body of the mandible or maxilla

Applications

The popularity of orthodontic implants, especially the mini-implants, stems from their ease of use with minimally invasive surgery as well as a high level of patient comfort and relatively low treatment costs. During treatment, they are supposed to provide stationary anchorage (i.e., remain rigid and resistant to load and momentum) and be easy to remove. The limited possibilities to find enough bone volume with sufficient cortical thickness and inter-radicular distance on the vestibular side of the jaws have made the palatal side and para-medial an attractive alternative. The mini-implants placed para-medially, however, sometimes require an additional laboratory construction. This step complicates and prolongs the clinical procedure and increases the cost compared to mini-implants on the vestibular site. However, those mini-implants have the advantage over traditional palatal implants in that they do not require healing time before loading and surgical removal. Palatal implants comparable with prosthodontic implants recommends loading after an appropriate healing period. Immediate loading has, however, been demonstrated to be successful [21]. The insertion and removable of palatal implants is more invasive because of their dimension and surface character. Lately however, devices have been presented that allows for removal of the palatal implants by an unscrewing technique making a second invasive surgical intervention unnecessary (Hänggi M, results not yet published).

The most invasive surgical procedure is needed for the mini-plates. Both palatal implants and mini-plates have though demonstrated higher success rates compared to mini-implants. The described three kinds of orthodontic implant types can be used depending on the clinical situation (i.e., orthodontic movement) and on the force required (i.e., direction and magnitude). The system of preference is also a matter of training, experience, and availability. The most commonly used systems today are mini-implants used both inter-radicular on the vestibular site and para-medial in the palate.

All three orthodontic implant types can be used for direct anchorage and indirect anchorage. Direct anchorage means pull or push directly to the active unit tooth or teeth to be moved, whereas indirect means that the reactive a group of teeth that are pushed or pulled against are supported and stabilized. Indications could be movements of teeth such as distalization, mesialization, intrusion and extrusion of tooth segments for space closure, uprighting of molars, impacted teeth, transversal expansions of palates, and protraction and retraction of the entire maxilla and mandible (Fig. 12.2).

Stability

Success and Failure Rate

The literature has presented results of the success/failure rates (ranging from 0 to 100 %) of orthodontic implants. The variation in success rate depends on many factors including type of orthodontic implant, study design, evaluation time, and criteria for success and failure. These variations also make it hard to compare results from different studies. In individual studies, a success rate of >80 % is the most frequently reported [22–31]. There are four systematic reviews [32–35] and two meta-analyses [36, 37] published on success failure of orthodontic implants so far, where one considers experimentally in vivo studies [33]. Reynders and co-workers and Chen and co-workers in their systematic reviews from 2009 presented a

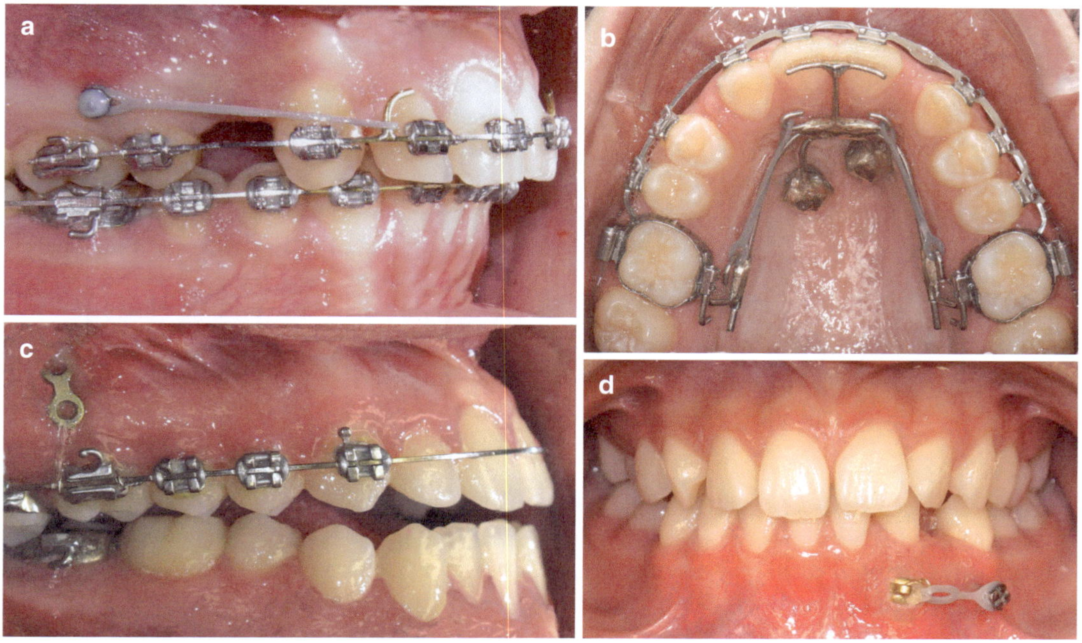

Fig. 12.2 Example of clinical applications. (**a**) Overbite reduction by distalization using mini-implant anchorage (Courtesy A. Ödman). (**b**) Space closure in a case with lateral agenesis using mini-implant anchorage. (**c**) Intrusion in an open bite using mini-plate anchorage (Courtesy M. Möller). (**d**) Extrusion of impacted canine using mini-implant anchorage

success rate for mini-implants being between 0 and 100 %; however, most rates were above 80 % [35] and between 85 and 100 % [32]. In a systematic review and meta-analysis from the same year, Schätzle and co-workers evaluated failure rates for different orthodontic implant types and presented a double failure rate for mini-implants compared to mini-plates and palatal implants according to the following figures: onplants, 17.2 % (95 % CI: 5.9–35.8 %); palatal implants, 10.5 % (95 % CI: 6.1–18.1 %); mini-implants, 16.4 % (95 % CI: 13.4–20.1 %); and mini-plates, 7.3 % (95 % CI: 5.4–9.9 %) [37]. In a more recent systematic review (2012), Tsui and co-workers also identified success rates: for mini-plates, 91.4–100 %; for palatal implants, 74–93.3 %; for mini-screws, 61–100 %; and for prosthodontic implants, 100 % [34]. In a meta-analysis from 2012, a mini-implant failure rate was found to be 13.5 % (95 % CI: 11.5–15.8) [36]. It could be concluded from the results presented here that orthodontic implants present a higher failure rate compared to prosthodontic implants. The almost 100 % success rate for the prosthodontic implants additionally represents a follow-up period over years, while orthodontic implants operate between 6 and 24 months. The consequence from a failed orthodontic implant, although not as harmful as loss of a prosthodontic tooth, could deteriorate the treatment totally and is inconvenient for both patient and clinician.

Primary and Secondary Stability

The overall stability of an implant depends initially on primary stability and later on secondary stability. Primary stability is the mechanical retention in the bone due to displacement and compression of surrounding tissue, and secondary stability is obtained by osseointegration [38]. A study regarding bone healing presented a critical period around the second to third week when the primary mechanical stability is replaced by the secondary biological stability (i.e., when inflammation and osteoclastic

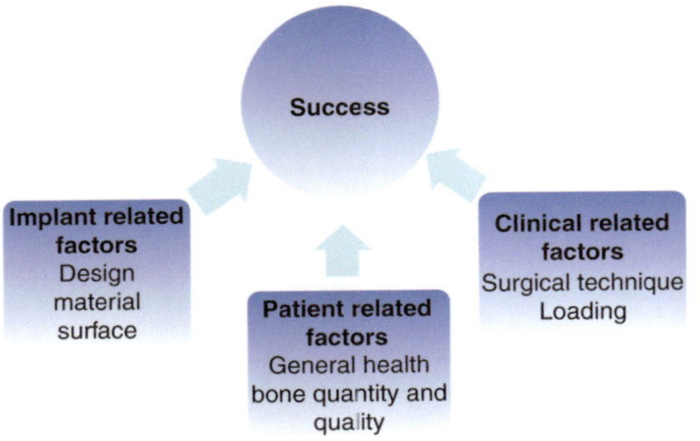

Fig. 12.3 Parameters of importance for orthodontic implant success

activity decreases, primary stability and new bone have not yet been formed) [39]. Insertion torque, an indicator of rotational resistance, and resonance frequency analysis (RFA) are the most often used evaluation methods to characterize primary stability, whereas removal torque, pullout tests, resonance frequency analysis, and histomorphometry are used to evaluate secondary stability.

A systematic review demonstrated that there is no evidence that associates specific maximum insertion torque levels with higher success rates [40]. This seems reasonable since primary stability alone is not responsible for the long-term success; it is only a prerequisite. This finding is supported in a systematic review that demonstrated that not only proper primary stability but also quality and quantity of loading is of importance [32, 41]. Many parameters are important for stability and success, and it is immensely tested and discussed in the scientific literature. In 1980, Albrektsson and co-workers suggested six factors as prerequisites for osseointegration related to the prosthodontic implants: (1) implant material, (2) implant design, (3) implant finish, (4) status of the bone, (5) surgical technique, and (6) implant loading conditions [42]. These factors could be categorized into three groups and be applied to orthodontic implant conditions: (A) factors related to the patient, (B) factors related to the clinical procedures, and (C) factors related to the implant (Fig. 12.3).

Patient-Related Factors

General and Local Health Status

Most important are factors that affect the bone and soft tissues surrounding the implant.

Bone quality and quantity are key factors in creating good primary stability, a precondition for implant success. Numerous studies demonstrate that bone with high density and more cortical bone present better primary stability. These results are supported by in vitro mathematical simulation, in vivo histomorphometrical evaluation, and clinical evaluation using micro-CT and CBCT [43–46]. Factors that affect bone quality and bone quantity include age, gender, location, and health. In some studies, young children have been identified as risk patients with higher probability of failure because they display less bone (i.e., both smaller volume and more immature and less mineralized bone) [47–49]. Moreover, when placing the implants palatally, the midpalatal suture is not ideal for implant insertion because of inadequate mineralization of the interposing connective tissue and the fact that areas of growth do not need to be distressed [50, 51]. However, in a recent meta-analysis, both age and gender have been demonstrated to be of no importance for implant success [36]. Although in vivo studies in general demonstrate higher primary stability for implants in the mandible compared to the maxilla due to more available cortical bone [52, 53], clinically implants in the maxilla have a presented higher success rate than the mandible over time [25, 30, 36, 47]. This differs though from the restorative implants. It might be explained by the increased osteogenic capacity in the maxilla due to the more reactive trabecular bone with better blood supply [38]. Greater stresses created at insertion in denser bone need to be considered as it might affect the success negatively over time [54]. The actual locations within the jaws are important [36], and there are several studies with guidelines of where to install implants optimally in the palatal [55–58] and vestibular [59–63] aspects of the jaws to receive stability and to avoid sinus perforations and root damages (Fig. 12.4). It has been recommended

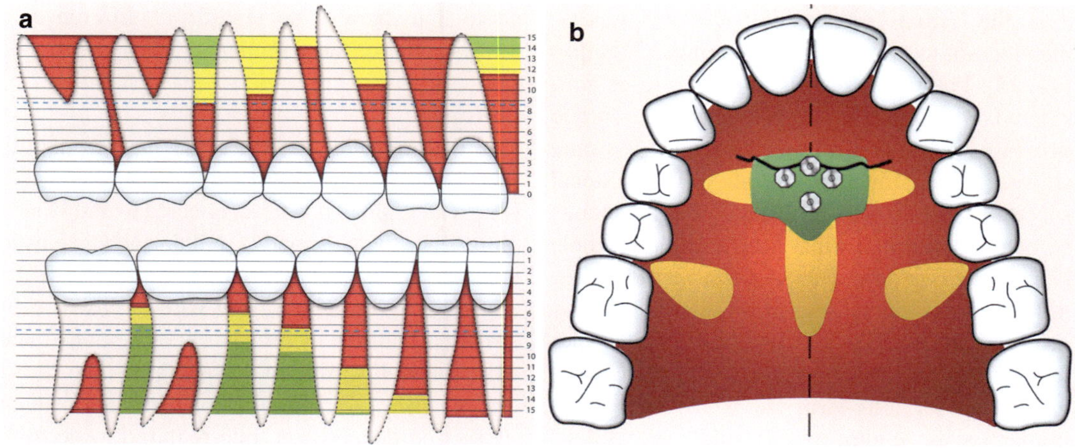

Fig. 12.4 (**a**) Green areas represent recommended places in the vestibular area to place mini-implants (Courtesy B. Ludwig). (**b**) Green areas represent recommended places in the palatal area (third palatal rugae) to place mini-implants (Courtesy B. Ludwig)

that at least 0.5–2 mm of bone should surround the mini-implant to avoid iatrogenic injury to the root and because close root approximates increase risk of failure [54, 64]. Anchorage from orthodontic implants is of interest not only for the treatment of children and adolescences but also for adults, e.g., as pre-prosthodontic treatment. Bone quality and bone quantity are compromised when a patient becomes old, but could also be a result of diseases or medications. Uncontrolled diabetes and smoking are significant relative contraindications for orthodontic implants as healing following surgical procedures is delayed due to impaired peripheral blood circulation [65]. Medications such as corticosteroids and long-term use of systemic bisphosphonates used for treatment of osteoporosis and certain forms of breast cancer may compromise healing [66].

The recommendations regarding soft tissue placement is to stay within the attached gingiva and out of the nonkeratinized mucosa facial [67] and in the palate when deviating from the midpalatal region not too far posteriorly [68]. Poor oral hygiene and inflammation of the tissue around the implants have been presented as a parameter for failure [30]; however, no specific pathogen has been associated with failure [69].

Factors Related to the Clinical Procedures

Surgical Technique

The basis for success is proper surgical technique (i.e., minimal damage during surgical installation, irrigation to prevent overheating, preservation of the periosteal tissue, and sterile working procedures). The "surgeon's experience" has been demonstrated to be a cornerstone for implant success [70] where stable installation without substantial wobbling is required [71]. All mini-implants are self-taping; as they turn, they create their own threads. Some of the mini-implants are additionally provided with a sharp cutting tip giving them the potential to be self-drilling. Usually, a self-drilling implant requires no predrilling. However, compared to non-self-drilling implants, experimental self-drilling implants can cause greater bone damage such as pressure necrosis and crack/ruptures in the bone [72]. To avoid these problems, predrilling has been recommended for implants with a larger diameter (≥1.8 mm) and additionally when the cortex is thicker than 2 mm. Predrilling decreases stresses in the bone and prevents fractures of the mini-implant [73–75]. When predrilling is needed, burs with diameters around 0.4–0.6 mm smaller than the actual implant diameter are recommended not to compromise the primary stability [44, 75]. Predrilling depths also have to be considered because maximal insertion torque decreases with predrilling depths [76]. Some studies demonstrate an overall higher clinical success rate with self-drilling mini-implants compared to implants that need a predrilled hole [77]. In vivo experiments confirm that drill-free mini-implants increases primary stability by insertion torque [78] and BIC values [79]. In a recent meta-analysis, however, the importance of predrilling for long-term survival of the mini-implants seemed to be of no significance [36].

The implants can be inserted either manually or with a mechanically (handpiece). Some clinicians prefer to place implants manually because of the tactile feedback such an approach provides; others believe that using a handpiece decreases the possibility of wobbling. Motor-driven insertion also guarantees a constant insertion speed. Because of the potential of the titanium-based implants to osseointegrate, battery-operated driver units with set torque limitation in both insertion and reverse mode have been suggested. Placement torques between 5 and 10 Ncm have been reported to be favorable [80]. However, precaution with battery-operated driver units with torque limitation devices is needed since the accuracy differs between the devices [81]. With respect to insertion depths and implant tightening, low values are insufficient for establishing primary stability as high values could generate excessive high stress and degeneration of interfacial bone and so-called relaxation. In addition, overtightening gives rise to enhanced microstructural damage of the bone [82]. The implant requires at least 1 mm of cortical thickness to avoid failure [83]. Available cortical bone thickness is often not more than 1 mm, so a change in the insertion angle has been suggested and results demonstrate an increase stability by means of bone-to-implant contact [84, 85] and insertion torque and pullout values [86]. A proper angulation might also prevent root damage and failures related to root contact [87]. If the mini-implant fails, there is a possibility to reinstall the implants, and results presented demonstrate that there is no significant difference in success rate for these implants [28].

Loading

The literature demonstrates that proper quality and quantity of loading is important for success [32]. The implant head is connected to and loaded either directly to the active unit through an elastic coil, chain, or springs unit or indirectly to the reactive unit through a rigid wire or casted construction. Indirect loading has been demonstrated experimentally to be more favorable than direct loading [88]. The duration of force application varies and depends on time required to perform the desired tooth movements. Studies present duration of loading time ranging from 3 to 37 months [35]. This survival rate might depend on whether or not the implants have had the possibility to osseointegrate as osseointegrated implants have higher potential to withstand load over time. The force magnitude is also important, and an increased load presents an increased risk of displacement and failure [89]. When the load is within physiologic limits (50–200 g), no correlation exists between the magnitude of force and effect on periodontal parameters [90]. Some studies demonstrated that the direction of the force (CV, CCV) is important [91], but others claim the force direction is not significant [92]. Furthermore, intermittent forces seem to do better than continuous forces in vivo [93].

Immediate loading is a topic of great interest. According to the Cochrane Review Group, early loading is defined as the initiation of implant loading between 1 week and 2 months after surgical insertion, whereas immediate loading is initiated within 1 week after surgical insertion. Others define immediate loading within 48 h or direct after implant placement. Over the last few decades, the proposed healing time before loading has been gradually decreased, but there are groups that still advocate a healing period of up to 3 months [68, 94, 95]. The perquisite for immediate loading is good primary stability. In 2007, a systematic review presented loading in experimental studies. At the time, only two studies were included that loaded the implants immediately. The success rate was higher for the implants that received a healing period compared to immediately loaded implants [33]. Since then, several experimental studies on immediate and early loading demonstrate no negative effect on the bone-healing pattern [53, 96–104]. Ohashi and co-workers in 2006 performed a systematic review on loading protocols for prosthodontic and palatal implants and mini-implants [105]. For the mini-implants, the healing time varied between 2 and 12 months (average of 4–6 months), and the mini-implants were loaded immediately or after 2 weeks. The prosthodontic implants were 100% successful, while the mini-implants demonstrated a failure rate of approximately 10–15 %. In a meta-analysis from 2012, no significant differences of the failure rates of mini-implants could be observed concerning the time of orthodontic force application (i.e., immediate loading (up to 2 weeks) or late loading (later than 2 weeks)) [36].

Although some studies claim increased osseointegration, no study so far has presented convincing evidence of increased early bone healing stimulated by load. This should not to be mixed with adaption mechanisms to physiological loading during remodeling [106, 107]. Parallels could be drawn to fracture healing where the role of mechanical stimuli and strain during the initial callus formation remains unclear. Experimental data has shown that maximal possible rigidity at the fracture site is advantageous until a mineralized callus is formed. After a mineralized callus is formed and the remodeling phase has started, mechanical strains could influence the remodeling and modeling phases of bone healing. The link between mechanical input and remodeling process is historically known as Wolff's law of bone. Why is it then that immediately loaded orthodontic implants demonstrate similar response as implants with delayed healing? Implant healing is sensitive to micromotion, and motion of less than 100 μm can cause tissue capsulation and failure. Because micromovement might be more harmful than load during the early phase [108], immediate and early loading techniques with light initial force can be applied at an early stage. Loading with a light force may not stimulate early healing, but it could prevent hazardous micromovements of surrounding tissues. This strategy could be compared with the specific guidelines for direct loaded prosthodontic implants that recommend initial splinting until osseointegration occurs to prevent micromotions and failure of immediately loaded implants [109]. Furthermore, it is recommended that if it is possible to have more than one implant in a unit.

Implant-Related Factors

Design (Dimensions and Form)

The lengths of mini-implants vary considerably, and manufacturers offer implant lengths from 4 to 15 mm. In vivo mechanical tests have demonstrated that longer mini-implants provide better primary stability [43, 110]. A too long mini-implant, however, may cause iatrogenic damage including root injury and sinus perforation [43]. Furthermore, increasing lengths decreases mechanical strength [111]. A longer mini-implant must be compensated by a greater diameter to withstand the equivalent mechanical requirements especially during insertion. An oblique insertion angle could be used to enhance contact between implant and cortical plate [84, 85]. Optimal lengths of the implant has been suggested to be approximately 8 mm, and lengths between 6–10 mm are the most commonly used lengths [112]. The length of the implant needs to be determined considering the bone available and the transmucosal thickness, screw angulation, and adjacent vital structures. Moreover, the part of the orthodontic and mini-implants inside the bone should be equal or longer as the part out of the bone.

The mini-implant diameter normally varies between 1.2 and 2.3 mm and is larger for palatal implants. Which diameter to choose is a compromise between the inter-radicular space available and mechanical strengths of the mini-implant. An implant with a smaller diameter (<1.5 mm) may bend or cause breakage of the implants [113]. A larger diameter (>1.7 mm) offers good mechanical stability, but there is not enough space between the roots. As reported before, studies recommend a large variation in the amount of bone required around an implant from 0.5 to

2 mm to be safe and stable [114]. For example, a mini- implant with a diameter of 1.6 mm requires as minimum a root distance from 2.6 mm over the whole length. This limits the potential places for inter-radicular placement to a small number [63]. Root contact during insertion can increase the failure rates compared with mini-screw implants without contact [29, 36, 115, 116]. Tooth position and mini-implant position changes during treatment also need to be considered. Although the mini-implants have proven to be perfectly stable, they are not perfectly stationary if loaded. Studies demonstrate displacement even with light forces [102, 103, 114, 117, 118]. A recent meta-analysis though demonstrated a displacement of 2.3 mm less than for conventional anchorage [119]. Implants smaller than 1.5 mm should be avoided because of the fracture risk especially in the thick cortical bone of the mandible [113, 120]. One study demonstrated that all mini-implants with a diameter less than 1 mm were lost prematurely [27]. This could be explained by the fact that the force required to remove the implant (removal torque) is directly proportional to the square of the implant diameter [79]. However, a larger diameter results in greater micro-damage [121]. Optimal diameters have been suggested to be 1.5–1.7; in vivo studies have demonstrated an increased insertion torque and primary stability with larger mini-implant diameters [45, 110, 121–123]. Some clinical studies demonstrate correlation between success rate and larger mini-implant diameter [25–27, 47], while others do not [29–31]. In a recent meta-analysis, both lengths and diameters have been demonstrated to be of no importance for mini-implant success [36].

Orthodontic implants are either a tapered/conical or a cylindrical shape. Tapered/conical implants have presented higher insertion torque than cylindrical implants [123, 124], and vice versa when tested by means of pull out tests [78, 122, 125]. With an increasing angle of insertion, pullout tests fail to demonstrate differences between the two designs [78]. Similar results have been demonstrated if predrilling is used in conjunction with the tapered implants [76]. Conical implants have a smaller diameter at the apex, which is beneficial in small inter-radicular spaces as they minimize root contact. Although from mechanical aspects, a thinner screw is a disadvantage. Cylindrical implants offer a more even stress distribution, and this helps prevent fracture during placement and removal.

The thread on the implant is the helical ridge, wrapped around the cylinder. The thread varies in design with respect to pitch, flute, and the angle of thread. Flutes are recessed areas in the screw's cross-sectional area, and pitch is the distance between the threads and angle and the angle of the threads in relation to the long axis. Increasing the dimensions of thread depths and decreasing thread pitch and flute will enhance primary stability in compromised bone; however, increased flutes and deeper threads create higher stresses and increased fracture risk [122, 126, 127]. A symmetric thread form has been proven to be better than an asymmetric thread form [120]. There are five head designs: hook, ball, hole, simple slot, and cross-slot and combinations (Fig. 12.1).

Conclusion Studies give contradictory results on optimal patient-related factors, clinical procedures, and implant design. In most studies, there are scatters of parameters evaluated at the same time, making it impossible to draw any evidence-based scientific conclusion. Studies need to be designed to provide proper information on independent variables. It might be that the relative importance of a single parameter is of no significance clinically; however, to determine this and to optimize implant design and clinical procedures, all other parameters need to be controlled. If all parameters are optimized independently, the synergetic effect might contribute to an increased clinical success rate.

Material

The first screws and wires used for the purpose of orthodontic anchorage were made of Vitallium and stainless steel [1]. They failed within 1 month and thereafter not much was presented regarding orthodontic bone anchors until three decades later. The first implant made of titanium used for orthodontic anchorage was the mandibular blade implants introduced by Linkow in the early 1970s. This treatment modality, however, never became a widespread treatment modality. Well into the 1980s, and after the invention of titanium, Vitallium implants were still used [3, 6]. Other materials presented were aluminum oxide implants [5] and vitreous carbon dental implants [4]. Also biodegradable materials including biodegradable polylactide acid have been anecdotally tested [128]. In the 1980s, Roberts and co-workers were among the first to use the prosthodontic restorative screw-shaped cp titanium implants [7]. Implants tailored for orthodontics use were made of either cp titanium or stainless steel when they were launched in the 1990s. Most implants today are made from titanium alloys because of its superior mechanical properties compared to cp titanium. Analysis of cp titanium has revealed that removal torque values were dangerously approaching yield stress values because of the small diameter used for mini-implants [129]. Today only one company markets mini-implants made of stainless steel.

The actual osseointegration of the mini-implants is controversial. Most researchers and clinicians categorize mini-implants as being "non-osseointegrated" devices that mainly rely on the mechanical interlocking established at installation (i.e., the primary stability) [130–133]. For mini-implants made of titanium alloy, these statements are questionable because titanium and titanium alloy implants by nature osseointegrate for some months during favorable conditions because of their biocompatibility properties, which have been known for several decades. This well-known fact dates back to the 1950s when Brånemark and co-workers by coincidence discovered that the titanium chambers used for studies of blood circulation in rabbits became permanently incorporated in the bone [134]. The concept of osseointegration was first described by Brånemark and co-workers [135] and originally defined with respect to histological criteria [42]. This definition was criticized for not defining the level of resolution and the amount of bone required to be in contact with the implant. A more recent definition is of a more clinical viewpoint and includes the biomechanical aspects of the implant: "A process whereby clinically asymptomatic rigid fixation of alloplastic materials is achieved, and maintained, in bone during functional loading" [136]. Before these findings, the idea was that only ceramic not metal could be in close contact with the bone and that capsule of connective tissue was developed around all metal implants placed in the body. Thereby the material used in the implant regulated the actual thickness of the capsule and the closeness of the bone to the implant. The material would thereby determine the amount of bone in contact with the implant and stability when the other parameters were controlled [137, 138].

There has been discussion regarding whether metals other than titanium – including Vitallium, tantalum, and stainless steel could osseointegrate. However, titanium differs from these metals by expressing a layer of oxide on its surface. This 100-Å-thick layer of oxide that forms on the surface in contact with air, mimicking ceramics, prevents the metal compounds from directly contacting the bone. Many studies of mini-implants also demonstrate osseointegration [102, 104, 139–141], whereas studies on Vitallium implants appeared to be completely enveloped by a capsule of fibrous connective tissue that varied in thickness [3]. A connective tissue capsule surrounding other implantable materials such as stainless steel does not rule out a functioning implant for limited periods. Bone-to-implant contact values (BIC), representing the magnitude of osseointegration, have been presented as low as 2 and 5 % with the implant still being stable [53, 97]. In addition, implants in dead avascular bone can withstand a load for long periods. Orthodontic stainless steel implants have demonstrated similar success, and bone contact in vivo as titanium alloy mini-implants after a short follow-up [142]. In vitro analysis of these implants suggests that some cells, the osteoblasts, are affected, while others, the fibroblasts, are not [143]. Furthermore, the detected concentrations of ions released have not reached toxic levels in in vivo experiments [129]. It could, however, be concluded that a fibrous capsule is more often expressed when using other materials than cp titanium because they are less corrosion resistant [144]. This results in an increased risk of inadequate long-term resistance of the peri-implant tissues due to mechanical, chemical, and microbial trauma.

The optimal scenario for implants is osseointegration that withstands orthodontic load and at the same time can be removed at the end of treatment with minimal trauma. Some studies claim that the osseointegration is a disadvantage and undesirable because of the risk of not being able to remove it after use [132–145]. Other studies, however, have demonstrated that even surface-modified cp titanium [141] and titanium alloy implants with bone-to-implant contact (BIC) of 75 % [139] could be removed safely. Some studies discuss this possibility to remove the implant as being due to partial osseointegration [139]. The term "partial" osseointegration is confusing and could be questioned since the implants at time of evaluation were functionally stable and demonstrated high values of bone-to-implant contact. Not even successful long-term prosthodontic implants present a 100 % BIC but rather a mean BIC around 75 % with a little higher values for the mandible than the maxilla [146]. "Full" osseointegration is probably disrupted and turned "no" osseointegration by the overload situation created when a force is applied to remove the implant. Secondary failure of osseointegration has been demonstrated due to overload [42]. The simplicity of removing the mini-implants is probably due to the small diameter. Studies have demonstrated that the stability, measured by means of removal torque values, is inversely correlated to the diameter of the implant [147].

Conclusion If orthodontic implants are made of titanium and titanium alloy, they have the potential to osseointegrate during favorable conditions. Osseointegration is advantageous for orthodontic implant stability and success rate, and it has though been demonstrated that they can be unscrewed without risks.

Implant Surface

The first Brånemark titanium implants launched had a turned comparatively smooth surface. However, since osseointegration depends on biomechanical bonding (i.e., ingrowth of bone into small irregularities of the implant), the topography and especially the roughness of the implants were areas of interest and the subject of numerous studies. Guidelines have been presented regarding how to perform and present parameters of topography in a standardized way to allow for comparisons [148]. Based on experimental evidence from the mid-1990s, a surface roughness of about 1.5-μm Sa (the average deviation in height from a mean plane) and Sdr (surface enlargement due to surface topography as compared with a flat reference area) of 50 % was defined as optimal for osseointegration [149]. This was rougher than the original: the turned Brånemark implant has a surface roughness (Sa) of about 0.9 μm and Sdr of 35 %. Surface orientation has been demonstrated to be of secondary importance for implant-bone integration compared to roughness [150]. A modified surface roughness results in altered protein absorption and subsequent inflammatory process cellular responses in vitro [151, 152]. There are several methods by which the titanium surface roughness can be modified to increase the surface area: physical (blasting), chemical (acid and alkali etching and electrochemical – electropolishing anodizing), deposition (plasma-spraying and solgel), and biochemical methods (proteins and other biomolecules) (Fig. 12.5). However, modifying the surface roughness will affect not only the topography but also the physical mechanical and chemical properties. Efforts have been made to modify the chemical composition to add a biochemical bonding to the biomechanical bonding. The theoretical benefit of a chemical bond would be earlier attachment because it is hypothesized to occur more rapidly than bony ingrowth. Materials that have the capacity to bond to living tissue are defined as "bioactive," and Hench and co-workers in the 1970s described the first bioactive material, bio-glass [153]. Jarcho and co-workers were the first to present indications of a possible direct bone bonding to hydroxyapatite (HA) [154]. The mechanism suggested was ion exchange resulting in an apatite layer that adsorbed proteins that serve as growth factors

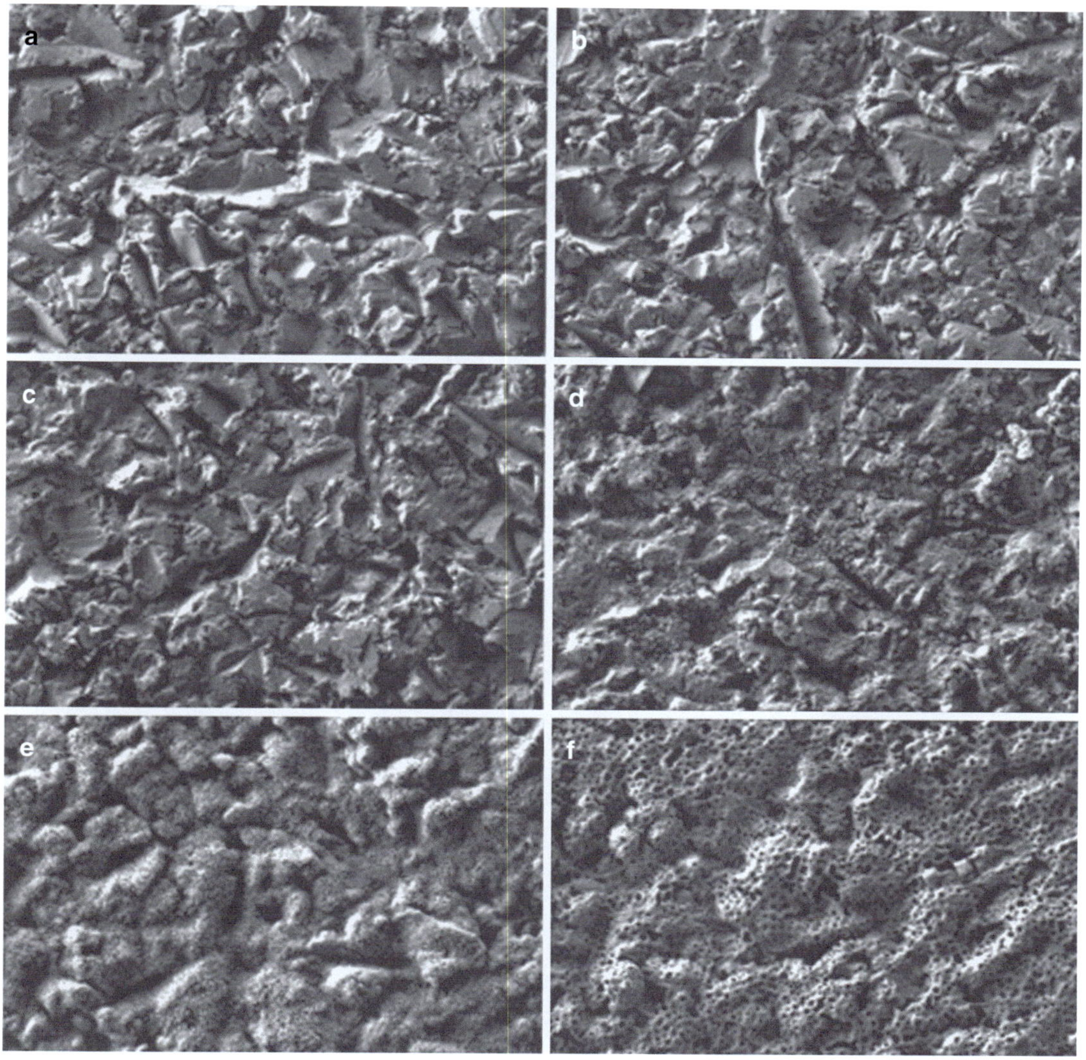

Fig. 12.5 SEM images (×1,000 magnification) demonstrating different surface modifications of titanium implants. (**a**) Blasted control surface. (**b**) Blasted surface treated in simulated body fluids (SBF) for 72 h. (**c**) Nano-hydroxyapatite (HA) surface. (**d**) Fluoride surface. (**e**) Alkali-heat-treated surface. (**f**) Anodized/Mg ion surface

for bone cells. The "bioactive" properties of these materials were based on morphological observations of the tissue coalescence by TEM and apatite formation in vitro and in vivo. However, bioactivity or chemical bonding is difficult to prove, and evidence presented is of an indirect nature. Poor mechanical properties of these materials make them unsuitable for load-bearing, clinical applications. To improve these properties, titanium surfaces were coated with calcium phosphates using the plasma-spraying technique. The surfaces showed rapid tissue response initially, but at later stages biodegradation and delaminating of the thick coating were frequently observed [155]. Additionally, the line-of-sight problem made the technique inappropriate to use for the coating of more complex shapes. To avoid these problems, alternative techniques – ultrathin coatings of calcium phosphates in solgels, etching with fluoride-containing acids, alkali-heat treatment, and anodization – have been used to make cp titanium bioactive [156]. Most commercial prosthodontic implants today have been subjected to either of these treatments in addition to the machining. Another possible approach to enhance the bone response is to immobilize organic biomolecules including proteins and pharmaceuticals [157]. There are, however, problems to overcome, and to date this is mostly on an experimental level. Nanotubes and mesoporous surfaces that produce systems for slow release of substances are state of the art.

Orthodontic Implant Surface

Early Vitallium and aluminum oxide implants were coated with bio-glass. Hench and co-workers at the time tried to create a biochemical bond for enhanced performance. The restorative prosthodontic implants used for orthodontic anchorage in the 1980s had an acid-etched surface [7]; however, these implants were also supposed to support crowns and bridgeworks lifelong.

The first orthodontic palatal implants were modifications similar to these prosthodontic implants, using an etched, and later, sandblasted large-grit and acid-etched surfaces (SLA). In accordance with their prosthodontic counterparts, the palatal implants traditionally use conventional loading protocols requiring a healing period of 3–4 months [15]. As such, the surface modifications were claimed to compensate for the short lengths of these implants. Because trephine burs are needed to remove the implants, materials could be collected for histological evaluations. Implants with only 3 mm of intrabony implant length expressed a BIC of approximately 60–70 % [158].

Other groups have increased the surface roughness of these implants by sintering two or three layers of titanium alloy particles to the surface, creating a porous region to approximately 65 % density and 0.3-mm total thickness. Loading these implants after 6 weeks of healing demonstrated significantly higher marginal bone levels and greater BIC in vivo than did the machined implants, a finding that suggests they would better withstand horizontal forces (i.e., rotational forces) [159] and displacement [160]. Moreover, they created less stress distribution according to finite element analysis [161]. Recently, improvements of surface and design of the palatal implants, resulting in increased BIC rates, have encouraged changes in conventional loading protocols in favor of early and immediate loading concepts. Experimental studies demonstrate that palatal implants show borderline reliability of osseointegration regarding histological findings for immediately loaded palatal implants [162]. A recent clinical study, however, demonstrates that immediately loaded palatal implants yield equivalent success rates as conventional loaded implants after 6 months [163]. This is also supported by histomorphometrically findings [164].

Regarding the orthodontic mini-implants of today, not much has been done to modify the surfaces of the orthodontic implants to improve osseointegration. Only one study could be found that compares surface characteristics regarding topography and chemistry of four commercially available orthodontic implant systems [165]. The implant systems presented smooth surfaces (Sa approximately 0.3 μ). There were statistically significant differences in hybrid (Sdr and Sds) and functional roughness parameters (Sci) although not for amplitude surface roughness parameters (Sa and Sz). This means that the surface area of the threaded part differed for the systems. Chemical analysis of the systems revealed differences in the thickness of the oxide layer, and it was speculated in possible surface modifications.

Although prosthodontic implants are marketed by their surface preparation, it is difficult to get information from most manufacturers about surface modifications on the orthodontic implants. Tailored orthodontic mini-implants are almost exclusively turned and polished without any additional treatment intended to enlarge surface or to modify their chemical composition. There are, however, a few exceptions with companies anodizing the surface. Arguments including the more temporary nature of these implants and the desire to enable removal have been posited. Clinical studies, however, have demonstrated that modified implants (SLA) could be removed without higher risk after use. For safe removal of surface-modified implants, a non-loading period of less than 6 months is recommended before removal [166]. If there are difficulties removing the implant, the patient can be dismissed for a period of 4–7 days after the screw has been manipulated, and then the bone remodeling will facilitate the unscrewing at the second attempt. The systems available on the market demonstrate acceptable survival rate although the success rate presented is lower than for the prosthodontic implants despite differences in expected survival time. Furthermore, considering the desire to load the implant as early as possible and by various forces, these implants would favor from improved surface properties to avoid tipping extrusion and failure. The same surface modification used restorative implants are tested for orthodontic purposes.

Experimentally, immediately loaded, implants prepared with sandblasted acid-etched surface (SAE and SLA) osseointegrate with a higher rate and reveal increased stability (RTQ) compared to machined implants [99]. The twice as high removal torque values for the SAE implants during immediate loading were suggested to give more freedom and would allow more variety in early force vector applications [99]. Furthermore, the SLA implants demonstrate lower insertion torque, lower angular momentum, and higher removal torque energy during removal compared to machined implants (i.e., SLA implants provide better rotational resistance) [167]. Although mini-implants with a SLA-prepared surface demonstrate good clinical stability [140, 168, 169], studies have not demonstrated increased survival rate compared to machined surfaces when loading immediately [170].

Except for SLA implant surfaces, anodic oxidation is a technique used for modifying commercially available implants. Experimentally, studies have been performed with implants prepared by sandblasted large-grit and anodic oxidation that gave an additional calcium and phosphorous reinforcement (SLAO). The results demonstrate improved performance for the SLAO implants compared to SLA and control-machined implants regarding higher removal torque values surface after 8 weeks of healing. In this study, there were no statistical differences in removal torque values between implants prepared with a machined and a SLA surface. As a result, these SLA implants could be used to reduce damage of surrounding bone tissue at insertion and to improve the mechanical stability of the orthodontic implants [171]. Implants with only an anodized surface demonstrate increased mechanical stability, a finding that suggests treatment would enhance their early-phase retention [172]. Clinical studies, however, need to verify this.

In vitro studies confirm the enhanced bone response in vivo to anodized surfaces with higher degree of osseoinduction by means of molecular bone marker PCR compared to machined surfaces. Although the calcium phosphate–reinforced grade 4 implants had a higher level of differentiation, the machined grade 5 implants also supported cell proliferation, matrix synthesis, and induced high expression of early differentiation markers [173].

Conclusion All orthodontic implants would benefit from having their surfaces modified for improved osseointegration. This might not only increase the success rate under favorable conditions but also maintain the success rate when compensating for other parameters being compromised in the clinical situation. This includes reduced bone quantity and quality, short and small diameter implants, and requirements on decreased healing time and immediate loading. It might be that orthodontic implant would favor from other surface modifications than prosthodontic implants; this is due partly to other requirements. Future studies need to explore the optimal surface modification for orthodontic implants.

Acknowledgements Dr. Thomas Lietz's valuable editorial comments.

References

1. Gainsforth BL, Higley LB. A study of orthodontic anchorage possibilities in basal bone. Am J Orthod Oral Surg. 1945;31(8):406–17.
2. Linkow LI. The endosseous blade implant and its use in orthodontics. Int J Orthod. 1969;7(4):149–54. Epub 1969/12/01.
3. Gray JB, Steen ME, King GJ, Clark AE. Studies on the efficacy of implants as orthodontic anchorage. Am J Orthod. 1983;83(4):311–7. Epub 1983/04/01.
4. Sherman AJ. Bone reaction to orthodontic forces on vitreous carbon dental implants. Am J Orthod. 1978;74(1):79–87. Epub 1978/07/01.
5. Turley PK, Shapiro PA, Moffett BC. The loading of bioglass-coated aluminium oxide implants to produce sutural expansion of the maxillary complex in the pigtail monkey (Macaca nemestrina). Arch Oral Biol. 1980;25(7):459–69. Epub 1980/01/01.
6. Creekmore TD, Eklund MK. The possibility of skeletal anchorage. J Clin Orthod. 1983;17(4):266–9. Epub 1983/04/01.
7. Roberts WE, Smith RK, Zilberman Y, Mozsary PG, Smith RS. Osseous adaptation to continuous loading of rigid endosseous implants. Am J Orthod. 1984;86(2):95–111. Epub 1984/08/01.
8. Roberts WE, Helm FR, Marshall KJ, Gongloff RK. Rigid endosseous implants for orthodontic and orthopedic anchorage. Angle Orthod. 1989;59(4):247–56. Epub 1989/01/01.
9. Linder-Aronson S, Nordenram A, Anneroth G. Titanium implant anchorage in orthodontic treatment an experimental investigation in monkeys. Eur J Orthod. 1990;12(4):414–9. Epub 1990/11/01.
10. Smalley WM, Shapiro PA, Hohl TH, Kokich VG, Branemark PI. Osseointegrated titanium implants for maxillofacial protraction in monkeys. Am J Orthod Dentofacial Orthop. 1988;94(4):285–95. Epub 1988/10/01.
11. Odman J, Lekholm U, Jemt T, Branemark PI, Thilander B. Osseointegrated titanium implants – a new approach in orthodontic treatment. Eur J Orthod. 1988;10(2):98–105. Epub 1988/05/01.
12. Higuchi KW, Slack JM. The use of titanium fixtures for intraoral anchorage to facilitate orthodontic tooth movement. Int J Oral Maxillofac Implants. 1991;6(3):338–44. Epub 1991/01/01.
13. Block MS, Hoffman DR. A new device for absolute anchorage for orthodontics. Am J Orthod Dentofacial Orthop. 1995;107(3):251–8. Epub 1995/03/01.
14. Wehrbein H, Glatzmaier J, Mundwiller U, Diedrich P. The Orthosystem–a new implant system for orthodontic anchorage in the palate. J Orofac Orthop. 1996;57(3):142–53. Epub 1996/06/01.
15. Wehrbein H, Merz BR, Diedrich P, Glatzmaier J. The use of palatal implants for orthodontic anchorage. Design and clinical application of the orthosystem. Clin Oral Implants Res. 1996;7(4):410–6.
16. Jenner JD, Fitzpatrick BN. Skeletal anchorage utilising bone plates. Aust Orthod J. 1985;9(2):231–3. Epub 1985/10/01.
17. Sugawara JD. Junji Sugawara on the skeletal anchorage system. Interview by Dr. Larry W. White. J Clin Orthod. 1999;33(12):689–96. Epub 2000/07/15.
18. Umemori M, Sugawara J, Mitani H, Nagasaka H, Kawamura H. Skeletal anchorage system for openbite correction. Am J Orthod Dentofacial Orthop. 1999;115(2):166–74. Epub 1999/02/11.
19. Kanomi R. Mini-implant for orthodontic anchorage. J Clin Orthod. 1997;31(11):763–7. Epub 1998/03/25.
20. Ludwig B, Baumgaertel S, Bowman J. Introduction in mini-implants in orthodontics innovative anchorage concepts. 1st ed. London: Quintessence Publishing Co Ltd; 2008. p. 1–4.
21. Jung BA, Wehrbein H, Hopfenmuller W, Harzer W, Gedrange T, Diedrich P, et al. Early loading of plalatal implants (ortho-type II) a prospective multicenter randomized controlled clinical trial. Trials. 2007;8(20):24. Epub 2007/09/22.
22. Cheng SJ, Tseng IY, Lee JJ, Kok SH. A prospective study of the risk factors associated with failure of mini-implants used for orthodontic anchorage. Int J Oral Maxillofac Implants. 2004;19(1):100–6.
23. Tseng YC, Hsieh CH, Chen CH, Shen YS, Huang IY, Chen CM. The application of mini-implants for orthodontic anchorage. Int J Oral Maxillofac Surg. 2006;35(8):704–7. Epub 2006/05/13.
24. Takaki T, Tamura N, Yamamoto M, Takano N, Shibahara T, Yasumura T, et al. Clinical study of temporary anchorage devices for orthodontic treatment–stability of micro/mini-screws and miniplates: experience with 455 cases. Bull Tokyo Dent Coll. 2010;51(3):151–63. Epub 2010/09/30.
25. Wiechmann D, Meyer U, Buchter A. Success rate of mini- and micro-implants used for orthodontic anchorage: a prospective clinical study. Clin Oral Implants Res. 2007;18(2):263–7. Epub 2007/03/14.
26. Berens A, Wiechmann D, Dempf R. Mini- and microscrews for temporary skeletal anchorage in orthodontic therapy. J Orofac Orthop. 2006;67(6):450–8. Epub 2006/11/25.
27. Miyawaki S, Koyama I, Inoue M, Mishima K, Sugahara T, Takano-Yamamoto T. Factors associated with the stability of titanium screws placed in the posterior region for orthodontic anchorage. Am J Orthod Dentofacial Orthop. 2003;124(4):373–8.
28. Baek SH, Kim BM, Kyung SH, Lim JK, Kim YH. Success rate and risk factors associated with miniimplants reinstalled in the maxilla. Angle Orthod. 2008;78(5):895–901. Epub 2008/02/27.
29. Kuroda S, Sugawara Y, Deguchi T, Kyung HM, Takano-Yamamoto T. Clinical use of miniscrew implants as orthodontic anchorage: success rates and postoperative discomfort. Am J Orthod Dentofacial Orthop. 2007;131(1):9–15. Epub 2007/01/09.
30. Park HS, Jeong SH, Kwon OW. Factors affecting the clinical success of screw implants used as orthodon-

tic anchorage. Am J Orthod Dentofacial Orthop. 2006;130(1):18–25. Epub 2006/07/20.
31. Wu TY, Kuang SH, Wu CH. Factors associated with the stability of mini-implants for orthodontic anchorage: a study of 414 samples in Taiwan. J Oral Maxillofac Surg. 2009;67(8):1595–9. Epub 2009/07/21.
32. Chen Y, Kyung HM, Zhao WT, Yu WJ. Critical factors for the success of orthodontic mini-implants: a systematic review. Am J Orthod Dentofacial Orthop. 2009;135(3):284–91. Epub 2009/03/10.
33. Cornelis MA, Scheffler NR, De Clerck HJ, Tulloch JF, Behets CN. Systematic review of the experimental use of temporary skeletal anchorage devices in orthodontics. Am J Orthod Dentofacial Orthop. 2007;131(4 Suppl):S52–8. Epub 2007/04/24.
34. Tsui WK, Chua HD, Cheung LK. Bone anchor systems for orthodontic application: a systematic review. Int J Oral Maxillofac Surg. 2012;41(11):1427–38. Epub 2012/06/19.
35. Reynders R, Ronchi L, Bipat S. Mini-implants in orthodontics: a systematic review of the literature. Am J Orthod Dentofacial Orthop. 2009;135(5):564 e1–19; discussion 564–5. Epub 2009/05/05.
36. Papageorgiou SN, Zogakis IP, Papadopoulos MA. Failure rates and associated risk factors of orthodontic miniscrew implants: a meta-analysis. Am J Orthod Dentofacial Orthop. 2012;142(5):577–95 e7. Epub 2012/11/03.
37. Schatzle M, Mannchen R, Zwahlen M, Lang NP. Survival and failure rates of orthodontic temporary anchorage devices: a systematic review. Clin Oral Implants Res. 2009;20(12):1351–9. Epub 2009/10/02.
38. Zhang Q, Zhao L, Wu Y, Wang H, Zhao Z, Xu Z, et al. The effect of varying healing times on orthodontic mini-implant stability: a microscopic computerized tomographic and biomechanical analysis. Oral Surg Oral Med Oral Pathol Oral Radiol Endod. 2011;112(4):423–9. Epub 2011/02/12.
39. Raghavendra S, Wood MC, Taylor TD. Early wound healing around endosseous implants: a review of the literature. Int J Oral Maxillofac Implants. 2005;20(3):425–31. Epub 2005/06/25.
40. Meursinge Reynders RA, Ronchi L, Ladu L, van Etten-Jamaludin F, Bipat S. Insertion torque and success of orthodontic mini-implants: a systematic review. Am J Orthod Dentofacial Orthop. 2012;142(5):596–614 e5. Epub 2012/11/03.
41. Ren Y. Mini-implants for direct or indirect orthodontic anchorage. Evid Based Dent. 2009;10(4):113. Epub 2009/12/22.
42. Albrektsson T, Branemark PI, Hansson HA, Lindstrom J. Osseointegrated titanium implants. Requirements for ensuring a long-lasting, direct bone-to-implant anchorage in man. Acta Orthop Scand. 1981;52(2):155–70. Epub 1981/01/01.
43. Lemieux G, Hart A, Cheretakis C, Goodmurphy C, Trexler S, McGary C, et al. Computed tomographic characterization of mini-implant placement pattern and maximum anchorage force in human cadavers. Am J Orthod Dentofacial Orthop. 2011;140(3):356–65. Epub 2011/09/06.
44. Wilmes B, Rademacher C, Olthoff G, Drescher D. Parameters affecting primary stability of orthodontic mini-implants. J Orofac Orthop. 2006;67(3):162–74. Epub 2006/06/01.
45. Holm L, Cunningham SJ, Petrie A, Cousley RR. An in vitro study of factors affecting the primary stability of orthodontic mini-implants. Angle Orthod. 2012;82(6):1022–8. Epub 2012/05/15.
46. Motoyoshi M, Inaba M, Ono A, Ueno S, Shimizu N. The effect of cortical bone thickness on the stability of orthodontic mini-implants and on the stress distribution in surrounding bone. Int J Oral Maxillofac Surg. 2009;38(1):13–8. Epub 2008/10/31.
47. Chen YJ, Chang HH, Huang CY, Hung HC, Lai EH, Yao CC. A retrospective analysis of the failure rate of three different orthodontic skeletal anchorage systems. Clin Oral Implants Res. 2007;18(6):768–75. Epub 2007/09/18.
48. Lee SJ, Ahn SJ, Lee JW, Kim SH, Kim TW. Survival analysis of orthodontic mini-implants. Am J Orthod Dentofacial Orthop. 2010;137(2):194–9. Epub 2010/02/16.
49. Ryu JH, Park JH, Vu Thi Thu T, Bayome M, Kim Y, Kook YA. Palatal bone thickness compared with cone-beam computed tomography in adolescents and adults for mini-implant placement. Am J Orthod Dentofacial Orthop. 2012;142(2):207–12. Epub 2012/08/04.
50. Jayakumar G, Biju T, George MA, Krishnaswamy NR. Quantitative assessment of palatal bone thickness in an ethnic Indian population: a computed tomography study. Indian J Dent Res. 2012;23(1):49–52. Epub 2012/07/31.
51. Asscherickx K, Wehrbein H, Sabzevar MM. Palatal implants in adolescents: a histological evaluation in beagle dogs. Clin Oral Implants Res. 2008;19(7):657–64. Epub 2008/05/22.
52. Luzi C, Verna C, Melsen B. A prospective clinical investigation of the failure rate of immediately loaded mini-implants used for orthodontic anchorage. Prog Orthod. 2007;8(1):192–201. Epub 2007/06/22.
53. Deguchi T, Takano-Yamamoto T, Kanomi R, Hartsfield Jr JK, Roberts WE, Garetto LP. The use of small titanium screws for orthodontic anchorage. J Dent Res. 2003;82(5):377–81. Epub 2003/04/24.
54. Motoyoshi M, Ueno S, Okazaki K, Shimizu N. Bone stress for a mini-implant close to the roots of adjacent teeth–3D finite element analysis. Int J Oral Maxillofac Surg. 2009;38(4):363–8. Epub 2009/03/10.
55. Baumgaertel S. Cortical bone thickness and bone depth of the posterior palatal alveolar process for mini-implant insertion in adults. Am J Orthod Dentofacial Orthop. 2011;140(6):806–11. Epub 2011/12/03.

56. Moon SH, Park SH, Lim WH, Chun YS. Palatal bone density in adult subjects: implications for mini-implant placement. Angle Orthod. 2010;80(1):137–44. Epub 2009/10/27.
57. Ludwig B, Glasl B, Bowman SJ, Wilmes B, Kinzinger GS, Lisson JA. Anatomical guidelines for miniscrew insertion: palatal sites. J Clin Orthod. 2011;45(8):433–41; quiz 67. Epub 2011/11/19.
58. Winsauer H, Vlachojannis C, Bumann A, Vlachojannis J, Chrubasik S. Paramedian vertical palatal bone height for mini-implant insertion: a systematic review. Eur J Orthod. 2012;36(5):541–9. Epub 2012/12/12.
59. Fayed MM, Pazera P, Katsaros C. Optimal sites for orthodontic mini-implant placement assessed by cone beam computed tomography. Angle Orthod. 2010;80(5):939–51. Epub 2010/06/29.
60. Lim JE, Lee SJ, Kim YJ, Lim WH, Chun YS. Comparison of cortical bone thickness and root proximity at maxillary and mandibular interradicular sites for orthodontic mini-implant placement. Orthod Craniofac Res. 2009;12(4):299–304. Epub 2009/10/21.
61. AlSamak S, Gkantidis N, Bitsanis E, Christou P. Assessment of potential orthodontic mini-implant insertion sites based on anatomical hard tissue parameters: a systematic review. Int J Oral Maxillofac Implants. 2012;27(4):875–87. Epub 2012/08/01.
62. Chun YS, Lim WH. Bone density at interradicular sites: implications for orthodontic mini-implant placement. Orthod Craniofac Res. 2009;12(1):25–32. Epub 2009/01/22.
63. Ludwig B, Glasl B, Kinzinger GS, Lietz T, Lisson JA. Anatomical guidelines for miniscrew insertion: Vestibular interradicular sites. J Clin Orthod. 2011;45(3):165–73. Epub 2011/07/26.
64. Asscherickx K, Vande Vannet B, Wehrbein H, Sabzevar MM. Success rate of miniscrews relative to their position to adjacent roots. Eur J Orthod. 2008;30(4):330–5. Epub 2008/07/18.
65. Hwang D, Wang HL. Medical contraindications to implant therapy: part II: Relative contraindications. Implant Dent. 2007;16(1):13–23. Epub 2007/03/16.
66. Hwang D, Wang HL. Medical contraindications to implant therapy: part I: absolute contraindications. Implant Dent. 2006;15(4):353–60. Epub 2006/12/19.
67. Lim WH, Lee SK, Wikesjo UM, Chun YS. A descriptive tissue evaluation at maxillary interradicular sites: implications for orthodontic mini-implant placement. Clin Anat. 2007;20(7):760–5. Epub 2007/06/23.
68. Motoyoshi M, Matsuoka M, Shimizu N. Application of orthodontic mini-implants in adolescents. Int J Oral Maxillofac Surg. 2007;36(8):695–9. Epub 2007/05/25.
69. Apel S, Apel C, Morea C, Tortamano A, Dominguez GC, Conrads G. Microflora associated with successful and failed orthodontic mini-implants. Clin Oral Implants Res. 2009;20(11):1186–90. Epub 2009/09/02.
70. Jung BA, Kunkel M, Gollner P, Liechti T, Wagner W, Wehrbein H. Prognostic parameters contributing to palatal implant failures: a long-term survival analysis of 239 patients. Clin Oral Implants Res. 2012;23(6):746–50. Epub 2011/05/07.
71. Cho IS, Baek SH, Kim YH. Effects of wobbling angle on the stability measures of orthodontic mini-implants during insertion and removal procedures. Angle Orthod. 2013;83:1009–14.
72. Yadav S, Upadhyay M, Liu S, Roberts E, Neace WP, Nanda R. Microdamage of the cortical bone during mini-implant insertion with self-drilling and self-tapping techniques: a randomized controlled trial. Am J Orthod Dentofacial Orthop. 2012; 141(5):538–46. Epub 2012/05/05.
73. Tachibana R, Motoyoshi M, Shinohara A, Shigeeda T, Shimizu N. Safe placement techniques for self-drilling orthodontic mini-implants. Int J Oral Maxillofac Surg. 2012;41(11):1439–44. Epub 2012/07/06.
74. Baumgaertel S. Predrilling of the implant site: is it necessary for orthodontic mini-implants? Am J Orthod Dentofacial Orthop. 2010;137(6):825–9. Epub 2010/08/06.
75. Wilmes B, Drescher D. Impact of bone quality, implant type, and implantation site preparation on insertion torques of mini-implants used for orthodontic anchorage. Int J Oral Maxillofac Surg. 2011;40(7):697–703. Epub 2011/04/05.
76. Cho KC, Baek SH. Effects of predrilling depth and implant shape on the mechanical properties of orthodontic mini-implants during the insertion procedure. Angle Orthod. 2012;82(4):618–24. Epub 2011/11/05.
77. Turkoz C, Atac MS, Tuncer C, Balos Tuncer B, Kaan E. The effect of drill-free and drilling methods on the stability of mini-implants under early orthodontic loading in adolescent patients. Eur J Orthod. 2011;33(5):533–6. Epub 2010/12/07.
78. Florvaag B, Kneuertz P, Lazar F, Koebke J, Zoller JE, Braumann B, et al. Biomechanical properties of orthodontic miniscrews. An in-vitro study. J Orofac Orthop. 2010;71(1):53–67. Epub 2010/02/06.
79. Kim JW, Ahn SJ, Chang YI. Histomorphometric and mechanical analyses of the drill-free screw as orthodontic anchorage. Am J Orthod Dentofacial Orthop. 2005;128(2):190–4. Epub 2005/08/17.
80. Motoyoshi M, Hirabayashi M, Uemura M, Shimizu N. Recommended placement torque when tightening an orthodontic mini-implant. Clin Oral Implants Res. 2006;17(1):109–14.
81. Pauls A, Nienkemper M, Drescher D. Accuracy of torque-limiting devices used for mini-implant placement–an in vitro study. J Orofac Orthop. 2013;74(2):124–36. Epub 2013/03/08.
82. Wawrzinek C, Sommer T, Fischer-Brandies H. Microdamage in cortical bone due to the overtightening of orthodontic microscrews. J Orofac Orthop. 2008;69(2):121–34. Epub 2008/04/04.
83. Motoyoshi M, Yoshida T, Ono A, Shimizu N. Effect of cortical bone thickness and implant placement

torque on stability of orthodontic mini-implants. Int J Oral Maxillofac Implants. 2007;22(5):779–84. Epub 2007/11/03.
84. Laursen MG, Melsen B, Cattaneo PM. An evaluation of insertion sites for mini-implants: a micro – CT study of human autopsy material. Angle Orthod. 2013;83(2):222–9. Epub 2012/08/28.
85. Inaba M. Evaluation of primary stability of inclined orthodontic mini-implants. J Oral Sci. 2009;51(3):347–53. Epub 2009/09/25.
86. Wilmes B, Su YY, Drescher D. Insertion angle impact on primary stability of orthodontic mini-implants. Angle Orthod. 2008;78(6):1065–70. Epub 2008/10/25.
87. Chen YH, Chang HH, Chen YJ, Lee D, Chiang HH, Yao CC. Root contact during insertion of miniscrews for orthodontic anchorage increases the failure rate: an animal study. Clin Oral Implants Res. 2008;19(1):99–106.
88. Holberg C, Winterhalder P, Holberg N, Rudzki-Janson I, Wichelhaus A. Direct versus indirect loading of orthodontic miniscrew implants-an FEM analysis. Clin Oral Investig. 2013;17(8):1821–7. Epub 2012/11/01.
89. Buchter A, Wiechmann D, Koerdt S, Wiesmann HP, Piffko J, Meyer U. Load-related implant reaction of mini-implants used for orthodontic anchorage. Clin Oral Implants Res. 2005;16(4):473–9. Epub 2005/08/25.
90. Justens E, De Bruyn H. Clinical outcome of mini-screws used as orthodontic anchorage. Clin Implant Dent Relat Res. 2008;10(3):174–80. Epub 2008/04/04.
91. Park KH, Lee EM, Shin SI, Kim SH, Park YG, Kim SJ. Evaluation of the effect of force direction on stationary anchorage success of mini-implant with a lever-arm-shaped upper structure. Angle Orthod. 2011;81(5):776–82. Epub 2011/05/28.
92. Lin TS, Tsai FD, Chen CY, Lin LW. Factorial analysis of variables affecting bone stress adjacent to the orthodontic anchorage mini-implant with finite element analysis. Am J Orthod Dentofacial Orthop. 2013;143(2):182–9. Epub 2013/02/05.
93. Wu Y, Xu Z, Tan L, Tan L, Zhao Z, Yang P, et al. Orthodontic mini-implant stability under continuous or intermittent loading: a histomorphometric and biomechanical analysis. Clin Implant Dentist Relat Res. 2013. doi:10.1111/cid.12090. [Epub ahead of print].
94. Zhang L, Zhao Z, Li Y, Wu J, Zheng L, Tang T. Osseointegration of orthodontic micro-screws after immediate and early loading. Angle Orthod. 2010;80(2):354–60. Epub 2009/11/13.
95. Wu J, Bai YX, Wang BK. Biomechanical and histomorphometric characterizations of osseointegration during mini-screw healing in rabbit tibiae. Angle Orthod. 2009;79(3):558–63. Epub 2009/05/06.
96. Luzi C, Verna C, Melsen B. Immediate loading of orthodontic mini-implants: a histomorphometric evaluation of tissue reaction. Eur J Orthod. 2009;31(1):21–9. Epub 2009/01/24.
97. Woods PW, Buschang PH, Owens SE, Rossouw PE, Opperman LA. The effect of force, timing, and location on bone-to-implant contact of miniscrew implants. Eur J Orthod. 2009;31(3):232–40. Epub 2008/12/17.
98. Freire JN, Silva NR, Gil JN, Magini RS, Coelho PG. Histomorphologic and histomophometric evaluation of immediately and early loaded mini-implants for orthodontic anchorage. Am J Orthod Dentofacial Orthop. 2007;131(6):704 e1–9. Epub 2007/06/15.
99. Mo SS, Kim SH, Kook YA, Jeong DM, Chung KR, Nelson G. Resistance to immediate orthodontic loading of surface-treated mini-implants. Angle Orthod. 2010;80(1):123–9. Epub 2009/10/27.
100. Owens SE, Buschang PH, Cope JB, Franco PF, Rossouw PE. Experimental evaluation of tooth movement in the beagle dog with the mini-screw implant for orthodontic anchorage. Am J Orthod Dentofacial Orthop. 2007;132(5):639–46. Epub 2007/11/17.
101. Serra G, Morais LS, Elias CN, Meyers MA, Andrade L, Muller CA, et al. Sequential bone healing of immediately loaded mini-implants: histomorphometric and fluorescence analysis. Am J Orthod Dentofacial Orthop. 2010;137(1):80–90. Epub 2010/02/04.
102. Chen Y, Lee JW, Cho WH, Kyung HM. Potential of self-drilling orthodontic microimplants under immediate loading. Am J Orthod Dentofacial Orthop. 2010;137(4):496–502. Epub 2010/04/07.
103. Chen Y, Kang ST, Bae SM, Kyung HM. Clinical and histologic analysis of the stability of microimplants with immediate orthodontic loading in dogs. Am J Orthod Dentofacial Orthop. 2009;136(2):260–7. Epub 2009/08/05.
104. Cha JY, Lim JK, Song JW, Sato D, Kenmotsu M, Inoue T, et al. Influence of the length of the loading period after placement of orthodontic mini-implants on changes in bone histomorphology: microcomputed tomographic and histologic analysis. Int J Oral Maxillofac Implants. 2009;24(5):842–9. Epub 2009/10/30.
105. Ohashi E, Pecho OE, Moron M, Lagravere MO. Implant vs screw loading protocols in orthodontics. Angle Orthod. 2006;76(4):721–7. Epub 2006/07/01.
106. Wehrbein H, Diedrich P. Endosseous titanium implants during and after orthodontic load–an experimental study in the dog. Clin Oral Implants Res. 1993;4(2):76–82.
107. Ohmae M, Saito S, Morohashi T, Seki K, Qu H, Kanomi R, et al. A clinical and histological evaluation of titanium mini-implants as anchors for orthodontic intrusion in the beagle dog. Am J Orthod Dentofacial Orthop. 2001;119(5):489–97. Epub 2001/05/09.
108. Szmukler-Moncler S, Salama H, Reingewirtz Y, Dubruille JH. Timing of loading and effect of micromotion on bone-dental implant interface: review of experimental literature. J Biomed Mater Res. 1998;43(2):192–203. Epub 1998/06/10.

109. Ghoul WE, Chidiac JJ. Prosthetic requirements for immediate implant loading: a review. J Prosthodont. 2012;21(2):141–54. Epub 2012/03/03.
110. Chatzigianni A, Keilig L, Reimann S, Eliades T, Bourauel C. Effect of mini-implant length and diameter on primary stability under loading with two force levels. Eur J Orthod. 2011;33(4):381–7. Epub 2010/11/11.
111. Pithon MM, Figueiredo DS, Oliveira DD. Mechanical evaluation of orthodontic mini-implants of different lengths. J Oral Maxillofac Surg. 2013;71(3):479–86. Epub 2013/01/01.
112. Lietz T. Mini-screws – aspects of assessment and selection among different systems. In: Ludwig B, Baumgaertel S, Bowman J, editors. Mini-implants in orthodontics: innovative anchorage concepts. London: Quintessence Publishing Co Ltd; 2008. p. 11–72.
113. Wilmes B, Panayotidis A, Drescher D. Fracture resistance of orthodontic mini-implants: a biomechanical in vitro study. Eur J Orthod. 2011;33(4):396–401. Epub 2011/02/12.
114. Liou EJ, Pai BC, Lin JC. Do miniscrews remain stationary under orthodontic forces? Am J Orthod Dentofacial Orthop. 2004;126(1):42–7. Epub 2004/06/30.
115. Kim SH, Kang SM, Choi YS, Kook YA, Chung KR, Huang JC. Cone-beam computed tomography evaluation of mini-implants after placement: is root proximity a major risk factor for failure? Am J Orthod Dentofacial Orthop. 2010;138(3):264–76. Epub 2010/09/08.
116. El-Beialy AR, Abou-El-Ezz AM, Attia KH, El-Bialy AM, Mostafa YA. Loss of anchorage of miniscrews: a 3-dimensional assessment. Am J Orthod Dentofacial Orthop. 2009;136(5):700–7. Epub 2009/11/07.
117. Alves Jr M, Baratieri C, Nojima LI. Assessment of mini-implant displacement using cone beam computed tomography. Clin Oral Implants Res. 2011;22(10):1151–6. Epub 2011/02/10.
118. Lifshitz AB, Munoz M. Evaluation of the stability of self-drilling mini-implants for maxillary anchorage under immediate loading. World J Orthod. 2010;11(4):352–6. Epub 2010/01/01.
119. Papadopoulos MA, Papageorgiou SN, Zogakis IP. Clinical effectiveness of orthodontic miniscrew implants: a meta-analysis. J Dent Res. 2011;90(8):969–76. Epub 2011/05/20.
120. Carano A, Lonardo P, Velo S, Incorvati C. Mechanical properties of three different commercially available miniscrews for skeletal anchorage. Prog Orthod. 2005;6(1):82–97.
121. Lee NK, Baek SH. Effects of the diameter and shape of orthodontic mini-implants on microdamage to the cortical bone. Am J Orthod Dentofacial Orthop. 2010;138(1):8 e1–8; discussion 8–9. Epub 2010/07/14.
122. Walter A, Winsauer H, Marce-Nogue J, Mojal S, Puigdollers A. Design characteristics, primary stability and risk of fracture of orthodontic mini-implants: pilot scan electron microscope and mechanical studies. Med Oral Patol Oral Cir Bucal. 2013;18(5):e804–10. Epub 2013/06/01.
123. Wilmes B, Ottenstreuer S, Su YY, Drescher D. Impact of implant design on primary stability of orthodontic mini-implants. J Orofac Orthop. 2008;69(1):42–50. Epub 2008/01/24.
124. Pithon MM, Nojima MG, Nojima LI. In vitro evaluation of insertion and removal torques of orthodontic mini-implants. Int J Oral Maxillofac Surg. 2011;40(1):80–5. Epub 2010/11/06.
125. Pithon MM, Nojima MG, Nojima LI. Primary stability of orthodontic mini-implants inserted into maxilla and mandible of swine. Oral Surg Oral Med Oral Pathol Oral Radiol. 2012;113(6):748–54. Epub 2012/06/09.
126. Brinley CL, Behrents R, Kim KB, Condoor S, Kyung HM, Buschang PH. Pitch and longitudinal fluting effects on the primary stability of miniscrew implants. Angle Orthod. 2009;79(6):1156–61. Epub 2009/10/27.
127. Chang JZ, Chen YJ, Tung YY, Chiang YY, Lai EH, Chen WP, et al. Effects of thread depth, taper shape, and taper length on the mechanical properties of mini-implants. Am J Orthod Dentofacial Orthop. 2012;141(3):279–88. Epub 2012/03/03.
128. Glatzmaier J, Wehrbein H, Diedrich P. Biodegradable implants for orthodontic anchorage. A preliminary biomechanical study. Eur J Orthod. 1996;18(5):465–9. Epub 1996/10/01.
129. Morais LS, Serra GG, Muller CA, Andrade LR, Palermo EF, Elias CN, et al. Titanium alloy mini-implants for orthodontic anchorage: immediate loading and metal ion release. Acta Biomater. 2007;3(3):331–9. Epub 2007/01/30.
130. Cousley R. Mini-implants principles and potential complications. In: Cousley R, editor. The orthodontic mini-implant clinical handbook. Hoboken: Wiley Blackwell; 2007. p. 1–6.
131. Melsen B. The Aarhus anchorage system. In: Cope JB, editor. OrthoTADs the clinical guide and atlas. Dallas: Under Dog Media, LP; 2007. p. 179–90.
132. Papadopoulos MA, Tarawneh F. The use of miniscrew implants for temporary skeletal anchorage in orthodontics: a comprehensive review. Oral Surg Oral Med Oral Pathol Oral Radiol Endod. 2007;103(5):e6–15. Epub 2007/02/24.
133. Cope J. Temporary anchorage devices in orthodontics: a paradigm shift. Semin Orthod. 2005;11:3–9.
134. Branemark PI. Vital microscopy of bone marrow in rabbit. Scand J Clin Lab Invest. 1959;11(Supp 38):1–82. Epub 1959/01/01.
135. Branemark PI, Adell R, Breine U, Hansson BO, Lindstrom J, Ohlsson A. Intra-osseous anchorage of dental prostheses. I. Experimental studies. Scand J Plast Reconstr Surg. 1969;3(2):81–100. Epub 1969/01/01.
136. Zarb G, Albrektsson T. Osseointegration– a requiem for the periodontal ligament?– An editorial. Int J Periodont Rest Dent. 1991;11:88–91.

137. Johansson CB, Sennerby L, Albrektsson T. A removal torque and histomorphometric study of bone tissue reactions to commercially pure titanium and Vitallium implants. Int J Oral Maxillofac Implants. 1991;6(4):437–41. Epub 1991/01/01.
138. Johansson CB, Albrektsson T. A removal torque and histomorphometric study of commercially pure niobium and titanium implants in rabbit bone. Clin Oral Implants Res. 1991;2(1):24–9. Epub 1991/01/01.
139. Vande Vannet B, Sabzevar MM, Wehrbein H, Asscherickx K. Osseointegration of miniscrews: a histomorphometric evaluation. Eur J Orthod. 2007;29(5):437–42. Epub 2007/11/03.
140. Seo W, Kim SH, Chung KR, Nelson G. A pilot study of the osseointegration potential of a surface-treated mini-implant: bone contact of implants retrieved from patients. World J Orthod. 2009;10(3):202–10. Epub 2009/11/04.
141. Favero LG, Pisoni A, Paganelli C. Removal torque of osseointegrated mini-implants: an in vivo evaluation. Eur J Orthod. 2007;29(5):443–8. Epub 2007/11/03.
142. Gritsch K, Laroche N, Bonnet JM, Exbrayat P, Morgon L, Rabilloud M, et al. In vivo evaluation of immediately loaded stainless steel and titanium orthodontic screws in a growing bone. PLoS One. 2013;8(10):e76223. Epub 2013/10/15.
143. Malkoc S, Ozturk F, Corekci B, Bozkurt BS, Hakki SS. Real-time cell analysis of the cytotoxicity of orthodontic mini-implants on human gingival fibroblasts and mouse osteoblasts. Am J Orthod Dentofacial Orthop. 2012;141(4):419–26. Epub 2012/04/03.
144. Harris B. Corrosion of stainless steel surgical implants. J Med Eng Technol. 1979;3(3):117–22. Epub 1979/05/01.
145. Maino BG, Bednar JR, Mura P. The spider screw. In: Cope JB, editor. OrthoTADs the clinical guide and atlas. Dallas: Under Dog Media LP; 2007. p. 201–12.
146. Albrektsson T. Hard tissue implant interface. Aust Dent J. 2008;53 Suppl 1:S34–8. Epub 2008/08/09.
147. Ivanoff CJ, Sennerby L, Johansson C, Rangert B, Lekholm U. Influence of implant diameters on the integration of screw implants. An experimental study in rabbits. Int J Oral Maxillofac Surg. 1997;26(2):141–8. Epub 1997/04/01.
148. Wennerberg A, Albrektsson T. Suggested guidelines for the topographic evaluation of implant surfaces. Int J Oral Maxillofac Implants. 2000;15(3):331–44. Epub 2000/06/30.
149. Wennerberg A. On surface roughness and implant incorporation. Gothenburg: Gothenburg University; 1995.
150. Goransson A, Wennerberg A. Bone formation at titanium implants prepared with iso- and anisotropic surfaces of similar roughness: an in vivo study. Clin Implant Dent Relat Res. 2005;7(1):17–23. Epub 2005/05/21.
151. Nygren H, Tengvall P, Lundstrom I. The initial reactions of TiO2 with blood. J Biomed Mater Res. 1997;34(4):487–92. Epub 1997/03/15.
152. Nygren H, Eriksson C, Lausmaa J. Adhesion and activation of platelets and polymorphonuclear granulocyte cells at TiO2 surfaces. J Lab Clin Med. 1997;129(1):35–46. Epub 1997/01/01.
153. Hench LL, Paschall HA. Direct chemical bond of bioactive glass-ceramic materials to bone and muscle. J Biomed Mater Res. 1973;7(3):25–42. Epub 1973/01/01.
154. Jarcho M, Kay JF, Gumaer KI, Doremus RH, Drobeck HP. Tissue, cellular and subcellular events at a bone-ceramic hydroxylapatite interface. J Bioeng. 1977;1(2):79–92. Epub 1977/01/01.
155. Rokkum M, Reigstad A, Johansson CB. HA particles can be released from well-fixed HA-coated stems: histopathology of biopsies from 20 hips 2–8 years after implantation. Acta Orthopaedica Scand. 2002;73(3):298–306. Epub 2002/07/30.
156. Göransson A. On possibly bioactive CP titanium implant surfaces. Gothenburg: Gothenburg University; 2006.
157. Malekzadeh B, Tengvall P, Ohrnell LO, Wennerberg A, Westerlund A. Effects of locally administered insulin on bone formation in non-diabetic rats. J Biomed Mater Res A. 2013;101(1):132–7. Epub 2012/07/25.
158. Wehrbein H, Gollner P, Diedrich P. Orthodontic load on short maxillary implants with reduced sink depth: an experimental study. Clin Oral Implants Res. 2008;19(10):1063–8. Epub 2008/10/03.
159. Oyonarte R, Pilliar RM, Deporter D, Woodside DG. Peri-implant bone response to orthodontic loading: part 2. Implant surface geometry and its effect on regional bone remodeling. Am J Orthod Dentofacial Orthop. 2005;128(2):182–9. Epub 2005/08/17.
160. Oyonarte R, Pilliar RM, Deporter D, Woodside DG. Peri-implant bone response to orthodontic loading: part 1. A histomorphometric study of the effects of implant surface design. Am J Orthod Dentofacial Orthop. 2005;128(2):173–81.
161. Pilliar RM, Sagals G, Meguid SA, Oyonarte R, Deporter DA. Threaded versus porous-surfaced implants as anchorage units for orthodontic treatment: three-dimensional finite element analysis of peri-implant bone tissue stresses. Int J Oral Maxillofac Implants. 2006;21(6):879–89. Epub 2006/12/28.
162. Borbely P, Dunay MP, Jung BA, Wehrbein H, Wagner W, Kunkel M. Primary loading of palatal implants for orthodontic anchorage–a pilot animal study. J Craniomaxillofac Surg. 2008;36(1):21–7. Epub 2007/11/09.
163. Jung BA, Harzer W, Wehrbein H, Gedrange T, Hopfenmuller W, Ludicke G, et al. Immediate versus conventional loading of palatal implants in humans: a first report of a multicenter RCT. Clin Oral Investig. 2011;15(4):495–502. Epub 2010/04/13.

164. Gollner P, Jung BA, Kunkel M, Liechti T, Wehrbein H. Immediate vs. conventional loading of palatal implants in humans. Clin Oral Implants Res. 2009;20(8):833–7. Epub 2009/06/11.
165. AlSamak S, Bitsanis E, Makou M, Eliades G. Morphological and structural characteristics of orthodontic mini-implants. J Orofac Orthop. 2012;73(1):58–71. Epub 2012/01/12.
166. Kim SH, Cho JH, Chung KR, Kook YA, Nelson G. Removal torque values of surface-treated mini-implants after loading. Am J Orthod Dentofacial Orthop. 2008;134(1):36–43. Epub 2008/07/12.
167. Kim SH, Lee SJ, Cho IS, Kim SK, Kim TW. Rotational resistance of surface-treated mini-implants. Angle Orthod. 2009;79(5):899–907. Epub 2009/08/27.
168. Calderon JH, Valencia RM, Casasa AA, Sanchez MA, Espinosa R, Ceja I. Biomechanical anchorage evaluation of mini-implants treated with sandblasting and acid etching in orthodontics. Implant Dent. 2011;20(4):273–9. Epub 2011/07/26.
169. Kim SH, Choi JH, Chung KR, Nelson G. Do sand blasted with large grit and acid etched surface treated mini-implants remain stationary under orthodontic forces? Angle Orthod. 2012;82(2):304–12. Epub 2011/08/13.
170. Chaddad K, Ferreira AF, Geurs N, Reddy MS. Influence of surface characteristics on survival rates of mini-implants. Angle Orthod. 2008;78(1):107–13. Epub 2008/01/16.
171. Cho IS, Kim SK, Chang YI, Baek SH. In vitro and in vivo mechanical stability of orthodontic mini-implants. Angle Orthod. 2012;82(4):611–7. Epub 2011/10/21.
172. Karmarker S, Yu W, Kyung HM. Effect of surface anodization on stability of orthodontic microimplant. Korean J Orthod. 2012;42(1):4–10. Epub 2012/11/01.
173. Galli C, Piemontese M, Ravanetti F, Lumetti S, Passeri G, Gandolfini M, et al. Effect of surface treatment on cell responses to grades 4 and 5 titanium for orthodontic mini-implants. Am J Orthod Dentofacial Orthop. 2012;141(6):705–14. Epub 2012/05/30.

Index

A. Wennerberg et al. (eds.), *Implant Surfaces and their Biological and Clinical Impact*,
DOI 10.1007/978-3-662-45379-7, © Springer-Verlag Berlin Heidelberg 2015

MIX
Papier aus verantwortungsvollen Quellen
Paper from responsible sources
FSC® C105338

If you have any concerns about our products,
you can contact us on
ProductSafety@springernature.com

In case Publisher is established outside the EU,
the EU authorized representative is:
Springer Nature Customer Service Center GmbH
Europaplatz 3, 69115 Heidelberg, Germany

Printed by Libri Plureos GmbH
in Hamburg, Germany